Modern Cardiovascular Physiology

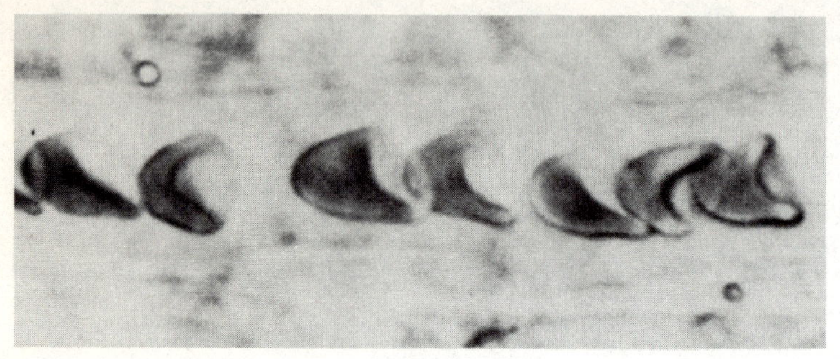

Modern Cardiovascular Physiology

Second Edition

Carl R. Honig, M.D. Professor of Physiology,
University of Rochester School of Medicine
and Dentistry, Rochester, New York;
Adjunct Professor of Physiology,
University of Hawaii, Honolulu

Little, Brown and Company
Boston/Toronto

Second Edition

Library of Congress Catalog Card No. 87-83644

Frontispiece Illustration: Red cells in a capillary are folded into streamlined shapes that decrease resistance to flow. (From R. Skalak and P.-I. Brånemark, *Science* 164:717, 1969. Copyright © 1969 by the American Association for the Advancement of Science.)

ISBN 0-316-37213-7

Printed in the United States of America

DON

To Betty, who made it possible

Contents

Preface

Modern Cardiovascular Physiology, Second Edition, is intended for both medical and graduate students. The latter may choose to ignore the material identified by the heading Clinical Application. The book should also be useful to residents and practitioners interested in updating their knowledge. It is assumed that the reader has been exposed to biochemistry and histology; cell physiology and anatomy are helpful but not essential.

Research continues to revitalize cardiovascular physiology and advance clinical practice. Discoveries of lasting value in cell physiology, microcirculation, regulation, and, most notably, O_2 transport must be incorporated into the thinking of physicians and scientists. The title reflects emphasis on these subjects in the revised text.

Two themes continue to pervade the book. The first is the concept of a factor of safety or reserve of function. The second is the systems concept. Care has been taken to develop factual material around these and other unifying concepts. The text is divided into five parts. The first two deal with the biophysical essentials: cardiac mechanics, electrophysiology, and hemodynamics. The third part is concerned with exchanges between blood and tissue, including new concepts in O_2 transport. The fourth part describes selected regional circulations. This idiosyncratic material has been simplified by use of a common approach. The final part develops the regulation of pressure, flow, and volume and the integration of cardiovascular controls with voluntary behavior.

It is essential to know the facts, but this is merely the first step in understanding. One must then organize the information and apply it to practical problems. If you cannot use it, you do not really know it! Text headings, summary tables, logic diagrams, and systems diagrams illustrate techniques for organizing causal and temporal relationships. Problem sets of graded difficulty are provided for self-evaluation.

Anatomy courses train students to think visually. Accordingly, illustrations are abundant; most are new or revised. Brief reference lists at the end of each chapter include at least one recent monograph or review. Those titles marked with an asterisk are particularly recommended. Normal values for cardiovascular variables are listed in the Appendixes to encourage quantitative thinking.

The Second Edition has been designed so that page or chapter assignments can be tailored to the length and content of a particular course. Students will find the additional material useful in pathophysiology and clinical studies. Each chapter has been thoroughly reworked. Material on cardiac mechanics has been expanded, and the chapters on O_2 transport and coronary circulation were rewritten completely. Most of the other chapters have been simplified and shortened. Finally, new problems permit self-testing at a level appropriate to the reader's preparation.

Comments on the Second Edition from students and faculty will be welcomed with sincere thanks.

C. R. H.

Acknowledgments

I deeply appreciate the continued support of the University of Rochester and the University of Hawaii. Colleagues who offered suggestions and criticism include Drs. Martha L. Blair, Giles Cokelet, Richard J. Connett, Thomas E. J. Gayeski, Robert S. Kass, Yu-Chong Lin, Camillo Peracchia, Lawrence P. Schramm, and the late Edward S. Kirk. I also thank the many authors and publishers who granted permission to use their material, often with considerable modification. Mrs. Wendy Keck and Miss Karen Vogt typed the entire manuscript, Mrs. Shari Harwell revised the illustrations, and the friendly staff at Little, Brown provided expert assistance throughout.

The book could not have been written — let alone revised — without my wife's help and encouragement. Working together on *our* book has been one of the most rewarding aspects of authorship.

C. R. H.

Overview, Concepts, and Themes

First things first: The circulation is a *transport system,* which delivers O_2, substrate, and nutrients to individual cells and conveys metabolic wastes to the environment. The circulation also serves as a major channel of intercellular communication by transporting hormones to the receptor sites. Most of this text is concerned with properties of cardiovascular muscles and the intricacies of hemodynamics and regulation — in other words, with how the circulation works. In considering these *means,* it helps to ask oneself how they contribute to transport *ends.*

Properties of the Heart

The first requirement for a transport system based on bulk flow is a suitable pump. The human heart performs about 10^5 strokes every day, without ever resting for more than a few hundred milliseconds. Daily, it lifts about 1000 kg (1 metric ton) 10 meters, and in the course of a lifetime performs about 1000 kilowatt-hours of external, useful work. This performance cannot be matched by any inanimate device. The reason, of course, is that the heart is constantly being renewed by turnover of its chemical components. The heart beating in your chest today is not the same one that served you a year ago.

The heart's reliability is due not only to metabolic repair, but also to its intrinsic physiological properties. It does not need the central nervous system to tell it what to do. It can beat rhythmically outside the body, if given proper support. Cardiac rhythmicity depends on electrical properties of the surface membrane that allow certain cells to act as pacemakers. Other membrane properties ensure that the stimulus is distributed so rapidly that all ventricular muscle cells contract in unison. This intercellular communication is essential for life: Only if contraction is coordinated can the heart develop tension in its walls and pressure on its contents. Diseases and many drugs alter cardiac rhythm, cell-to-cell conduction, or both. Rational management demands thorough understanding of the underlying ionic mechanisms.

The salient mechanical property of the heart is its response to stretch. If distended by an increase in venous return, it automatically contracts more strongly and empties itself of the larger volume. In this way an isolated heart can regulate its own contractility. Nevertheless, cardiac nerves play an essential role. Nerves create no new mechanism; they merely amplify, suppress, or change the rate of processes already present. For example, nerves control tension by modifying the heart's intrinsic response to stretch and change heart rate by modifying the normal pacemaker. The main effect is to extend greatly the *range* of cardiac output under conditions of stress.

According to the National Center for Health Statistics, diseases of the heart account for roughly half of the deaths from all causes in the United States and other "developed" countries. If the heart is so powerful and reliable, why this epidemic? The answer is that disease of the coronary vessels can limit transport of O_2 and metabolites to the myocardium.

Adequacy of Transport

What constitutes "adequate" transport? On first thought, one might judge the circulation a success if each and every cell were as free of transport constraints as a unicellular organism in sea water. This ideal might have been attempted early in evolution; but as animals became larger, literally billions of minute vessels were required. Perfect order in such populations was impossible, and large (though highly local) differences in blood flow and microvascular geometry appeared.

The simplest way nature could have dealt with this heterogeneity would have been to set *mean* blood flow and the number of perfused capillaries high enough to ensure delivery to each and every site at all times, no matter where it was located. To do this, however, the vast majority of tissue loci would have to be overperfused, and the size and energy cost of circulation would be enormous. Nature opted for economy; transport was set to the minimum required by the bulk of the cell population, and carte blanche for all cells and bodily functions simultaneously was abandoned.

Local transport is modified by *active vasomotion*. The arterioles, which are the principal sites of resistance to flow, constrict and dilate, often rhythmically. Consequently, local blood flow varies with time. Diffusion between blood and tissue also varies, because only a fraction of the available capillaries are perfused with erythrocytes under normal circumstances. By rotating the location of sites at which transport is curtailed, active vasomotion permits *mean* flow and capillarity to be much lower than would be possible otherwise. Other functions of active vasomotion will be developed in Part III. In view of the heterogeneity of the microcirculation, judgments about the adequacy of transport must be based on large cell populations. The simplest and most practical criterion is the ability to perform a physiological function. For example, circulatory adequacy for a contracting muscle can be judged by its ability to sustain tension.

Conflicting Functions and Circulatory Priorities

The mammalian circulation permits an incredible range of activity: In world-class athletes the rate of O_2 consumption ($\dot{V}O_2$) may briefly increase 25-fold! Maximal function of all organs cannot be supported simultaneously, however, so a system of priorities is required. These priorities are based on the metabolic needs of the individual organs, as determined locally, and the requirements of the whole animal, as determined by the brain.

The organs are connected in parallel, so each organ can vary its flow independently by constricting or dilating its arterioles. Intraorgan resistances are controlled by nerve mediators, which are released at rates set by the brain. Arterioles also respond to vasodilator substances produced locally at rates coupled to tissue metabolism. Neural and metabolic controls operate as a system of checks and balances. If the brain "throttles" flow to an organ, metabolic controls can override the brain's instructions and prevent tissue injury. Conversely, local controls can be restrained in the interests of the whole animal. Some examples should clarify these ideas.

A built-in local mechanism independent of the brain dilates vessels in skeletal muscle when work begins. This increases flow. However, the extent of the increase depends not only on the vessels, but also on the output of the heart and the fraction of that output available to muscle. Initially, the central nervous system stimulates the heart and limits flow to skin, kidney, and gastrointestinal tract. These organs are concerned with exchanges with the external environment that need not be maintained at all times. Thus extrinsic and intrinsic controls act together to increase muscle flow.

As work goes on, body temperature rises, because heat production is high and heat transport to the environment is decreased by low skin flow. The rise in temperature is detected by the brain, which now must choose between support of muscle contraction and defense of body temperature. Temperature has the higher priority; cutaneous vessels are dilated, flow is diverted from muscle to skin, and maximal muscle work can no longer be sustained. The reverse situation (neural controls overridden in the interest of local metabolism) is also important, not only in the normal animal, but also in the development of shock.

The two most flow-dependent organs are heart and brain. They are continuously active, have a high metabolic rate, and are essential for life. Coronary and cerebral vessels have exceptionally powerful metabolic controls, whereas extrinsic neural controls are comparatively weak. This imbalance implements their high priority for flow; in adversity, the heart and brain have the first crack at the cardiac output.

Reserves and Safety Factors

Priorities are necessitated by limits or maxima. However, physiological systems seldom operate "flat out," and then only briefly; recall our discussion of heavy exercise. The difference between the usual value of some parameter or function and its maximum should be regarded as a *reserve*, which can be called on to compensate for stress or disease. For example, an athlete's cardiac output may be 5 liters per minute at rest and 25 liters per minute during brief effort. The 20-liters-per-minute difference is the athlete's reserve of cardiac output. Often it is preferable to express the reserve in relative terms, that is, the cardiac output can be expanded fourfold relative to its value at rest. Expansion factors for cardiovascular parameters are provided in Appendix 2.

A related concept is that of a *factor of safety*. This refers to the ability of a system to function well over a wide range of some parameter. O_2 transport in blood is a good example. About 99 percent of the O_2 is bound to hemoglobin. The extent to which hemoglobin is saturated with O_2 depends on the O_2 partial pressure (PO_2): Hemoglobin is about 95 percent saturated at 100 mm Hg PO_2 and 90 percent saturated at 60 mm Hg. Thus PO_2 can fall 40 mm Hg because of respiratory insufficiency with little effect on O_2 transport to tissue. The range 60 to 100 mm Hg is a *factor of safety* for PO_2. The concept implies that disaster may follow if the factor of safety is exceeded, and this is often the case.

The effect of a stimulus, drug, or disease is strongly conditioned by the available reserves and safety factors. For example, the larger the cardiac output reserve, the longer an increase in cardiac output can be maintained, as explained in Chapter 13. One of the principal tasks of a physician is to estimate a patient's reserves. Diagnosis includes not only identification of the cause of an illness, but also a semiquantitative estimate of how much function remains. Prognosis is an estimate of the rate at which reserves may disappear. Finally, therapy is designed to increase the reserves and to prevent or eliminate stresses that might compromise them.

Physiological Systems

Concepts related to systems pervade modern science and medicine. A system is a set of interacting components with special properties that arise from the interactions. For example, a watch is a set of interacting gears and springs that has the property of telling time. The same components are not a system if interaction is prevented; a pile of watch parts will not tell time. To use a system we need not identify its components or know how it works; we can consider it a "black box" that does something. For example, we can use a watch without knowing whether it contains a spring or battery.

Physiologists are mainly concerned with temporal and causal relations: A stimulus (cause, input to a system) produces a certain response (effect, output). The output of many physiological systems is an appropriate value of some parameter, such as blood pressure, despite the tendency of extraneous factors to cause inappropriate change. Variables appropriately adjusted by a system are said to be *regulated*. Regulatory systems consist of a *controller*, an *effector*, and a *detector*. The cardiovascular effectors are muscle cells. The controller is usually the brain and autonomic nerves, and the detector is generally a bioelectric transducer that converts the value of the regulated quantity into action potentials in a sensory nerve. Not all systems depend on nerves, however. The important *autoregulatory* system discussed in Chapter 1 depends instead on built-in properties of the heart that serve as transducer and controller.

It is convenient to summarize the organization of systems with diagrams, as in the accompanying figure. The arrows mean "leads to" or "has an effect on." Notice that the regulated variable is influenced by the output of other systems and by disturbances. Consequently, the controller must know the value of the variable in order to keep it constant. This is why the detector (more often called receptor) is so important. It measures the regulated variable and feeds this information back to the controller. Notice in the figure that this results in a closed loop. *Feedback* of information is considered negative if it acts to minimize disturbances. All physiological regulations are based on

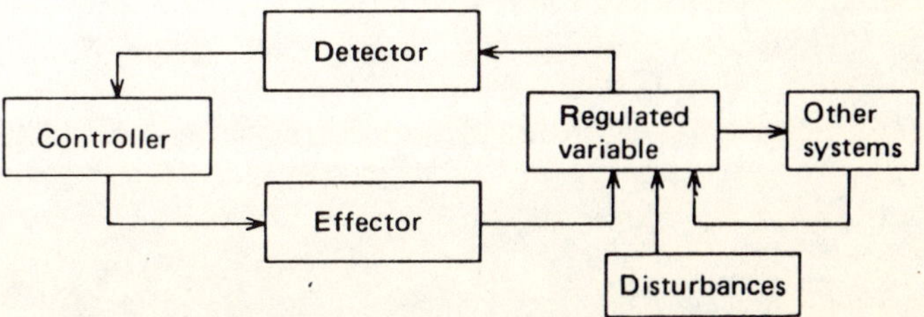

Conceptual diagram of a regulatory system based on negative feedback.

closed-loop, negative feedback systems. We shall see that the performance of the neural systems that regulate circulation is often limited by the properties of the receptor and feedback signal.

Certain drugs and diseases produce their effects by opening negative feedback loops. Alternatively, disease (or an experimental maneuver) may create a system where none normally exists. In most such instances, feedback is positive — it tends to promote disturbance. This in turn causes an even larger disturbance, and so on. Such conditions progress rapidly and are often fatal unless the positive feedback can be eliminated.

Reserves, safety factors, and concepts related to systems are themes that recur throughout this book. They should become part of your thinking, not only about circulation, but about medicine and research generally.

I : Properties of Cardiac Muscle

1 : Cardiac Mechanics

> . . . the mechanical energy set free on passage from the resting to the contracting state depends on the area of chemically active surfaces, i.e., on the length of the muscle fiber. This simple formula serves to "explain" the whole behavior of the isolated mammalian heart . . .
>
> — S. W. Patterson, H. Piper, and E. H. Starling
> *J. Physiol.* (Lond.) 48:465, 1914.

And so we believe today. The formula is by no means simple, however, if we wish to substitute ultrastructural and chemical understanding for the word *explain*. (Notice that Starling et al. qualified that word with quotation marks.) We begin at the molecular level, where some of the most basic properties of the heart are encoded in the structure and arrangement of the contractile proteins.[1]

The Cardiac Myocyte

Each cardiac muscle fiber is a single cell, about 100 μm long. Bundles of thick and thin filaments are interspersed between long rows of mitochondria. The mitochondria account for about one-third of cell volume in humans, reflecting the high and constant aerobic metabolism that supports cardiac function. The filaments are arranged in linearly repetitive arrays called *sarcomeres,* delineated by a Z disc at either end; see Figure 1-1.

The Sarcomere

The length of every sarcomere in a fiber is almost exactly the same, so the macroscopic fiber length (and muscle length) correspond to a unique microscopic sarcomere length. These lengths vary with cardiac filling and emptying. The Z disc consists of a fine mesh of filaments, rather like a hemp rope. The thin filament, about 2 μm long, traverses and is anchored to the Z disc. The thick filaments interdigitate with the thin ones. The thick filaments are fixed in a hexagonal three-dimensional array by spacers (M-line filaments) located at the center of the sarcomere. The thin filaments lie at the trigonal points of the array.

[1]The following "refresher" should be familiar to those who have studied histology. Others would be wise to consult reference 6 at the end of this chapter, or a standard histology text.

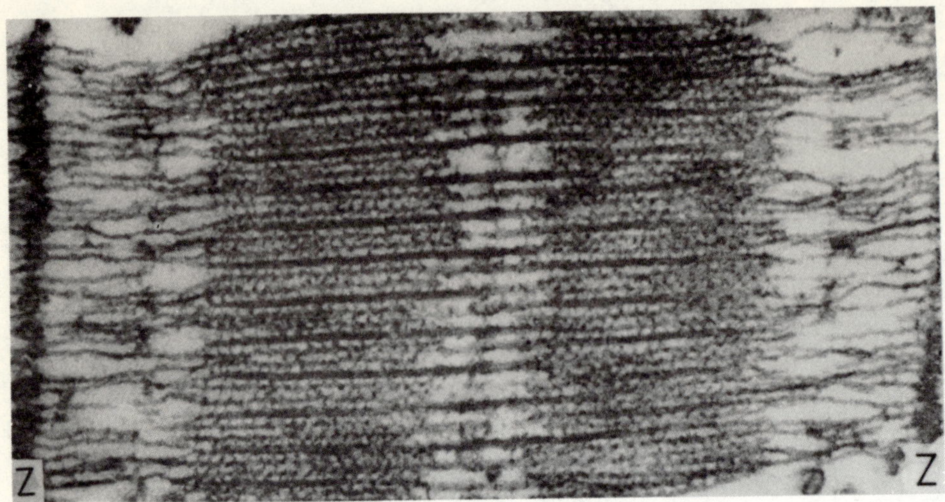

Figure 1-1
Electron photomicrograph of one sarcomere, showing interdigitated array of filaments. Myosin heads and the bare central zone of the thick filaments are noteworthy. Magnification ×75,000. (From H. Huxley, *J. Biophys. Biochem. Cytol.* 3:631, 1957.)

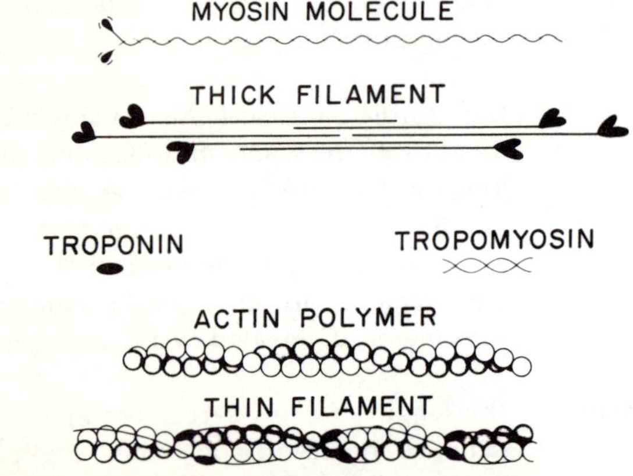

Figure 1-2
Organization of thick and thin filaments of striated muscles. (Modified from I. Danishefsky, *Biochemistry for Medical Sciences*. Boston: Little, Brown and Co., 1980.)

Chemical Anatomy

The chemical composition of the filaments is diagrammed in Figure 1-2. The thick filament is composed almost exclusively of myosin. A myosin molecule consists of an inert tail 0.12 μm long (!) and two globular heads. Myosin molecules aggregate spontaneously into a sheaf about 1.6 μm long. The heads project from the sheaf in a regular pattern. They possess an actin-binding site and an adenosine triphosphatase (ATPase) responsible for energy transduction. Myosin molecules aggregate with their heads facing in opposite directions. This mode of aggregation results in a central zone about 0.3 μm long devoid of myosin heads.

Under physiological conditions the globular actin molecules exist as a linear polymer. A thin filament contains two helically wound actin strands. Each actin monomer possesses a binding site for myosin and another for tropomyosin. The latter is a rodlike protein that is also linearly aggregated in vivo. A strand of tropomyosin lies in each of the grooves of actin helix. Finally, one troponin molecule is attached near the end of each tropomyosin. Tropomyosin and troponin are regulatory proteins that switch the mechanochemistry on and off. This molecular switch is tripped by Ca^{++} binding to troponin, as described in Chapter 4.

Micro-contraction and Macro-contraction

When the cell is activated[2] by a suitable stimulus, a myosin head can attach to an adjacent actin molecule to form a cross-bridge between the thick and thin filaments. Attachment causes a conformational change that tends to draw the thin filaments and Z discs toward the center of the sarcomere. After this microcontraction, actin and myosin dissociate, a process that requires ATP. The myosin head then reattaches at another site on the thin filament. The cycle is repeated until the muscle is deactivated. The total tension developed by the whole cell is the sum for all its cross-bridges pulling in parallel. If actively developed tension exceeds the resistance to shortening, the interdigitated filaments slide past each other in a smooth, telescoping motion. Since each bridge moves a minute force through a distance, it performs work. Much of the rest of this chapter is concerned with how this "miniwork" at the cross-bridges is coupled to the movement of blood.

The precise mode of operation of the cross-bridges is not fully understood, though there is general agreement that one molecule of ATP is split per turn of the mechanochemical cycle. Tension reflects the number of cross-bridges activated, or "turned on," by Ca^{++}. This depends in part on sarcomere length at the onset of activation, which takes us back to Starling's prescient insight: His "area of chemically active surfaces" corresponds to the *number* of Ca^{++}-activated cross-bridges.

Relation between Sarcomere Length and Active Tension

The active tension that a *skeletal* fiber can develop from various fixed sarcomere lengths is shown as a dashed line in Figure 1-3. Notice that tension in skeletal muscle is maximal and constant between 2.2 and 2.0 μm. This follows directly from the position

[2]We use this term intuitively for now; the mechanism is described in Chapter 4.

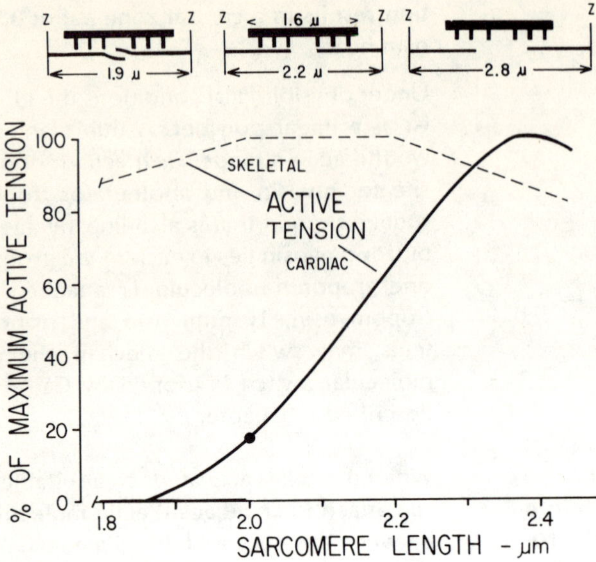

Figure 1-3
Top, arrangement of thick and thin filaments in heart and skeletal muscles at three sarcomere lengths. Bottom, relation between normalized tension and sarcomere length for strips of cardiac muscle (*solid line*) and skeletal muscle (*dashed line*). The experimental apparatus prevented any change in muscle length.

of the filaments. At 2.2 μm the tips of the thin filaments are at the edge of the central zone of the thick filament, where there are no myosin "heads"; see schematic, Figure 1-3. With further shortening, actins adjacent to the central zone cannot "find" a head, but an equal number of actins become exposed to myosin heads at the opposite ends of the thin filaments. Thus the number of possible bridges is constant between 2.2 and 2.0 μm. Since every skeletal-muscle actin is fully activated during contraction, tension in a skeletal fiber is constant and maximal in that range. Active tension decreases at shorter lengths because of steric hindrance caused by overlap of thin filaments. Active tension falls at lengths greater than 2.2 μm because some myosin heads are out of range of actin. It is truly remarkable that gross and molecular architecture are so matched that the bony attachments of a skeletal muscle constrain it to the plateau of its length–active tension curve.

Contractility may be defined as the ability of a fiber to develop tension; it depends largely on the number of activated cross-bridges. Notice in Figure 1-3 that the active tension that a cardiac fiber develops from an initial length of 2.0 μm is about 20 percent of that obtained from a skeletal fiber, even though sarcomere structure in the two muscles is almost identical. The reason for this low contractility is that *the sarcomeres in the unstressed heart are not completely activated* by an electrical stimulus, so some actins in proximity to myosin cannot react. Active tension increases almost linearly between 1.9 and 2.3 μm because of recruitment of additional cross-bridges. This intrinsic *reserve of contractility* ensures that the heart would develop the extra tension needed to empty itself if more blood were returned to it. Many of the symptoms of cardiac failure are due to loss of contractile reserve.

Passive Tension and Resistance to Stretch

It is essential to distinguish between active tension during contraction and passive tension when the muscle is at rest. That part of the cardiac cycle during which the heart is at rest is called *diastole*. During diastole cardiac muscle behaves like a spring: If we fix one end and apply a force to the other, the length will increase until the passive tension balances the stretching force. The length of resting cardiac fibers in vivo depends on the volume in the chamber. This volume also determines the ventricular pressure at the end of diastole.

End-Diastolic Pressure as Index of Sarcomere Length

Thus far we have been concerned with the behavior of muscle strips. To apply the ideas to hearts in situ we need a measurable quantity proportional to sarcomere length. Fibers in the wall are stretched passively by inflowing blood throughout diastole. Ventricular volume at the end of diastole is a major determinant of cardiac performance because it sets sarcomere length, and hence active tension, in the next contraction. Measurements of ventricular volume require invasive radiological techniques and are subject to considerable error. However, the resting heart, like an automobile tire, exhibits a highly reproducible relation between volume and pressure, as shown in Figure 1-4. Pressure can be monitored readily; it is expressed in millimeters of mercury, or *torr*. Sarcomere length is derived from measurements in canine hearts fixed in situ at various end-diastolic pressures and volumes. Notice that the scale for sarcomere length is not linear.

The ratio of change in volume to change in pressure ($\Delta V/\Delta P$) is called *compliance*. Over the normal range of sarcomere lengths the ventricle is very compliant: Large changes in volume and sarcomere length are accompanied by small changes in end-diastolic pressure. The upper limits of normal for end-diastolic pressures are 6 torr and 12 torr for right and left ventricles, respectively. The ventricles become very noncompliant (stiff) at end-diastolic pressures greater than normal. This behavior prevents surges in venous inflow from pulling actins out of range of myosin heads. Were this to happen, the heart would have fewer

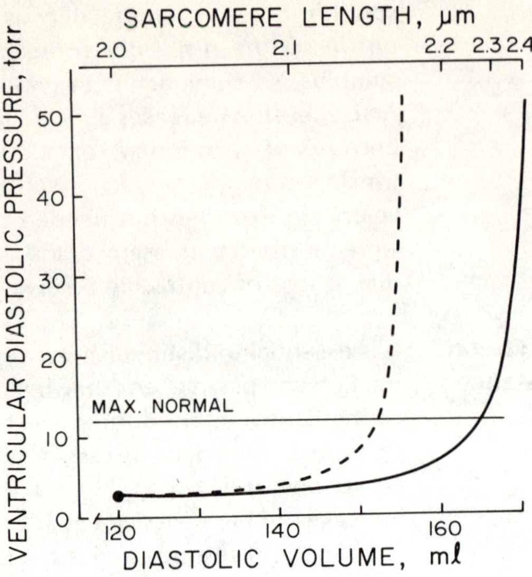

Figure 1-4
Solid line: Compliance curve for relaxed human left ventricles. Note non-linear scale for sarcomere length. Dashed line: effect of hypertrophy of muscle fibers, or replacement of injured fibers by collagen.

contractile units and would empty itself less completely in the next beat. Further inflow would stretch the heart still more, so it would be even weaker, and so on.[3] The heart's principal *factor of safety* against such a disaster is its very low compliance when the ventricle is filled to capacity. Indeed, it is almost impossible to stretch cardiac sarcomeres beyond 2.4 μm. The cost of exercising this safety factor is high pressure in the ventricle and in the veins from which it fills. High pulmonary venous pressure can be life-threatening, as explained in Chapter 15.

Resistance to passive stretch is due to a connective tissue "skeleton" that surrounds and interconnects myocytes; see Figure 1-5. A weave of collagen envelops each myocyte. The weave is braided into "struts" that prevent myocytes from slipping with respect to one another. Elastic fibers wound around the myocytes store potential energy during systole. Elastic recoil promotes lengthening in diastole. Growth of collagen matrix in disease can decrease ventricular compliance. The consequence is shown by the dashed curve in Figure 1-4. The less compliant ventricle requires a higher end-diastolic pressure to achieve a given sarcomere length and active tension.

[3] Notice that we have just described a case of positive feedback — the effect of a disturbance (decreased active tension) promotes the cause (increased ventricular volume), and vice versa.

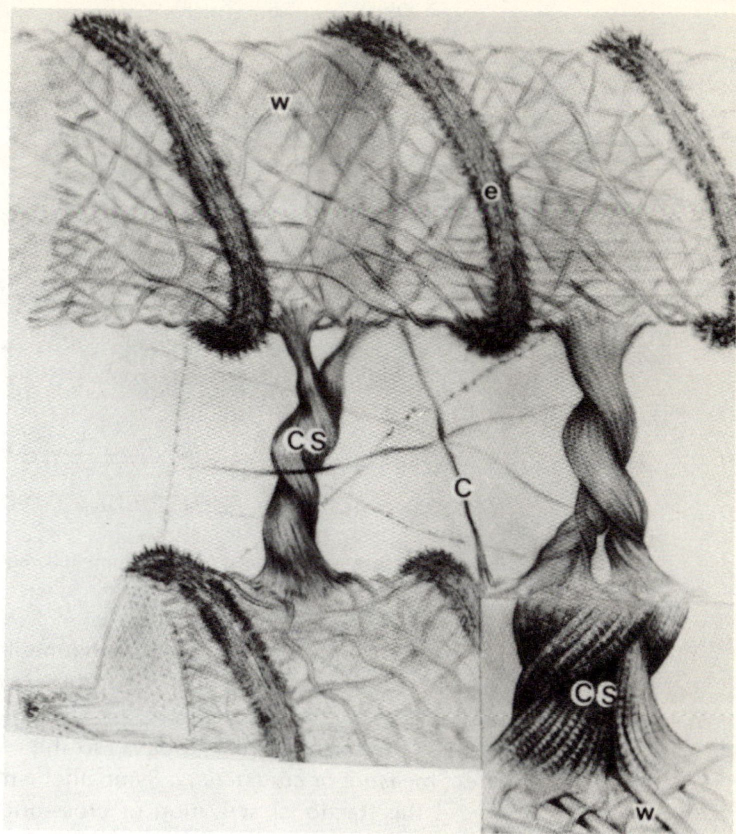

Figure 1-5
Diagram of a myocyte enmeshed in a weave (*w*) of collagen fibers (*C*) and a coil of elastic fibers (*e*). Inset shows braiding of the collagen weave into struts (*CS*) that connect adjacent myocytes. (From T. F. Robinson, L. Cohen-Gould, and S. Factor. *Lab. Invest.* 49:482, 1983.)

The Heart as a Pump: The Systolic Elastance Concept

The period when the heart contracts is called *systole*. Systolic performance is described in Figure 1-6. If the aorta is clamped to prevent ejection, miniwork at the cross-bridges appears as potential energy (increased intraventricular pressure), but no external work is done on the vascular system. The extent of the isovolumic pressure rise depends on the end-diastolic volume. This volume is often termed *preload* because it is a load applied to the muscle fibers before they contract. At a preload of 150 ml, human heart may develop a peak isovolumic pressure of 200 torr (point I_1 in Figure 1-6). At a preload of only 50 ml (shorter sarcomere length), peak isovolumic pressure falls to 50 torr (point I_2). Peak isovolumic pressure at various preloads falls along a straight line that intercepts the abscissa at V_o. At volume V_o the contracting ventricle cannot increase its pressure at all.

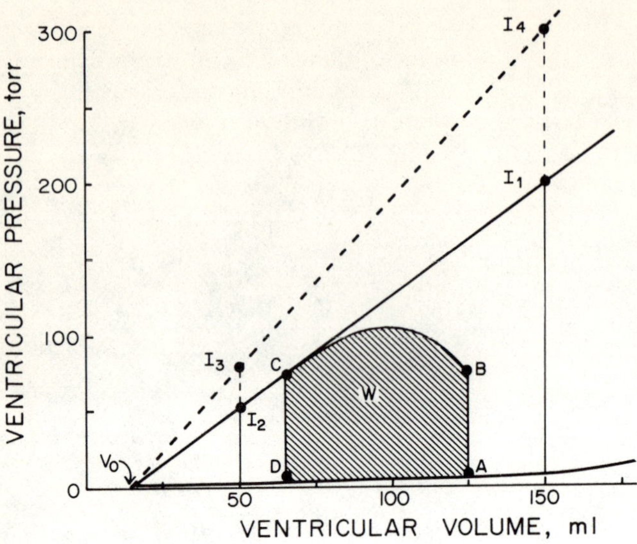

Figure 1-6
Systolic pressure–volume relations for canine left ventricle. See text for explanation.

The slope of the *systolic* pressure–volume line is the ratio $\Delta P/\Delta V$, the reciprocal of compliance, or the *elastance*. The greater the elastance, the stiffer the wall.[4] Stiffness depends on the number of attached cross-bridges, so the *elastance slope is a direct measure of contractility*. Sympathetic nerve mediators increase the fractional activation of cross-bridges and the elastance slope; see I_3, I_4, and dashed line. Conversely, the elastance slope decreases if contractility is impaired by a drug or disease (not shown in Figure 1-6).

The above concepts can be applied to hearts allowed to eject normally. At point *A* in the figure, systole begins, and at point *B* intraventricular pressure exceeds aortic pressure, the aortic valve opens, and ejection begins. At *C* ventricular pressure falls below aortic pressure, the aortic valve closes, and ejection ends. Ventricular pressure drops below atrial pressure at *D*, the mitral valve opens, and filling begins, completing the cycle. The upper left "corner" of a pressure-volume loop corresponds to peak systolic elastance for that beat.

The corners of loops from various preloads define the same elastance line that is obtained with the aorta clamped. This fact illustrates the principal advantage of the systolic elastance concept: It affords a measure of contractility uninfluenced by the resistance to outflow that the ventricle must overcome. This

[4]Note that this is the reverse of the common use of the word *elastic*.

resistance is termed the *afterload*, since it is applied after contraction is initiated. The above concepts have proved extremely useful in clarifying cardiac energetics and contractility. There is intense interest in applying them to clinical medicine using imaging procedures to evaluate ventricular volume.

External Cardiac Work

The pressure-volume loop *ABCD* in Figure 1-6 represents the integral of pressure with respect to volume, or the external stroke work (W_s). This integral cannot be determined in patients, so W_s is approximated as the product of the volume ejected per stroke (*S.V.*) and the difference between mean aortic pressure ($\overline{Pa}$) and ventricular end-diastolic pressure (*EDP*):

$$\underset{\text{gm}\cdot\text{m}}{W_s} \cong \underset{\text{gm}}{S.V.} \times (\underset{\text{mm Hg}}{\overline{Pa} - EDP}) \times 0.0136$$

Since the density of blood is about one, *S.V.* can be expressed in gm; 0.0136 converts millimeters of mercury to meters of blood.

The Intrinsic Reserve of Contractility

In the Navy important matters aboard ship are announced by a "Now hear this!" The ideas in Figure 1-7 well deserve a "Now read this!" because they are the principal frame of reference for describing cardiac performance.

A plot of external cardiac work as a function of end-diastolic pressure is called a Starling, or ventricular function, curve. The examples in Figure 1-7 are for human hearts. Application of the ventricular function curve requires a method for determining ventricular end-diastolic pressure. This key variable is estimated in humans by passing a catheter from a peripheral vein through the right heart into a branch of the pulmonary artery. A balloon near the catheter tip is inflated to occlude the vessel. This catheter creates a closed, continuous column of blood between the tip of the catheter and the left heart. In effect, the pulmonary capillaries and venules become an extension of the catheter. Pressure is measured via a catheter lumen distal to the balloon. This pressure, called the *pulmonary capillary wedge pressure* (PCWP), closely approximates LVEDP under most circumstances. The normal range is 4–15 torr. When combined with a determination of stroke work and Starling curves like those in Figure 1-7, PCWP permits an evaluation of the performance and contractile reserve.

Preload (i.e., end-diastolic volume) varies with the balance between venous return and stroke volume. If preload increases, sarcomeres are stretched, more cross-bridges are recruited, and stroke work increases. The increase is greatest at the low end-diastolic pressures characteristic of normal, unstressed hearts

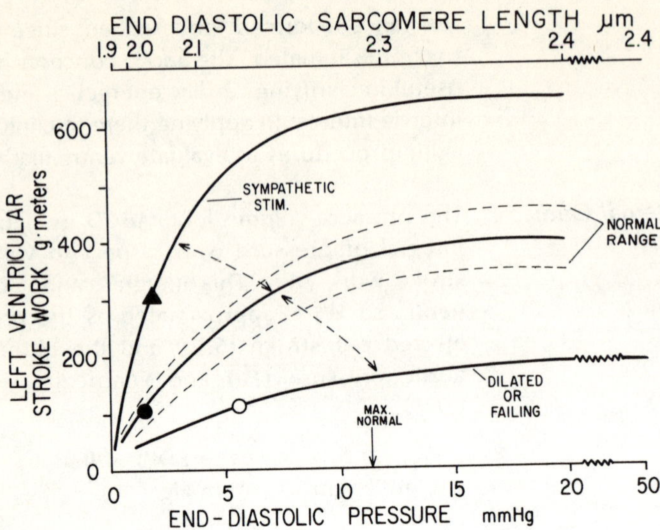

Figure 1-7
Hypothetical ventricular function curves for human left ventricle. Filled circle indicates normal operating point at rest. See text for explanation of symbols.

(*filled circle* in Figure 1-7). This "built-in" contractile reserve normally provides for a threefold increase in stroke work. Above the normal range for end-diastolic pressure (>12 mm Hg), smaller increments in ventricular volume produce large increases in end-diastolic pressure, but stroke work changes hardly at all. Figure 1-7, including its quantitative features, should be learned for permanent retention.

The Extrinsic Contractile Reserve

The heart's performance is strongly modified by nerves and hormones that adjust its output to events in the external environment. Thus one should visualize a family of ventricular function curves, one for each steady state of neuroendocrine drive. Increased drive permits the ventricle to perform more work at any preload; see, for example, the triangle in Figure 1-7. The mechanism is considered in Chapter 5. Thus stroke work can change in two ways. The heart can utilize its *intrinsic* reserve by "moving" up or down a particular function curve, as the difference between inflow and outflow may dictate. Alternatively, *extrinsic* modifiers may switch it to a new curve. Together, the intrinsic and extrinsic contractile reserves can increase stroke work five- or sixfold.

Application to Pumps in Series

The heart is actually two pumps in series, with the all-important pulmonary capillary bed in between. If the right ventricle were to eject only 1 ml per beat more than the left, the volume of the pulmonary reservoir would increase about 1000 ml in 15 minutes! The rise in pulmonary capillary pressure produced by that

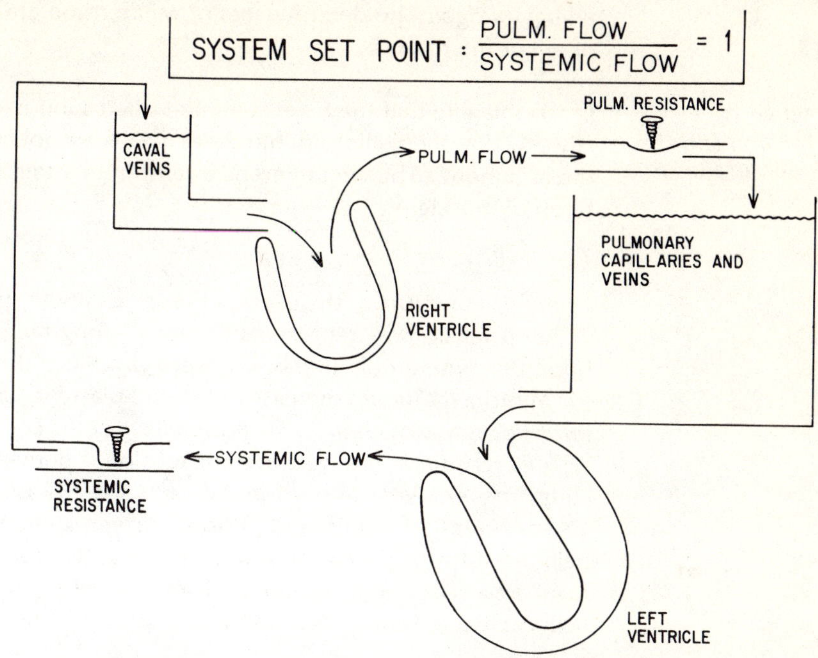

Figure 1-8
System for matching pulmonary and systemic blood flows.

increment in volume would squeeze an ultrafiltrate of plasma into the alveoli. One would literally drown. This cannot happen in the absence of disease, because of the continual operation of Starling's law. The situation is shown in Figure 1-8, as a system designed to keep the ratio of pulmonary to systemic flow equal to one.

The two ventricles fill from reservoirs that buffer changes in venous return. If the right ventricle is stretched by a surge in inflow, its output increases and the level in the pulmonary reservoir rises. This raises the end-diastolic pressure in the left ventricle, and systemic flow increases to match pulmonary flow. Since the total volume remains the same, an increase in pulmonary volume lowers the level of the right ventricular reservoir, so right ventricular output falls. Thus Starling's law and reciprocal changes in reservoir volumes ensure equal output of the two ventricles on a time scale of a few heart beats.

Cardiac Energetics

The energy consumed during each beat is used to create active tension in the ventricular wall. Only a small fraction of this energy is converted to useful work. The ratio of useful work to the total energy turnover is the *mechanical efficiency*. Like most machines, the heart's mechanical efficiency is about 15 percent. Thus *active tension in the wall is the principal item in the heart's energy budget*. The determinants of wall tension are therefore of major importance.

Active Wall Tension and the Law of Laplace

Let us imagine that the heart is a thin-walled sphere. (It is actually a thick-walled ellipsoid, but these details are not essential to the argument.) The circumferential tension in a thin equatorial hoop of muscle is

$$T_h = \tfrac{1}{2} P \cdot r$$

where P is pressure in the cavity, r the radius of the sphere, and T_h hoop tension. T_h represents the force along the axis of the hoop that would pull it apart if it were cut. Since the radius of the ventricular lumen increases with end-diastolic volume, *the intrinsic reserve of contractility is mobilized at the cost of greater systolic tension in the wall*. Systolic tension is derived from cycling cross-bridges, so dilation increases the ATP turnover and O_2 consumption required to perform a given amount of externally useful work. A rise in arterial pressure (increase in afterload) also raises wall tension and myocardial O_2 demand. Finally, active tension in the wall varies with heart rate.

Influence of Heart Rate

A significant increase in heart rate above the normal value is called *tachycardia*. Tachycardia can be produced by electrophysiological disturbances in an otherwise normal heart. More commonly heart rate increases in defense of cardiac output. The cost is greater stress on the heart itself. A large increase in active wall tension occurs early in systole as intraventricular pressure rises isovolumically from a few torr to the pressure in the aorta. Only then do ejection and external work begin. Since a larger fraction of each minute is spent in isovolumic contraction during tachycardia, total active tension per minute increases. O_2 demand increases proportionately.

Effect of Sympathetic Drive

Recruitment of cross-bridges by sympathetic mediators depends on release of additional Ca^{++} into the myoplasm during systole. This Ca^{++} must be sequestered in diastole to allow relaxation. Transport of extra Ca^{++} into storage depots costs ATP and O_2, over and above the O_2 consumption obligated by the actomyosin cross-bridges. Consequently, sympathetic stimulation increases O_2 demand and decreases the overall mechanical efficiency of the heart.

Clinical Application

Cardiac Dilation and Failure

If some muscle fibers are damaged, others must take up the load. They do this by increasing length, so the heart dilates and both active and passive wall tension increase. In animal models of severe chronic cardiac dilation, sarcomere lengths averaged 2.2 μm. Though the intrinsic contractile reserve was almost completely lost, the end-diastolic volumes were far greater than could be accounted for by the 10 percent increase in sarcomere length. Disruption of collagen struts with slippage of whole fibers appears to be the principal mechanism. The tension applied to collagen fibers increases with ventricular radius, so dilation tends to progress.

The ratio of the change in ventricular volume during systole to end-diastolic volume is called the *ejection fraction;* the normal range is 0.6 to 0.8. Ejection fraction is a useful clinical measure of ventricular performance that can be determined by echocardiography. The percent change in ventricular radius in systole is normally about the same as the percent rise in aortic pressure, so active tension — the product of pressure and radius — remains nearly constant throughout ejection. The dilated heart loses this advantage because its stroke volume is accompanied by only a small change in ventricular radius. For example, if the ejection fraction were 0.3, peak active tension would double during ejection even though stroke volume and arterial pressure were normal. The rates of energy turnover and O_2 consumption of a dilated heart are therefore greater for the same external work. Low mechanical efficiency is a salient characteristic of the dilated heart.

Ventricular failure may be defined as inability to perform sufficient work to meet systemic demands despite maximum normal end-diastolic pressure. Thus a heart may not be in failure at rest but may go into failure during exercise or emotional stress. On the lower curve in Figure 1-7, for example, normal stroke work at rest requires an end-diastolic pressure of 6 torr. Though this pressure is within normal limits, the intrinsic reserve of contractility is strongly engaged. Consequently, if the heart were stressed, the intrinsic reserve could not increase stroke work by more than 50 percent. Even with additional sympathetic drive, stroke work and cardiac output would be limited. If systemic demands cause end-diastolic pressure to exceed acceptable limits, the ventricle is said to be failing.

References

*1. Caro, C. G., Pedley, T. J., Schroter, R. C., and Seed, W. A. *The Mechanics of the Circulation*. New York; London: Oxford University Press, 1978. Pp. 190–230.

2. Chapman, C. B., and Mitchell, J. H. *Starling on the Heart: Facsimile Reprints*. London: Dawsons of Pall Mall, 1965.

3. Ciba Foundation Symposium. *The Physiological Basis of Starling's Law of the Heart*. Amsterdam: Associated Scientific Publishers, 1974.

4. Gibbs, C. L., and Chapman, J. B. Cardiac mechanics and energetics: Chemomechanical transduction in cardiac muscle. *Am. J. Physiol.* 249: H199, 1985.

5. Jewell, B. R. A reexamination of the influence of muscle length on myocardial performance. *Circ. Res.* 40:221, 1977.

6. Langner, G. A., and Brady, A. J. (eds.). *The Mammalian Myocardium*. New York: Wiley, 1974. Pp. 1–104.

7. Robinson, T. F., Cohen-Gould, L., and Factor, S. M. Skeletal framework of mammalian heart muscle. *Lab. Invest.* 49:482, 1983.

8. Ross, J., Jr., Sonnenblick, E. H., Taylor, R. R., Spotnitz, H. M., and Covell, J. W. Diastolic geometry and sarcomere lengths in the chronically dilated canine left ventricle. *Circ. Res.* 28:49, 1971.

*9. Sagawa, K. The end-systolic pressure-volume relation of the ventricle: Definition, modifications and clinical use. *Circulation* 63:1223, 1981.

2 : Resting and Action Potentials

The biophysical basis of the heart's electrical activity is directly applicable to pathophysiology and therapeutics and must be understood by the modern physician. We begin with a brief summary of electrophysiological essentials. Readers who have never been exposed to these ideas should consult reference 1 or 4 or an equivalent source before continuing. Those confident of their background can proceed directly to Electrical Anatomy, page 20.

The Resting Potential

The tendency of ions to diffuse in or out of cells down concentration gradients is opposed by the electrical potential generated by the inward or outward movement of charge. When the chemical and electrical forces acting on an ion are equal and opposite there is no net flux, and the system is in equilibrium. The potential E required for equilibrium if only one ion species is present is given by the Nernst equation:

$$E = \frac{RT}{zF} \ln \frac{[C_o]}{[C_i]},$$

where R is the gas constant, T the absolute temperature, F the Faraday, and z the valance of the ion. RT/F amounts to 26 mV at 37°C. C is ion concentration, and subscripts o and i denote outside and inside, respectively. Table 2-1 shows concentrations and equilibrium potentials for cat heart.

Thus far we have assumed that the cell membrane is no barrier, whereas ionic distribution — and hence the transmembrane potential, E_m — strongly depends on membrane permeability. Assuming a constant electrical field, E_m may be approximated by the Goldman-Hodgkin-Katz equation:

$$E_m = \frac{RT}{F} \ln \frac{P_K [K^+]_o + P_{Na} [Na^+]_o + P_{Cl} [Cl^-]_i}{P_K [K^+]_i + P_{Na} [Na^+]_i + P_{Cl} [Cl^-]_o},$$

where P is the permeability for a particular ion species, defined as the number of ions traversing a unit area per unit concentration gradient when the electrical potential difference is zero. E_m can be measured with an intracellular microelectrode and a ref-

Table 2-1
Ion Concentrations and Equilibrium Potentials in Cat Heart*

Ion	Concentrations (mEq/L) Out	In	Equilibrium Potential (mV)
Na^+	145	32	+40
K^+	5.3	172	−90
Ca^{++}	5.2	~.00007	+205
Cl^-	87	30	−28

*$[Ca^{++}]_i$ is too low to measure. Value shown is in the range required to prevent interaction of actin and myosin.

erence electrode considered to be at zero potential. E_m varies somewhat from cell to cell. An average value in canine ventricle is −85 mV. As E_m becomes smaller (less negative), the cell is said to become *depolarized.*

Except for nodal tissue, cardiac "resting" potentials are not far from the K^+ equlibrium potential, E_{K^+}, and distinctly different from equilibrium potentials for other ions. This means that the "resting" membrane is most permeable to K^+. Though the overall permeability of the "resting" membrane is low, ions continually diffuse in or out down their electrochemical gradients. These gradients are maintained by cell metabolism, coupled to a Na^+-K^+ ion pump.

The Action Potential

If E_m is not equal to the equilibrium potential, there will be a net flow of ionic current, I. For example:

$$I_{K^+} = g_{K^+}(E_m - E_{K^+}).$$

This is simply a statement of Ohm's law, where g is the reciprocal of resistance, or the *conductance,* and $(E_m - E_{K^+})$ is the driving force. The conductance depends on ionic concentrations, the number of available channels, the properties of each channel, membrane potential, and time. When E_m is depolarized to a critical, or *threshold* value, a characteristic series of changes in ionic conductances is brought about. The resulting time course of E_m is called the *action potential.*

It helps to recognize that a resting potential of −85 mV across 10 nm is equivalent to 8500 V across 1 cm! This enormous gradient controls the position of charged groups within and at the entrance to ion-specific transmembrane channels. Small wonder that conductances are highly voltage-dependent. Most are also time-dependent. To measure conductances at various times and voltages, it is necessary to prevent the action potential from running its course. This can be done in the relatively large Purkinje fibers by inserting two electrodes into the fiber — one to record, the other to pass current equal and opposite to net transmembrane current. By connecting the two electrodes in a feedback circuit, E_m can be "clamped" at a specified value and the transmembrane current can be measured.

The voltage clamp technique requires control of voltage over a considerable length. Good control can be achieved in the giant axon of squid by passing a wire longitudinally into the fiber. We shall therefore consider excitation in this nerve and then deal with the specializations that have evolved in the heart.

Conductance changes measured by Hodgkin and Huxley during an action potential of squid axon are shown in Figure 2-1. To account for the changes, they imagine that each channel is controlled by one to four charged molecules. These act as *gates* that are either open or closed, depending on E_m. The Na^+ gates open much more rapidly than K^+ gates. Consequently, as E_m is depolarized (made less negative), more g_{Na^+} than g_{K^+} is turned on (*activated*). When g_{Na^+} exceeds g_{K^+}, net positive charge accumulates inside and decreases E_m. This further increases g_{Na^+},

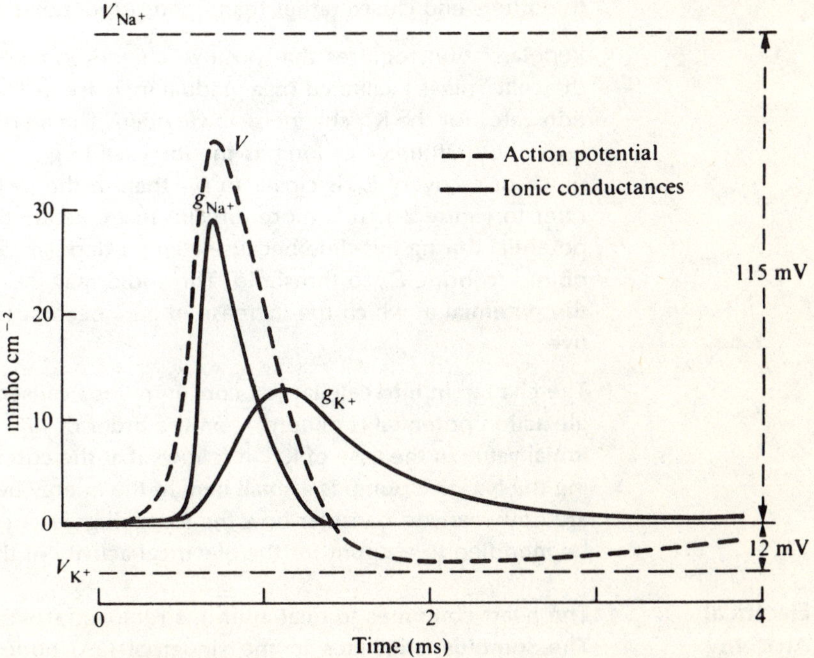

Figure 2-1
Action potential and ionic conductances in squid giant axon bathed in seawater. (From A. L. Hodgkin and A. F. Huxley, *J. Physiol.* [Lond.] 117:500, 1952.)

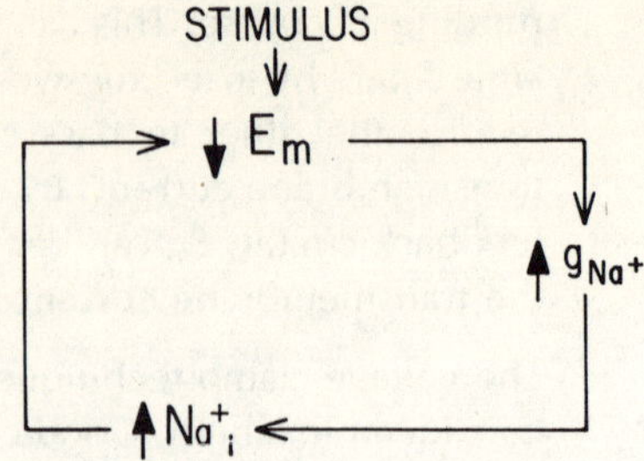

Figure 2-2
Depolarization as positive feedback. Filled arrows mean "increases" or "decreases," open arrows mean "causes," or "leads to."

and the process becomes self-accelerating, or *regenerative*. Notice in Figure 2-2 that this is an example of positive feedback. Nature uses positive feedback to transmit signals reliably. In this case it ensures that all Na^+ channels will open every time an adequate stimulus is applied. Na^+ activation takes less than 1 msec and is complete at about −45 mV. The resulting high I_{Na^+} drives E_m toward E_{Na^+} (see Figure 2-1); g_{Na^+} then decays exponentially over 1 to 2 msec. This *inactivation* can be accounted for by assuming that one of the Na^+ gates moves more slowly than the others and closes rather than opens on depolarization.

Repolarization requires that positive charge be carried out of the cell. This is facilitated by a gradual increase in I_{K^+} as activation gates for the K^+ channels slowly open. The increase in g_{K^+} lasts about 10 times as long as the increase in g_{Na^+}, so during much of recovery E_m is closer to E_{K^+} than in the resting state; refer to Figure 2-1. It is more difficult to excite another action potential during this time because a larger depolarization is required to bring E_m to threshold. Threshold may be defined as the potential at which the increase in g_{Na^+} becomes regenerative.

The change in intracellular ion concentrations caused by a single action potential is minute — on the order of 10^{-6} times the initial value in the case of K^+. It follows that the cost of operating the Na^+-K^+ pump is a small item in the energy budget. We are now ready to consider how the foregoing description must be modified to account for the electrical activity of the heart.

Electrical Anatomy

The heart continues to beat after it is removed from the body. The stimulus originates in the sinoatrial (SA) node near the superior vena cava and spreads throughout the myocardium. The basis for this intercellular conduction is considered in Chapter 3. The sequence of excitation and representative action potentials are diagrammed in Figure 2-3. Excitation reaches the

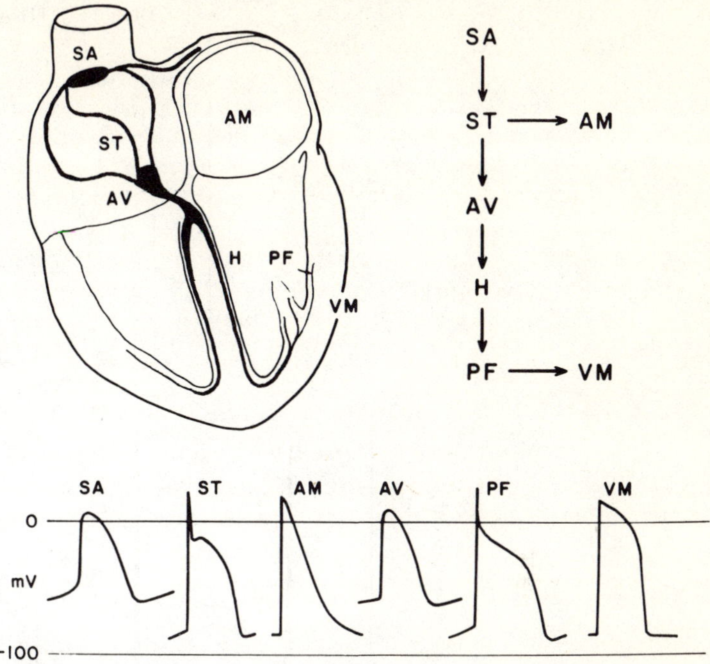

Figure 2-3
Sequence of spread of excitation and corresponding action potentials. (*SA* = sinoatrial node; *ST* = specialized atrial tracts; *AM* = atrial muscle; *AV* = atrioventricular node; *H* = bundle of His; *PF* = Purkinje fibers; *VM* = ventricular muscle.) Differences in rate of phase 0 depolarization cannot be observed on the time scale of these recordings. (From R. W. Tsien and S. Siegelbaum, Excitable Tissues: The Heart. In T. E. Andreoli, J. F. Hoffman, and D. Fanestil [eds.], *The Physiological Basis for Disorders of Biomembranes.* New York: Plenum, 1978.)

atrioventricular (AV) node over fast-conducting tracts much like ventricular Purkinje fibers. It spreads more slowly over the atria, where it must travel from one atrial muscle cell to another. The AV node is specialized for slow unidirectional conduction and is the only electrical connection between the atria and ventricles. Its principal function is to delay ventricular excitation and ventricular contraction until after the atria have contracted. When the excitation escapes from the AV node, it enters the Purkinje system, which is highly specialized to distribute the excitation rapidly to small groups of true muscle cells. Within these groups, conduction occurs slowly, but over very small distances. Consequently, all ventricular fibers are excited almost simultaneously and contract in unison. Synchronous contraction is essential for mechanical function.

All cardiac muscle cells contract, conduct excitation, and are capable of rhythmic beating. Nevertheless, each is specialized

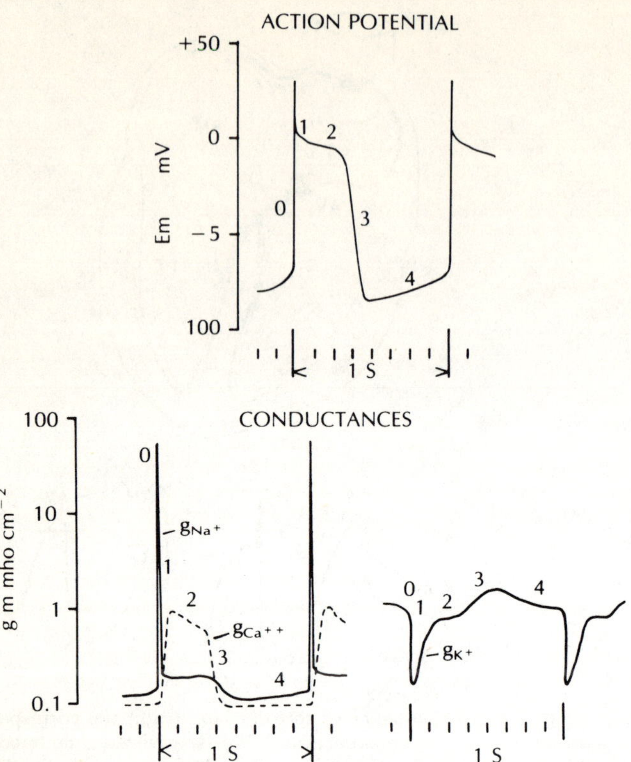

Figure 2-4
Purkinje fiber action potential and time courses of ionic conductances. Note log scale in lower panel. (Modified from D. Noble, *The Initiation of the Heart Beat.* New York, London: Oxford University Press, 1975.)

for one of these functions. Specialization depends largely on unique features of the action potential.

Action Potential in Purkinje Fibers: A Prototype

It is convenient to divide the action potential into five phases. These are shown for a Purkinje fiber in Figure 2-4, together with estimated time courses of ionic conductances.

Contribution of Fast Na^+ Channels

Maximum g_{Na^+} is almost two orders of magnitude greater than peak g_{K^+} or $g_{Ca^{++}}$. The large rapid change in g_{Na^+} generates a rapidly rising action potential and a positive overshoot in phase 0. We shall see in Chapter 3 that these features greatly facilitate spread of excitation along the fiber.

Phase 1 of the action potential reflects the abrupt fall in g_{Na^+} as the Na^+ inactivation gates close. Up to this point things are qualitatively and quantitatively the same as in nerve or skeletal muscle. Subsequent events, however, are different. In nerve the Na^+ inactivation gates reopen after only 1 to 2 ms, thus "repriming" the Na^+ channels for a new excitation. Repriming cannot occur until repolarization is almost complete. In the heart this is delayed for hundreds of milliseconds.

Mechanism of the Plateau

The salient feature of a cardiac action potential is its duration, which is perhaps 100 times longer than in squid axon. In Chapter 4 we learn that signals initiated by the action potential switch active tension on and off. Since ventricular emptying requires about 300 ms at normal heart rate, sustained depolarization is essential for maintenance of active tension. A long action potential is also necessary for ventricular filling, for if repolarization were as fast as in nerve or skeletal muscle a rapid succession of action potentials could tetanize the heart and prevent entry of blood. Finally, the duration of the action potential is a major factor in the genesis of arrhythmias.

To understand the mechanism of phase 2 (the so-called plateau), consider a uniform patch of membrane in which there is no propagation of excitation. For this special case the *net* ionic current I_i is equal and opposite to I_c, the current flowing into the membrane capacity

$$I_c = C_m \frac{dV}{dt} = -I_i,$$

where C_m is membrane capacity and V is voltage. Since E_m changes very slowly during the plateau (about 0.1 percent of the maximum rate in phase 0), the net ionic current must be very small. Thus delayed repolarization depends on a *delicate balance of inward and outward* currents.[1] I_c is small in phase 2 because the electrical resistance of the membrane is about 300 times that in phase 0. High resistance (low permeability) minimizes the changes in ion concentrations that must be restored by metabolic work after the action potential is over.

Role of K^+ Channels

Two properties of the K^+ channels largely account for high resistance during the plateau. First, the K^+ activation gates open about 100 times more slowly than in nerve, so the number of channels available to carry outward current remains almost constant in phase 1 and increases very slowly in phase 2. In addition, the outward conductance of each K^+ channel decreases as E_m becomes appreciably less negative than E_{K^+}. This is reflected in the plot of inward and outward currents shown in Figure 2-5. If the K^+ channels were simple ohmic resistors, the current-voltage relation would be a straight line that intersects the abscissa at E_{K^+}. Instead, the channels act like rectifiers that, in the

[1] Inward current means inflow of positive charge or outflow of negative charge. Outward current means the reverse.

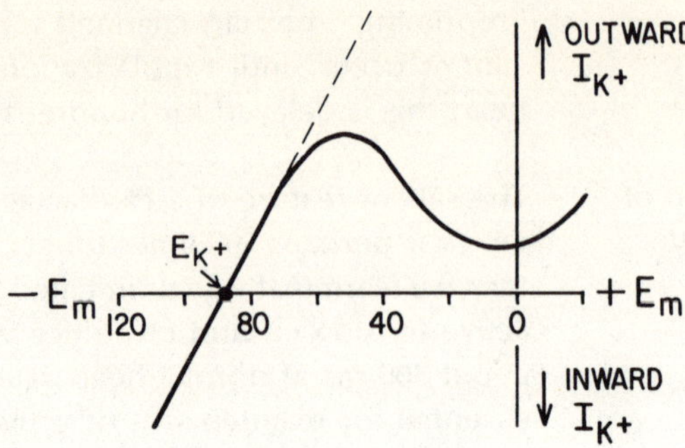

Figure 2-5
Effective current-voltage relation for K^+ channels. Dashed line indicates expected behavior if the channels obeyed Ohm's law.

range of voltages characteristic of the plateau, limit flow of outward current. Inward rectification accounts for the sharp fall in g_{K^+} in phase 1, and keeps g_{K^+} relatively low in phase 2.[2]

The Ca^{++} Channel

A slow inward current (I_{si}) opposes the outward K^+ current during the action potential plateau. This important current activates at about −40 mV, a potential at which Na^+ channels are completely inactivated. It is not much affected by removal of Na^+ or by tetrodotoxin (TTX), a substance that blocks Na^+ channels specifically and completely. In the experiment shown in Figure 2-6, a Purkinje fiber was exposed to graded doses of TTX. The initial spike attributable to fast Na^+ channels decreases progressively and is abolished in panel *E*. The action potential generated by unblocked I_{si} closely matches the time course of the normal plateau. I_{si} is almost abolished by removal of Ca^{++} or by Ca^{++} channel antagonists such as Mn^{++} or verapamil. The specificity of the channels for I_{si} varies among species and in different regions of the heart. In ventricular cells the ratios $P_{Ca^{++}}/P_{Na^+}$ and $P_{Ca^{++}}/P_{K^+} \cong 1/0.01$, so the term *$Ca^{++}$ channel* seems appropriate. The Ca^{++} inactivation gates must move about 100 times more slowly than Na^+ gates to account for the conductance changes shown in Figure 2-4.

Rapid Phase of Repolarization

Several factors act in concert to terminate the plateau. Late in phase 2, closure of Ca^{++} inactivation gates turns off a depolarizing current, while at the same time the K^+ activation gates continue to open. This tips the balance toward outward currents, and E_m begins to drift negative. Were this the entire story re-

[2]The matter is actually much more complicated. There are several categories of K^+ channels, and the current-voltage relation is not independent of time and K^+_o, as assumed in Figure 2-5. Thus one should visualize a family of current-voltage curves.

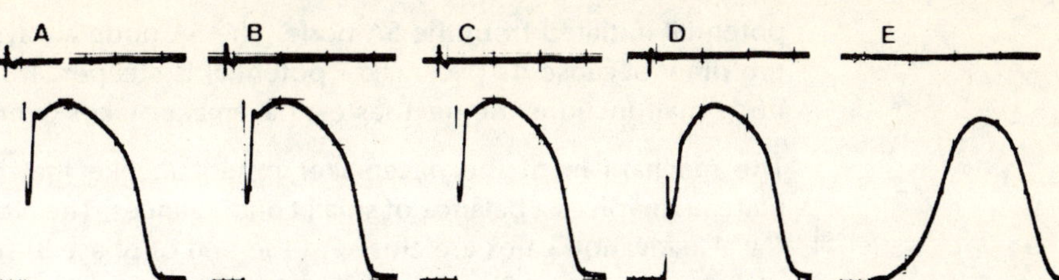

Figure 2-6
Progressive blockade of I_{Na^+} in calf Purkinje fiber by increasing doses of TTX. The experiment was performed in the presence of epinephrine, which enhances I_{si}. (Modified from E. Carmeliet and J. Vereecke, *Pflügers Arch.* 313:303, 1969.)

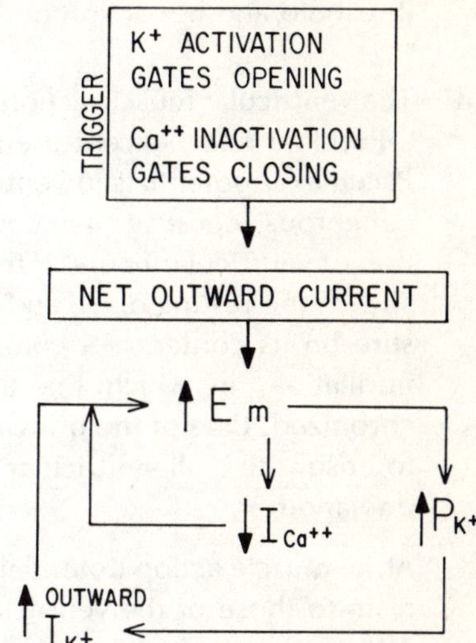

Figure 2-7
Repolarization as positive feedback. Filled arrows mean "increases" or "decreases"; open arrows mean "causes" or "leads to." An increased E_m is more negative and closer to the K^+ equilibrium potential.

polarization would be prohibitively slow. In fact, it accelerates and becomes regenerative in phase 3, partly because $g_{Ca^{++}}$ inactivates more rapidly as E_m becomes more negative. In addition, the amount of outward current per K^+ channel increases between about -20 and -60 mV because of the current-voltage relation shown in Figure 2-5. A plausible scheme for regenerative repolarization is shown in Figure 2-7.

The Pacemaker Potential

In the Purkinje fiber, E_m gradually drifts toward threshold during phase 4. This slow depolarization is called the *pacemaker potential*. Similar potentials exist in cells of the atrial tracts and the SA and AV nodes. The one in the Purkinje fiber is a backup system. Long before it reaches threshold it is extinguished by an action potential initiated from the SA node. The SA node always wins the draw because its pacemaker potential is steeper. If the SA node malfunctions the next fastest pacemaker takes over.

The mechanism of the pacemaker potential, like that of the plateau, involves a balance of small conductances. The Na^+ and Ca^{++} activation gates are closed at the end of phase 3, so g_{Na^+} and $g_{Ca^{++}}$ are low. Since more of the K^+ activation gates have opened, and the conductance of each channel is relatively high, g_{K^+} reaches a maximum; refer again to Figure 2-4. As the K^+ activation gates slowly close in phase 4, g_{K^+} steadily decreases. This allows inward leak of positive charge, probably carried by Na^+, to depolarize the membrane gradually. If E_m reaches threshold another action potential begins.

Modifications in Ventricles and Atria

The ventricular muscle action potential closely resembles that of a Purkinje fiber, except there is no depolarization in phase 4. Pacemaker potentials in ventricular muscle would be extremely dangerous, because they could initiate asynchronous contraction of ventricular fibers. If this happens, the active cells merely stretch the resting ones, and the ventricle fails to develop pressure on its contents. A common cause of death is ventricular fibrillation, in which the fibers become completely desynchronized. One of the principal functions of the Purkinje net is to ensure that all ventricular muscle fibers remain in step with one another.

Atrial muscle action potentials are identical in form and mechanism to those of the ventricle except that phase 2 is short and often inseparable from phase 3. Ventricular action potentials with comparably short plateaus are observed at very rapid heart rates.

Ca^{++}-Dependent Slow Action Potentials

The slow time course of action potentials in the SA and AV nodes resembles that in a Purkinje fiber treated with TTX; compare AV in Figure 2-3 with Figure 2-6. This is to be expected, because the fast Na^+ channels are almost fully inactivated at the low "resting" (or maximum diastolic) potentials characteristic of nodal tissue. Ca^{++} is chiefly responsible for phase 0 depolarization in the SA and AV nodes. The mechanism of the SA nodal pacemaker potential is the same in principle as described for Purkinje fibers, except that I_{si} makes a substantial contribution.

It is difficult to overestimate the importance of I_{si}. Apart from functions already considered, we shall see that it influences AV conduction, excitation-contraction coupling, tension development, and the effects of neurohumoral mediators.

References

1. Armstrong, C. M. Sodium channels and gating currents. *Physiol. Rev.* 61:644, 1981.

2. Brown, H. F., Giles, W., and Noble, S. J. Membrane currents underlying activity in frog sinus venosus. *J. Physiol.* (Lond.) 271:783, 1977.

*3. Kass, R. S. The Ionic Basis of Electrical Activity in the Heart. In N. Sperelakis (ed.), *Physiology and Pathophysiology of the Heart*. Boston: Nijhoff, 1984. Pp. 83–96.

4. Katz, B. *Nerve, Muscle and Synapse*. New York: McGraw-Hill, 1966. Pp. 12–96.

5. Noble, D. *The Initiation of the Heart Beat*. New York, London: Oxford University Press, 1979. Pp. 10–84.

6. Reuter, H., and Scholz, H. A study of the ion selectivity and the kinetic properties of the calcium dependent slow inward current in mammalian cardiac muscle. *J. Physiol.* (Lond.) 264:17, 1977.

7. Stein, W. D. *Ion Channels: Molecular and Physiological Aspects*. New York: Academic, 1985.

3 : Conduction, Excitation, and Arrhythmias

Cell-to-Cell Communication

Action potentials spread throughout the heart even though each cell is a discrete anatomical unit. The ultrastructural basis for this behavior is the *nexus,* which connects two adjacent cells electrically. It is generally associated with an intercalated disc that connects the cells mechanically; see Figure 3-1. At a nexus the plasma membranes of two cells come into close proximity but do not fuse. Figure 3-2 is a schematic of the ultrastructure of a nexus. If the adjacent cells are analogous to water tanks, the nexus is a system of short connecting pipes 1 to 2 nm in diameter and flared at each end like a rivet. Tracer molecules up to about 800 daltons can diffuse across the nexus when injected intracellularly. This means that cardiac cells exchange not only ions but small organic molecules as well. Calculations indicate that transnexus channels add only about 1 percent to the longitudinal resistivity of a cardiac fiber, and that even one open channel should suffice to couple two cardiac myocytes. Thus from the electrical point of view the atria can be thought of as one big "cell" and the ventricles another. However, these virtual cells are extremely large, so time is required for excitation to spread from one part to another.

Permeability of the nexus is controlled by intracellular Ca^{++} and H^{+}. If the transmembrane Ca^{++} and H^{+} gradients cannot be maintained because of injury or anoxia, the resistance of the nexus increases and the cell is electrically sealed off. This prevents flow of excitatory current from the injured, depolarized cell to its normal neighbors. Sealing off requires 10 to 30 minutes. It may not be coincidence that fatal arrhythmias are most common in the first few minutes after a coronary occlusion.

Fibers as Cables

When an action potential propagates along a fiber, the regenerative response is preceded by subthreshold current flow, which acts as a stimulus to the unexcited membrane. This stimulus depends on the properties of the fiber as a cable. The effect of a *subthreshold* square pulse of current is shown in Figure 3-3. Current was injected intracellularly at one end of the fiber. E_m was measured at increasing distances from the elec-

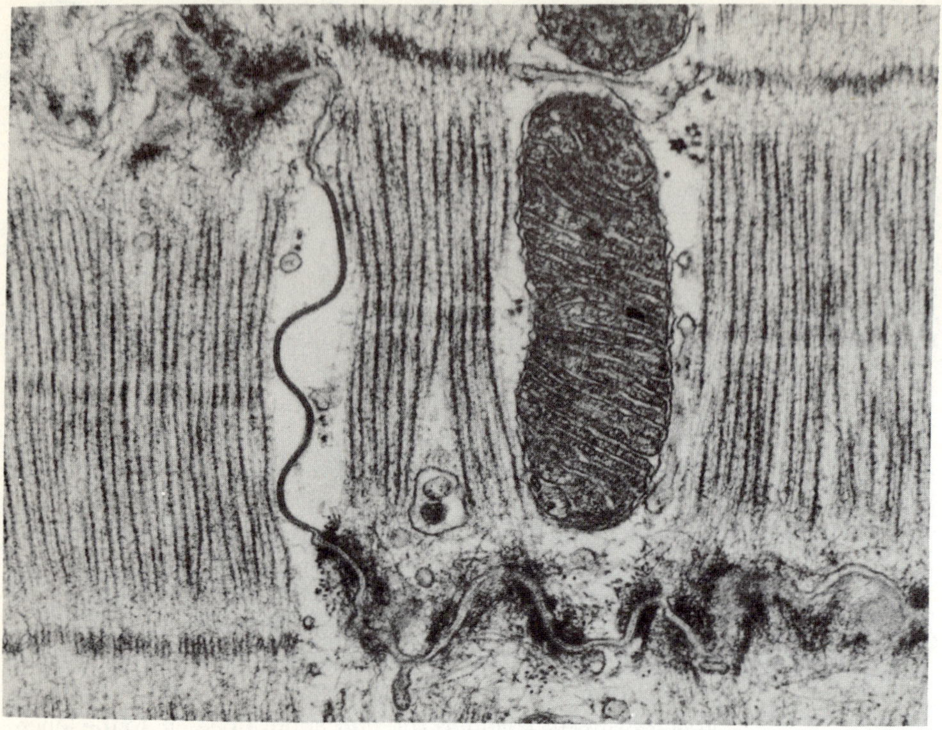

Figure 3-1
Longitudinal section through an intercalated disc, which includes a nexus. The disc exhibits a typical zigzag course with patches of dark-staining anchoring filaments. The nexus runs parallel to the long axis of the myofibrils. Because of a fortuitous artifact it is surrounded by clear cytoplasm. Magnification × 60,000 (before 21% reduction). (From J. R. Sommer, R. L. Steere, E. A. Johnson, and P. H. Jewett, Ultrastructure of Cardiac Muscle. In *Hibernation and Hypothermia. Perspectives and Challenges*. Amsterdam: Elsevier, 1972.)

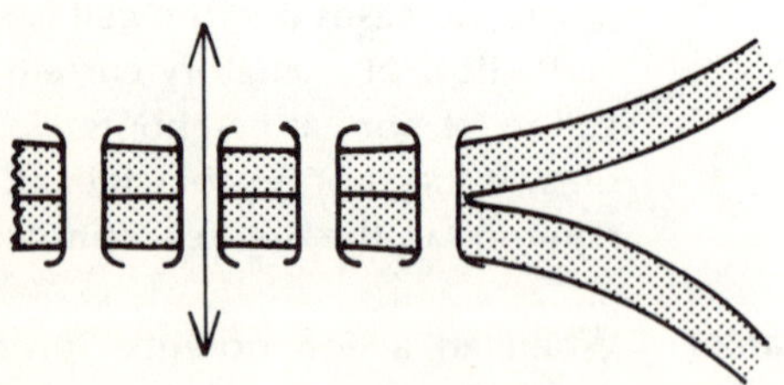

Figure 3-2
Nexus, showing aqueous intercellular channels.

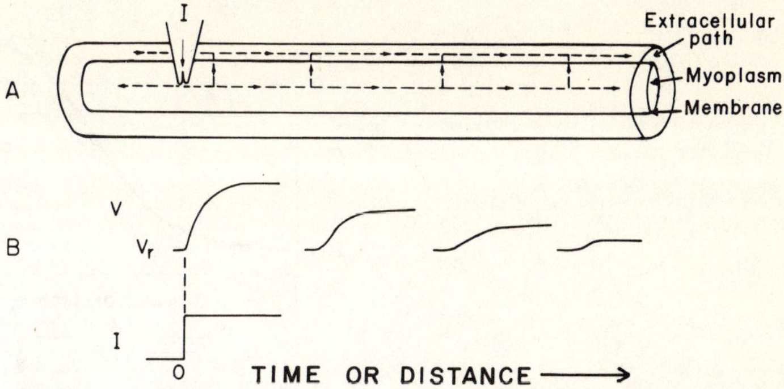

Figure 3-3
A. Subthreshold current is injected through an intracellular electrode. Dashed arrows indicate paths of current flow. B. Change in E_m at increasing distances from microelectrode. (Modified from A. J. Brady, In G. A. Langer and A. J. Brady [eds.], *The Mammalian Myocardium*. New York: Wiley, 1974.)

trode. The decrease in E_m with distance from the stimulation site is defined by the space constant:

$$\lambda = \sqrt{R_m/R_i},$$

where R_m is the transmembrane resistance and R_i is the resistance of the interior of the fiber. A large space constant facilitates conduction. Thanks to the nexus, λ is about 10 cell lengths throughout the heart except for the atrioventricular (AV) node. R_i can be increased by lack of O_2 and by drugs such as halothane and digitalis, probably by affecting the nexus. The decrease in λ so produced can halve the speed of propagation of an action potential.

Propagation of the Action Potential

In contrast to passive spread of subthreshold current, an action potential generally propagates without decrement, because it is reamplified at every point by positive feedback; recall Figure 2-2. The spread of a Purkinje fiber action potential is diagrammed in Figure 3-4. At *1*, a battery symbolizes a regenerative inward current carried by Na^+ (or Ca^{++}). Positive charge (mostly K^+) flows through the interior of the fiber from right to left. The resistor at *2* represents R_i. This passive current spread depolarizes adjacent patches of membrane to threshold. Current that escapes through the membrane capacity at *3* returns through the resistance of the extracellular fluid *4* to complete the circuit. Local currents that accompany repolarization flow in the reverse direction. Phase 0 of the action potential is shown above. If the conduction velocity is 2 meters per second, E_m changes from about -80 to $+30$ mV within 1 mm and in 0.5 ms.

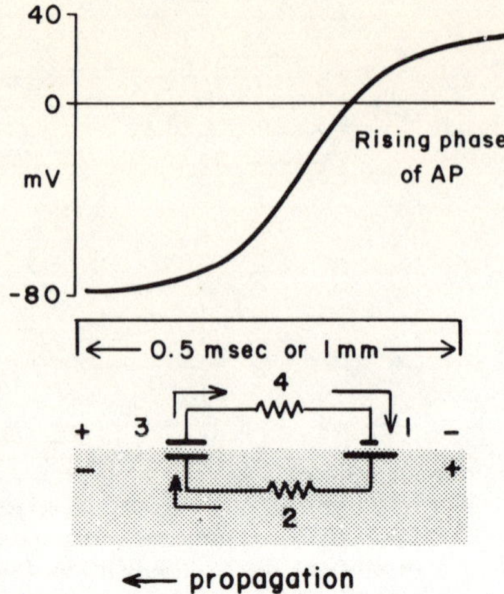

Figure 3-4
Top, Rising phase of a propagating Purkinje fiber action potential (*AP*), if conduction velocity is 2 m/s. Bottom, Simplified diagram of local circuit current and action potential propagation. (Modified from R. W. Tsein and S. Siegelbaum, Excitable Tissues: The Heart. In T. E. Andreoli, J. F. Hoffman, and D. Fanestil [eds.], *The Physiology of Membrane Disorders*. New York: Plenum, 1978.)

Recall from Chapter 2 that

$$-I_i \cong C_m \frac{dV}{dt}.$$

Consequently, the amount of excitatory current that can spread passively down a fiber depends on $\frac{dV}{dt}$. The ability of this current to excite adjacent patches of membrane also depends on $\frac{dV}{dt}$: If E_m changes too slowly, the Na^+ inactivation gates begin to close and a regenerative response becomes more difficult to produce. Thus the rate of rise of the action potential is a major determinant of the rate at which an action potential propagates along a fiber.

The influence of resting potential on channel availability, I_{Na^+}, and $\frac{dV}{dt}$ in a Purkinje fiber is shown in Figure 3-5. Almost all Na^+ channels are available at the normal resting potential. Consequently, I_{Na^+} and the rate of rise of the action potential ($\frac{dV}{dt}$) are almost at a maximum. If the membrane is depolarized to -70 mV, however, the number of available Na^+ channels is only half normal. The resulting action potential is small and propagates slowly. No fast Na^+ channels whatever are available if E_m is

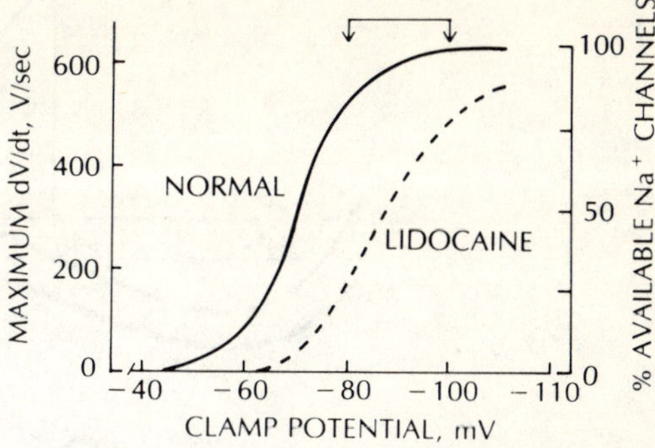

Figure 3-5
Data for a Purkinje fiber in which action potentials were initiated from various resting potentials. Ordinates are proportional to I_{Na^+}. Depolarization, a local anesthetic, or both inactivate Na^+ channels, decrease the rate of change of E_m, and slow conduction. Arrows indicate range of normal resting potential.

clamped in the range of the plateau, and no action potential can be evoked. The arrows in Figure 3-5 indicate that the normal resting or end-diastolic potential is at the shoulder of the steep Na^+ inactivation curve. Therefore high serum K^+, ischemia, and other conditions accompanied by depolarization profoundly affect conduction velocity. Local anesthetics such as lidocaine inactivate Na^+ channels even without depolarization. Lidocaine also slows removal of inactivation ("repriming"). Both these effects are used therapeutically to control arrhythmias. The ideas in Figures 3-4 and 3-5 are particularly important and practical; take enough time to be sure you understand them thoroughly.

Conduction Through the AV Node

Most conduction disorders in clinical medicine occur at the AV node. This is hardly surprising, for nodal conduction is slow and precarious even under normal circumstances. Almost the entire AV delay occurs over 1 mm at the atrial end. Conduction velocity in these cells is about 20 microns per second, as compared with 2 meters per second in the much larger diameter Purkinje fibers. AV nodal cells possess few nexuses, and the calculated electrical conductance from cell to cell is three orders of magnitude less than for other cardiac tissues. To make matters worse, the action potential rises very slowly because it depends on I_{si}. The action potential therefore generates much less excitatory current than the fast-rising Na^+ spike in Purkinje fibers. It is easy to see how conduction might fail if $g_{Ca^{++}}$ were partly inactivated, or g_{K^+} were enhanced, or both. Examples of such effects are considered in Chapter 5.

Excitability

The rate at which an action potential propagates depends not only on local circuit current and cable properties, but also on

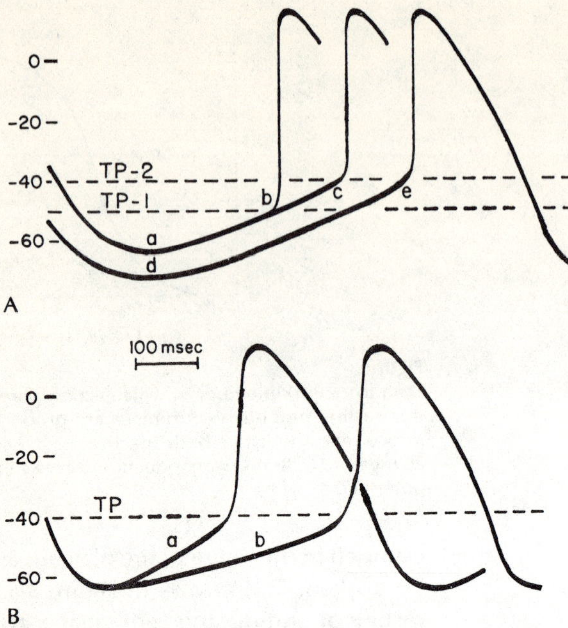

Figure 3-6
Heart rate can be controlled by changing excitability (*A*) or the slope of the pacemaker potential (*B*). Dashed lines and *TP* denote threshold potential. (From B. F. Hoffman and P. F. Cranefield, *Electrophysiology of the Heart.* Copyright © 1960, McGraw-Hill Book Company. Used with permission of McGraw-Hill Book Company.)

the ability of the membrane to respond. For pacemaker potentials, excitability during phase 4 may be defined as the difference between the maximum diastolic potential and threshold for a regenerative response; see Figure 3-6A. Raising threshold without changing E_m (curves *a, b,* and *c*) decreases excitability. This delays the action potential at c and lowers heart rate. If, in addition, the pacemaker is hyperpolarized (curve *d*), excitability and heart rate decrease further. Heart rate can be markedly altered without changing excitability by varying the slope of the pacemaker potential, as in Figure 3-6B.

If the heart is injured, or a premature beat arises, local currents may flow at any time. It is therefore essential to learn how excitability varies during the course of the action potential. The amount of current that must be delivered through a stimulating electrode is a measure of excitability; see Figure 3-7.

A regenerative response cannot be elicited between phase 1 and early phase 3, no matter how intense the stimulus. This is called the *effective refractory period* (ERP). The membrane is not completely unresponsive, for cathodal current delays repolarization, and anodal current accelerates it. At a critical time (and

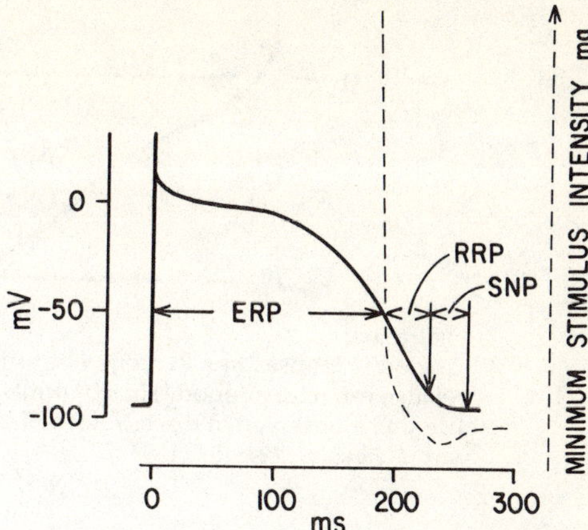

Figure 3-7
Normal relationship between action potential of ventricular muscle fiber and excitability to a depolarizing stimulus. Dashed line shows stimulus intensity required for excitation. (*SNP* = supernormal period; *RRP* = relative refractory period; *ERP* = effective refractory period.) (Modified from B. F. Hoffman and P. F. Cranefield, *Electrophysiology of the Heart*. Copyright © 1960, McGraw-Hill Book Company. Used by permission of McGraw-Hill Book Company.)

E_m) a sufficiently intense stimulus will evoke a small, slowly rising action potential. The interval during which the stimulus must be greater than in phase 4 is termed the *relative refractory period* (RRP). The stimulus intensity required for excitation (*dashed line*, Figure 3-7) falls very steeply during that time. Late in phase 3, E_m is greater than the normal threshold potential but less than the resting potential, so a smaller than normal stimulus will excite. This is called the *supernormal period*.

Variations in excitability in non-nodal tissue depend mainly on availability of Na^+ channels. During the ERP Na^+ channels are completely inactivated. The RRP reflects reactivation as progressively more Na^+ channels become available.

Clinical Application

Genesis of Arrhythmias

Cardiac rhythm can be disturbed if normal sinoatrial (SA) nodal impulses fail to conduct to the atria or ventricles. These arrhythmias are classified as passive. With the advent of electronic pacemakers, they are no longer life-threatening. Active arrhythmias, that is, those caused by ectopic excitation, are far more important. We shall use ventricular fibrillation as a prototype. Experimental evidence exists for two distinctly different mechanisms for active arrhythmias, namely, automaticity and reentry. Both can be initiated by premature beats.

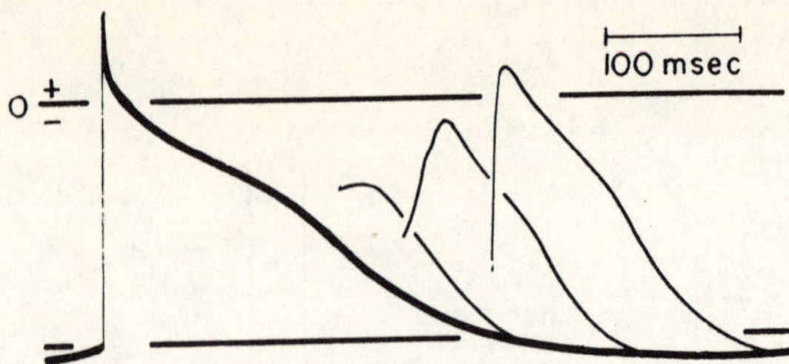

Figure 3-8
Graded responses in a Purkinje fiber stimulated at various times during the relative refractory period. The abnormal action potentials so produced simulate those observed in disease. (Modified from C. Y. Kao and B. F. Hoffman, *Am. J. Physiol.* 194:187, 1958.)

Extrasystoles and Graded Responses

Ventricular fibrillation is almost always preceded by one or more premature beats. The earlier they occur in phase 3 the greater the danger. Detection and elimination of extrasystoles are among the objectives of patient monitoring. The effect of induced extrasystoles on a Purkinje fiber is shown in Figure 3-8. One side of a double-barreled microelectrode was used to stimulate, the other to record. A second electrode monitored potential at a distance from the stimulus site. The more premature the response, the smaller its amplitude, rate of rise, and duration. Moreover, the earlier responses decreased in amplitude with distance from the site of origin. Normal action potentials are, of course, invariant. Premature responses differ from true all-or-none action potentials because the regenerative Na^+ and Ca^{++} mechanisms cannot supply depolarizing current fast enough in the face of high g_{K+} "left over" from the previous beat. Only a few milliseconds separate the relative and effective refractory periods. Consequently, small local differences in the duration of the plateau may allow some cells to respond with a decremental action potential, whereas adjacent ones are inexcitable or respond normally. The resulting desynchronization may die out or progress to ventricular fibrillation.

Automaticity

If a Purkinje fiber is sufficiently depolarized, it may exhibit low-amplitude, rhythmic oscillations that, if conducted to adjacent normal cells, can act as an ectopic pacemaker. An example is shown in Figure 3-9. Panel A is a control recording at normal "resting" potential. When the cell was depolarized to −65 mV, spontaneous, repetitive discharges appeared. The frequency of these oscillations in-

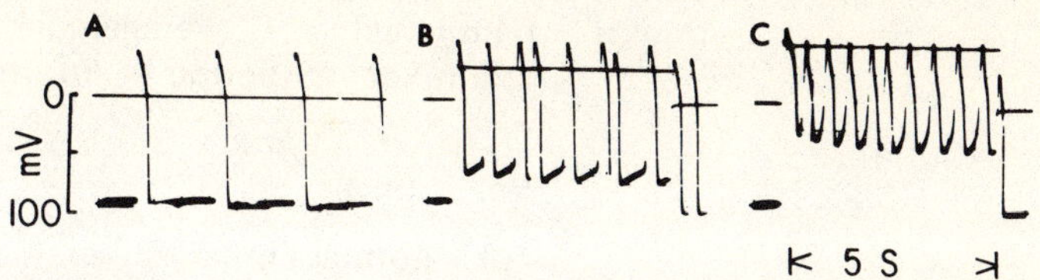

Figure 3-9
A. Recording from a normal Purkinje fiber, electrically driven. B, C. Depolarizing current was applied extracellularly as indicated by the steps in the upper baseline. Frequency of oscillation increased with depolarization. (Modified from S. Imanishi, *Jpn. J. Physiol.* 21:443, 1971.)

creased with the degree of depolarization, as in *C*. Oscillations are strongly dependent on Ca^{++} and only slightly on Na^{+}, indicating that a slow channel is responsible. Consequently, *dV/dt* and local circuit currents are small. Oscillations are therefore conducted very slowly — about 10 microns per second — and fade out over short distances.

The most common cause of local depolarization in humans is ischemia (insufficient blood supply). O_2 gradients in myocardium can occur over distances comparable to one space constant. Thus passive electrotonic spread can couple a normoxic cell to a hypoxic, partly depolarized oscillatory cell to produce an ectopic pacemaker. Coupled cells can follow rapid oscillations because one of the earliest effects of ischemia is to shorten the refractory period. Action potentials emanating from an ectopic focus can be disseminated by the Purkinje net. Normal cells at a distance from the ectopic focus that are "caught" in their effective refractory periods would not respond, but others with shorter refractory periods may. The next ectopic stimulus would excite a different population, and the heart would become more and more desynchronized. Ischemia is not the only means which oscillations may arise. Since they depend on a balance of small inward and outward currents, they may be initiated or modified by $[K^{+}]_o$, nerve mediators, or drugs, as explained in Chapter 5.

Reentry

Local circuit currents arise if some cells are less polarized, or have shorter action potentials than others, or both. Such currents — induced, for example, by ischemia — can be intense enough to arouse aberrant action potentials like those in Figure 3-8. Such action potentials may conduct slowly over a circuitous path and return to the site of origin. If cells there are not refractory they may fire again, so that a repetitive cycle of reexcitation is produced. If path length = L, average conduction velocity = Θ, and refractory period = Rp, reentry requires

$$\underset{(m)}{L} > \underset{(m/s)}{\Theta} \cdot \underset{(s)}{Rp}.$$

For a normal Purkinje fiber

$$0.5 \text{ m} = 2 \text{ m/s} \times 0.25 \text{ s}.$$

A cardiac cell 0.5 m long is obviously impossible. Rapid conduction in the Purkinje net and factors that maintain the plateau prevent reentry in the normal heart. The situation is different in a partly depolarized region in which action potentials depend on I_{si}, the refractory period is short, and conduction is slow. Then path length can be on the scale of heterogeneities of local O_2 supply:

$$0.001 \text{ m} = 0.01 \text{ m/s} \times 0.1 \text{ s}.$$

Though slow conduction is essential for reentry, fast conduction is required to disseminate the excitation beyond the reentry path. Availability of fast-conducting pathways is assured by the steep dependence of I_{Na^+} on E_m (and hence distance from site of injury). Computer modelling indicates that fibrillation caused by reentry is greatly facilitated in a nonhomogeneous myocardium in which Θ and Rp vary substantially from point to point. Thus fibrillation can be induced in experimental animals by clamping a small coronary artery, but seldom occurs if O_2 supply is reduced uniformly by lowering the O_2 content of arterial blood.

Though automaticity and reentry are conceptually different, both depend on local heterogeneities of E_m, conduction velocity, and refractory period. Moreover, both generally (though not invariably) involve I_{si}. The many clinical factors that predispose to fibrillation and their modes of action are informatively discussed in reference 10.

References

1. Bean, B. P., Cohen, C. J., and Tsien, R. W. Lidocaine block of cardiac sodium channels. *J. Gen. Physiol.* 81:613, 1983.
2. Cranefield, P. F. *The Conduction of the Cardiac Impulse: The Slow Response and Cardiac Arrhythmias.* Mt. Kisco, N.Y.: Futura, 1975.
3. Estápe-Wainwright, E., and DeMello, W. C. Cyclic nucleotides and calcium: Their roles in the control of cell communication in the heart. *Cell Biol. Int. Rep.* 7:91, 1983.

*4. Fozzard, H. A. Conduction of the Action Potential. In *Handbook of Physiology,* Section 2: The Cardiovascular System — The Heart, Vol. I. Bethesda, Md.: American Physiological Society, 1979.

5. Hauswirth, O., and Singh, B. N. Ionic mechanisms in heart muscle in relation to the genesis and the pharmacologic control of cardiac arrhythmias. *Pharmacol. Rev.* 30:5, 1979.
6. Hoffman, B. F., and Rosen, M. R. Cellular mechanisms for cardiac arrhythmias. *Circ. Res.* 49:69, 1981.
7. Kass, R. S., and Tsien, R. W. Fluctuations in membrane current driven by intracellular calcium in cardiac Purkinje fibers. *Biophys. J.* 38:259, 1982.
8. Noble, D. *The Initiation of the Heartbeat.* New York, London: Oxford University Press, 1979. Pp. 43–52, 150–163.
9. Peracchia, C., and Girsch, S. J. Functional modulation of cell coupling: Evidence for a calmodulin-driven channel gate. *Am. J. Physiol.* 248:H765, 1985.
10. Surawicz, B. Ventricular fibrillation. *J. Am. Coll. Cardiol.* 5:43B, 1985.

4 : Excitation-Contraction Coupling and Control of Tension

This chapter is concerned with the mechanisms by which tension is developed and controlled. Each skeletal-muscle cell always develops maximum tension in vivo; it has no contractile reserve. Tension in a whole skeletal muscle is graded by varying the number of cells recruited by the motor nerve. In contrast, all cardiac cells contract in unison on every beat, and no nerves are required at all. Tension developed by each cardiac cell is graded by recruiting or deleting actomyosin cross-bridges. The principle — recruitment of units in parallel — is the same for all muscles, even though the mechanisms are very different.

Ca^{++} and the Molecular Switch

Chemical interaction of actin in the thin filaments with myosin in the thick filaments is switched on and off by changes in the intracellular concentration of ionized Ca^{++}. The mechanism illustrates how an organ response can be accounted for at the molecular level; see Figure 4-1. At rest $[Ca^{++}]_i$ is less than 0.1 μM, and very little Ca is bound to troponin. Under these conditions one end of the troponin complex attaches to actin and holds tropomyosin in a position that physically blocks the actin binding site for myosin. The action potential initiates an abrupt rise in $[Ca^{++}]_i$ to approximately 1 μM. Each skeletal-muscle troponin has four high-affinity Ca^{++}-binding sites. Binding produces a conformational change that detaches troponin from actin. This allows the troponin-tropomyosin complex to "roll" to a more thermodynamically favorable position nearer the groove of the actin helix. The movement uncovers the myosin binding site and allows cross-bridge formation. Removal of Ca from troponin restores troponin and tropomyosin to the blocking position and switches off contraction.

Enough Ca^{++} is made available in contracting skeletal muscle to saturate all troponin binding sites, so every actin monomer is free to combine with myosin. In cardiac muscle, however, *troponin is not fully saturated under normal circumstances*. This fact accounts for the striking difference in the length–active tension relations of cardiac and skeletal muscles shown in Figure 1-3, p. 6. It follows that anything that increases Ca^{++} avail-

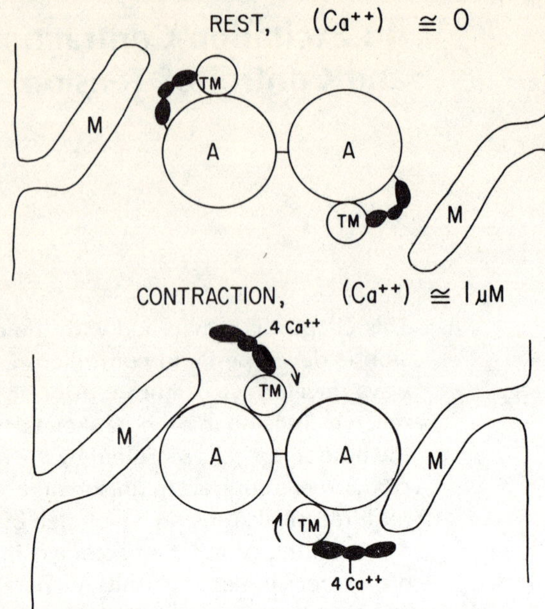

Figure 4-1
Molecular control of contraction. (*M* = myosin; *A* = actin; *TM* = tropomyosin; *black ovals* = troponin.) (Modified from J. D. Potter and J. Gergely, *Biochemistry* 13:2697, 1974.)

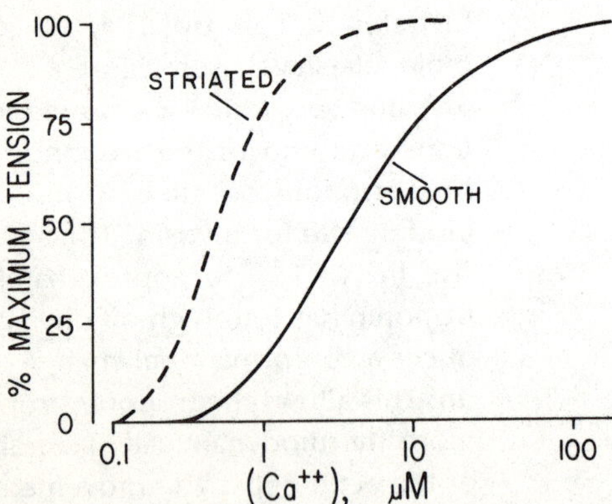

Figure 4-2
Ca^{++} dependence of tension development. (Modified from K. Saida and Y. Nonomura, *J. Gen. Physiol.* 72:1, 1978.)

ability will increase the number of cross-bridges and active tension.

A typical Ca^{++} concentration–effect curve for striated muscle is shown as the dashed line in Figure 4-2. Half-maximal tension and cross-bridge cycling require about 0.7 μM Ca^{++} at normal intracellular pH. Since the heart operates on the steep slope of the curve, small changes in $[Ca^{++}]_i$ produce large changes in tension.

Role of Slow Inward Current

An isolated heart stops beating within seconds if a Ca^{++}-chelating agent is added to the perfusate. Thus excitation-contraction coupling in the heart depends on extracellular Ca^{++} on a beat-to-beat basis. The source of extracellular Ca^{++} is the slow inward Ca^{++} current that flows during the action potential plateau. Cardiac tension and Ca^{++} conductance ($g_{Ca^{++}}$) exhibit exactly the same voltage dependence; both activate near −40 mV and are fully developed at 0 mV. Relationships among E_m, tension, and inactivation of $g_{Ca^{++}}$ are also congruent. The dependence of tension on I_{si} is illustrated in Figure 4-3. If a small ventricular fiber bundle is exposed to diltiazem, a Ca^{++}-channel-blocking agent, phase 2 of the action potential becomes more negative and its duration decreases, reflecting a new balance of inward and outward currents. Tension developed by the bundle decreases progressively as the concentration of the blocker is raised. Though contraction is initiated and terminated by $I_{Ca^{++}}$, the amount of Ca^{++} that enters during the action potential is about 100 times less than is required to activate the myofilaments. $I_{Ca^{++}}$ is simply the *trigger* for release of Ca^{++} from a large internal store.

The time course of change of $[Ca^{++}]_i$ can be observed by injecting the protein aequorin into a muscle cell. Aequorin emits a flash of light when it binds Ca^{++}; see Figure 4-4. Maximum light intensity coincides with the maximum rate of change of tension and precedes peak tension by about 30 ms. Under favorable conditions an initial, rapidly rising component of the aequorin signal can be distinguished from a slower, longer-lasting component. The former may be due to Ca^{++} entry, the latter to release from the internal store. Reuptake of Ca^{++} back into the

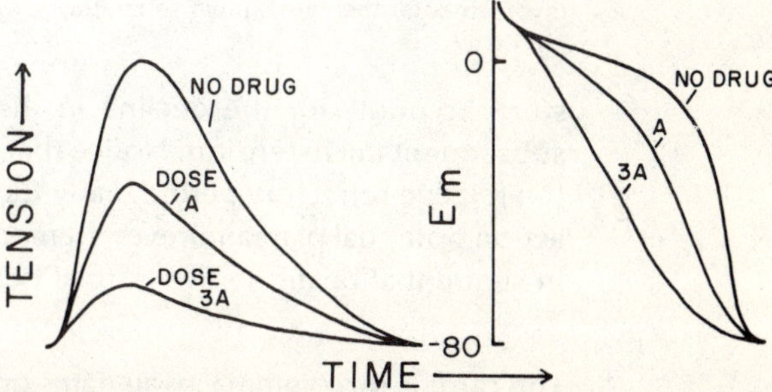

Figure 4-3
Effect of 10-mM and 30-mM diltiazem, a Ca^{++}-channel-blocking drug, on action potential and tension in ventricular fibers. (Based on data of C. Hirth, U. Borchard, and D. Hafner, *J. Mol. Cell. Cardiol.* 15:799, 1983.)

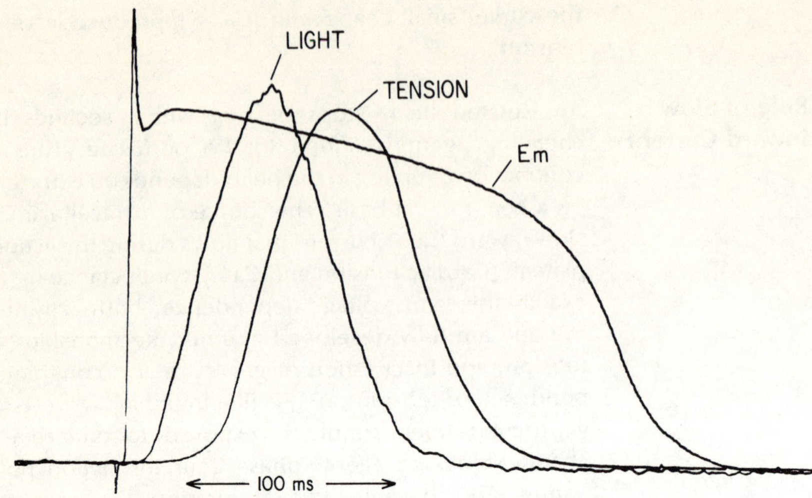

Figure 4-4
Temporal relations among E_m, $[Ca^{++}]_i$ (indicated by light signal), and tension in a Purkinje fiber injected with aequorin. The negative deflection that precedes the action potential is the stimulus artifact. (Recording courtesy W. G. Wier, Mayo Graduate School of Medicine, Rochester, Minn.)

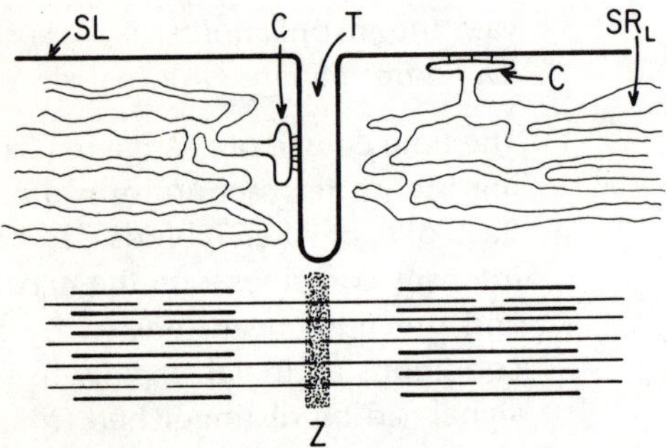

Figure 4-5
Relation of cardiac sarcoplasmic reticulum to surface membrane and myofibrils. (*SL* = sarcolemma; *C* = cisterna; *T* = transverse tubule; SR_L = longitudinal sarcoplasmic reticulum; *Z* = Z disc.) The SR_L and C overlie the myofilaments; they are shown separately for illustrative purposes.

store accounts for the decline in the light signal and for the subsequent fall in tension. Notice that tension is almost 0 during the relative refractory period. Early Ca^{++} reuptake and the long action potential plateau prevent temporal summation of tension in sequential beats, so the normal heart cannot be tetanized.

The Sarcoplasmic Reticulum

The cardiac sarcolemma invaginates opposite the Z discs to form a wide, transversely oriented tubule; see Figure 4-5. Its lumen is an extension of the extracellular space. A loose, anastomosing network of longitudinally oriented tubules — sarcoplasmic reticulum, or SR — envelops the myofilaments. The lumen of these tubules is in continuity with transversely oriented sacs called the terminal cisternae. These are closely applied to the transverse tubules or the sarcolemma. The SR never communicates with the extracellular space.

Radioautographs demonstrate that a large amount of Ca is stored in the cisternae. This Ca is released on signal from the action potential and diffuses to troponin binding sites. Ca is removed from troponin by the tubules of the SR and travels along the tubules back to the cisternae for rerelease. The cisternae are less than half full under ordinary circumstances. Since cardiac troponin is not fully saturated, the *unused Ca storage capacity of the SR represents a major reserve of contractility.*

How do the cisternae "know" when to release Ca? A tentative answer has been obtained by removing the sarcolemma, much as one would peel a banana. The $[Ca^{++}]$ can then be fixed at a desired value with Ca^{++} buffers. Experiments on such skinned fibers demonstrate that Ca^{++} can trigger its own release. Threshold for Ca^{++}-induced Ca^{++} release is exceeded when Ca^{++} enters during the action potential. Ca^{++}-induced Ca^{++} release depends on (1) the amount of "trigger" Ca^{++}, (2) the amount in the cisternal store, and (3) sarcomere length. The amount of trigger Ca^{++} is increased by adrenergic mediators and decreased by acetylcholine. It is also affected by E_m, transmembrane ion gradients, and heart rate. The electrophysiological basis for these effects is considered in Chapter 5.

The Cisternal Store and Transmembrane Transport

The cell gains a small amount of Ca^{++} with each heart beat. Overload of the SR is prevented by a transport mechanism in the sarcolemma; see Figure 4-6. A carrier with two negative charges (X^{2-}) can be occupied by two Na^+ or one Ca^{++}. Competitive loading of X^{2-} depends on the internal and external concentra-

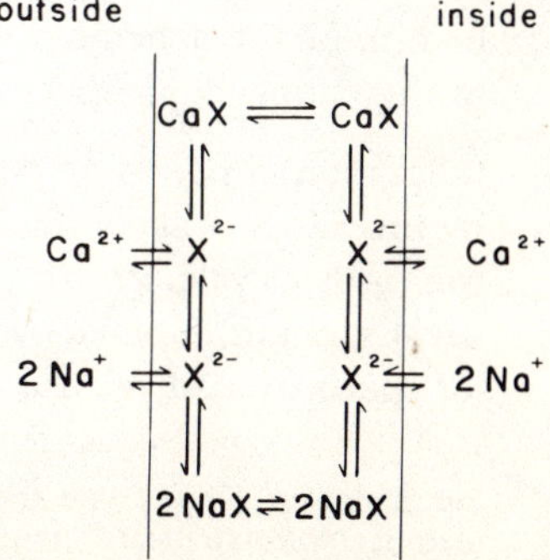

Figure 4-6
Carrier scheme for Na^+-Ca^{++} exchange. (Modified from H. Reuter, *Circ. Res.* 34:599, 1974. By permission of the American Heart Association, Inc.)

tions of Na^+ and Ca^{++}. Energy for an electroneutral exchange of two Na^+ for one Ca^{++} is provided by Na^+-K^+ ATPase (the Na^+ pump). Thus any change in the Na^+ gradient also affects the Ca^{++} gradient. The beat-to-beat balance between Ca^{++} influx during the action potential and outward Ca^{++} transport in exchange for Na^+ largely determines the content of the cisternal store and hence tension. Na^+-Ca^{++} exchange per se appears to account for the positive inotropic effect* of digitalis, a drug that inhibits the Na^+-K^+ ATPase.

Starling's Law and Cardiac Contractility

The strong length dependence of tension development considered in Chapter 1 can now be understood as length-dependent Ca^{++} availability. Since the sarcomere length–active tension relation is the same for intact and skinned fibers, factors related to the surface membrane (action potential and Na^+-Ca^{++} exchange) are not involved. Sarcomere length does not affect the steady-state Ca content of the SR but does control the amount of Ca^{++} released by the Ca^{++}-triggered process. This highly specific effect grades tension without changing the rates of contraction or relaxation; see Figure 4-7A. The positive inotropic effects of heart rate and norepinephrine, on the other hand, depend on the action potential. Both are accompanied by increased rate of contraction; Figure 4-7B and 4-7C. Norepinephrine also stimulates Ca^{++} reuptake by the SR and thereby accelerates relaxation. Thus the intrinsic and extrinsic reserves of contractility discussed in Chapter 1 are manifestations of cardiac excitation-contraction coupling.

A Complete Cycle

Cardiac excitation-contraction coupling is summarized in Figures 4-8 and 4-9. Beginning at the left in Figure 4-8, $I_{Ca^{++}}$ increases during phases 1 and 2 of the ventricular action potential. Influx of trigger Ca^{++} releases a much larger quantity from the cisternal store. These two steps are modified by nerve mediators. The amount of Ca^{++} in the cisternal store strongly influences the amount released. This amount depends on the beat-to-beat balance between Ca^{++} entry and active transport to the extracellular space.

Relaxation depends on Na^+-Ca^{++} exchange and Ca^{++} uptake by the SR. It is likely that both processes continue throughout the cardiac cycle. When $I_{Ca^{++}}$ inactivates late in the plateau (Figure 4-9, at left), uptake by the SR and transport to the extracellular space exceed release from the cisternae. As the $[Ca^{++}]$ in

*Physiologists' jargon; you are going to hear the word, so you may as well learn it. *Inotropic* means "modifying the strength of contraction"; *chronotropic* means "modifying heart rate." *Positive* or *negative* before either term means "increase" or "decrease," respectively.

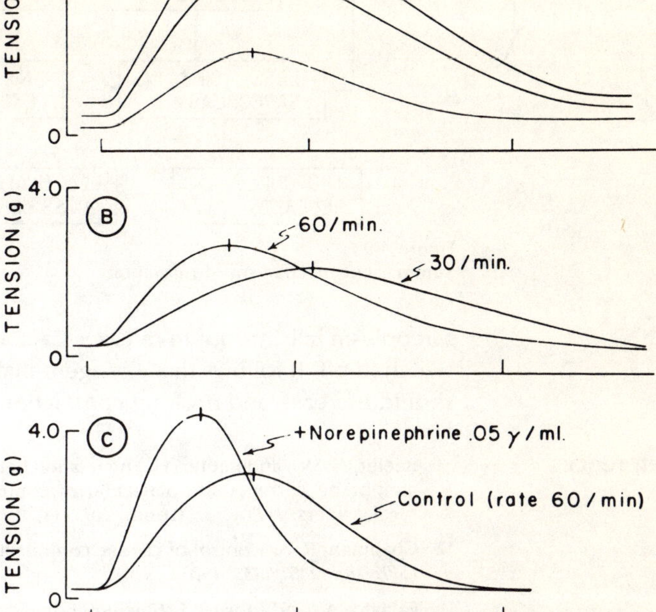

Figure 4-7
Comparison of inotropic effects of stretch (*A*), frequency (*B*), and norepinephrine (*C*). Norepinephrine- and frequency-induced changes take several beats to become established. (Reprinted with permission from E. Sonnenblick, *Fed. Proc.* 21:975, 1962.)

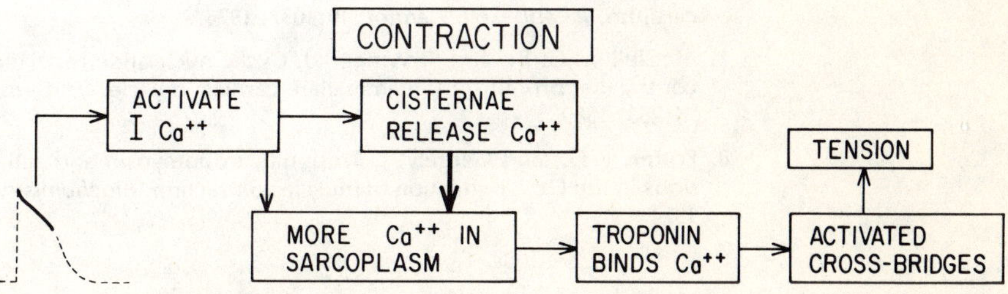

Figure 4-8
Summary of events during excitation and contraction.

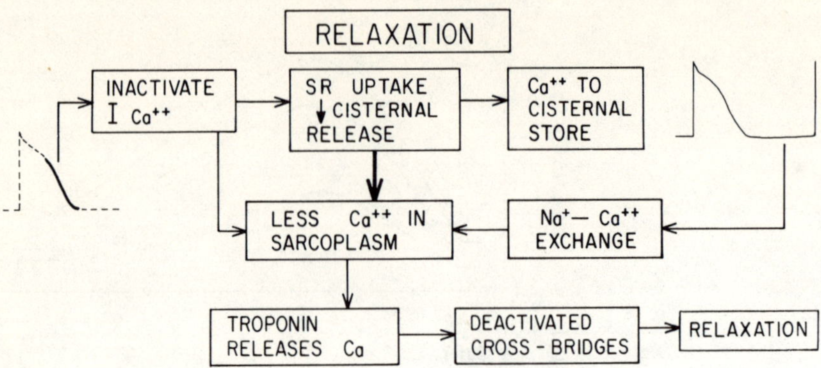

Figure 4-9
Summary of mechanism of relaxation.

sarcoplasm falls, troponin releases Ca, and the cross-bridges are switched off. It follows that any agent that lengthens the plateau should increase and prolong contraction.

References

1. Beeler, G. W., and Reuter, H. The relation between membrane potential, membrane currents and activation of contraction in ventricular myocardial fibers. *J. Physiol.* (Lond.) 207:211, 1970.

*2. Chapman, R. A. Control of cardiac contractility at the cellular level. *Am. J. Physiol.* 245:H535, 1983.

3. Fabiato, A., and Fabiato, F. Calcium-induced release of calcium from the sarcoplasmic reticulum. *Am. J. Physiol.* 245:C1, 1983.

4. Gadsby, D. C., and Cranefield, P. F. Effects of Electrogenic Sodium Extrusion on the Membrane Potential of Cardiac Purkinje Fibers. In A. Paes de Carvalho, B. F. Hoffman, and M. Lieberman (eds.), *Normal and Abnormal Conduction in the Heart.* Mt. Kisco, N.Y.: Futura, 1982.

5. Jewell, B. R. A reexamination of the influence of muscle length on myocardial performance. *Circ. Res.* 40:221, 1977.

6. Kohlhardt, M., and Mnich, Z. Studies on the inhibitory effect of verapamil on the slow inward currents in mammalian ventricular myocardium. *J. Mol. Cell. Cardiol.* 10:1037, 1978.

7. McClellen, G. B., and S. Winegrad. Cyclic nucleotide regulation of the contractile proteins in mammalian cardiac muscle. *J. Gen. Physiol.* 75:283, 1980.

8. Potter, J. D., and Gergely, J. Troponin, tropomyosin and actin interactions in the Ca^{2+} regulation of muscle contraction. *Biochemistry* 13:2697, 1974.

5 : Modifiers of Cardiac Function

The most important circulatory variable is the amount of blood pumped per minute, or the cardiac output (*C.O.*).

C.O. = stroke volume (*SV*) × frequency.

SV depends on contractility, and frequency is set by the pacemaker. In this chapter we apply the mechanisms thus far described to learn how *C.O.* is controlled by humoral agents.

Autonomic Nerves

Survival requires large, rapid changes in *C.O.*, geared to what is happening in the external environment. Such changes depend almost exclusively on the autonomic nerves. To a large extent *C.O.* reflects the balance between sympathetic stimulation and parasympathetic (vagal) inhibition. This autonomic reciprocal innervation is unique to the heart. A summary of the cardiac effects of autonomic nerves is provided in Table 5-1.

The Cardiac Vagus

The vagus releases acetylcholine from endings in the atria, the SA node and the AV node. Few vagal fibers reach the ventricle, and acetylcholine has no effect on ventricular action potentials. Vagal stimulation hyperpolarizes cells in the sinus node, suppresses the pacemaker potential, and slows the heart. Vagal hyperpolarization is shown in Figure 5-1. During prolonged stimulation, E_m closely approximates E_{K^+}, which suggests that P_{K^+} is increased. This is confirmed by experiments showing an increased rate of ^{42}K efflux from cells preloaded with the isotope. P_{K^+} also increases in atrium and AV node and accounts, directly or indirectly, for all the effects of the vagus on the heart.

The extent of hyperpolarization induced by acetylcholine is much less in atrial muscle than in the nodes. The salient change in the atrium is faster repolarization, as shown in Figure 5-2. Increased P_{K^+} shortens or abolishes phase 2 of the action potential and accelerates phase 3, thereby decreasing the refractory period. Shortening the action potential also decreases $I_{Ca^{++}}$. This accounts for the negative inotropic effect of the vagus on the atrium, and indirectly on the ventricle as well. The ventricles are affected because the atria serve as a booster pump. They

Table 5-1
Effects of Autonomic Mediators on the Heart

Physiological Effect		Major Cellular Mechanism
Epinephrine and Norepinephrine		
Electrical		
↑ Firing rate	In SA node	↑ I_{si}
	In Purkinje fiber	Altered I_{K^+} kinetics during pacemaker potential
↑ Conduction velocity in nodal tissue		↑ I_{si}
Faster repolarization		Altered I_{K^+} kinetics during plateau*, ↑ I_{K^+}
Mechanical		
↑ Peak tension		↑ I_{si}, larger store in SR
↓ Time to peak tension		↑ I_{si}, larger store in SR
↑ Relaxation rate		↑ Ca uptake by SR
Acetylcholine		
Electrical		
↑ Maximum diastolic potential		↑ Resting g_{K^+}
↓ Firing rate in SA node		↓ I_{si}; ↑ resting g_{K^+}
↓ Conduction velocity in nodal tissue		↓ I_{si}; ↑ g_{K^+}
↓ Action potential duration		↓ I_{si}
↓ Plateau height		↑ Resting g_{K^+}
Mechanical		
↓ Peak tension		↓ I_{si}

*Different set of K^+ channels than those responsible for increased firing rate.
SR = sarcoplasmic reticulum.
Source: Modified from R. W. Tsien and S. Siegelbaum, Excitable Tissues: The Heart. In T. E. Andreoli, J. F. Hoffman, and D. D. Fanestil (eds.), *The Physiological Basis for Disorders of Biomembranes*. New York: Plenum, 1978.

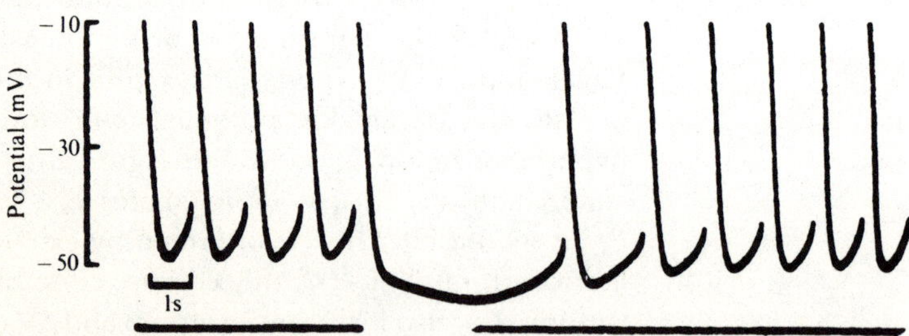

Figure 5-1
Membrane potentials in frog sinus venosus (homologous with SA node in mammals). The vagus was stimulated at 10/s during break in baseline. (From O. F. Hutter and W. Trautwein, *J. Gen. Physiol.* 39:715, 1956.)

give the ventricle a quick stretch, thereby increasing sarcomere length and active tension in the ventricular fibers.

Acetylcholine decreases the height and rate of rise of the action potential, particularly in the nodes. This effect is due to a large outward K^+ current, which opposes I_{si}. Acetylcholine also inhibits I_{si} directly in some species. Slow rate of rise of the action

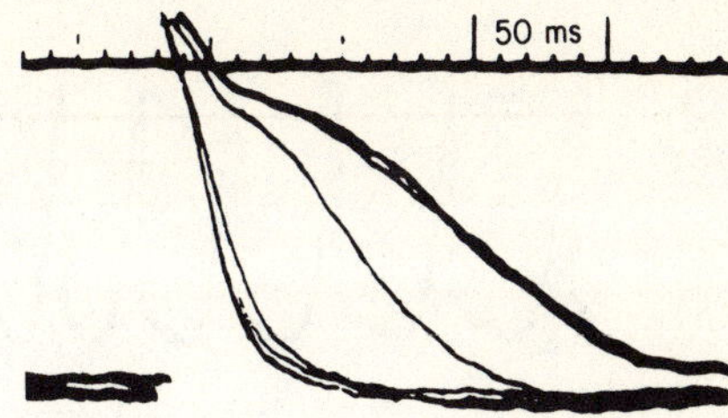

Figure 5-2
Superimposed action potentials from dog atrium before and during vagal stimulation. (From B. F. Hoffman and E. E. Suckling, *Am. J. Physiol.* 173:312, 1953.)

potential and decreased excitability (because of hyperpolarization) impede propagation of the action potential. Consequently, conduction across the AV node is slowed by vagal stimulation and may fail completely. The cardiac vagus may be stimulated reflexly, notably during changes in arterial pressure, in gastrointestinal and coronary artery disease, and in the presence of certain drugs. Disturbances of AV transmission occur commonly in such situations. Moreover, the combination of very short refractory period and slow conduction in the atria favors reentrant arrhythmias. Atrial fibrillation, for example, may be induced by endogenous vagal stimuli. Fortunately, the AV node prevents spread of fibrillation to the ventricles, and direct vagal innervation of ventricular muscle fibers appears to have been eliminated during millennia of evolution. Specific blocking agents that can eliminate undesirable vagal reflexes are available.

Norepinephrine and Epinephrine

Sympathetic nerves release norepinephrine, and small amounts of epinephrine and norepinephrine circulate in the blood. The principal effect of these mediators throughout the heart is to increase I_{si} (mainly Ca^{++}). The Ca^{++} that enters adds to the cisternal store, and within a few beats tension begins to rise. A typical response of the SA node to norepinephrine is shown in Figure 5-3. The dramatic increase in heart rate is due solely to the steeper pacemaker potential. The rate of rise and height of the action potential are also increased. The larger, faster-rising action potentials facilitate conduction. This effect can be used therapeutically in certain types of AV block. One would think that epinephrine would lengthen the action potential, because of its effect on I_{si}. (More outward current would have to be activated for repolarization.) If this were the case, mechanical systole would lengthen because the action potential controls contraction. Longer systole in the face of faster heart rate would not allow enough time for the heart to fill. This is avoided by a separate effect of adrenergic mediators on the K^+ current that

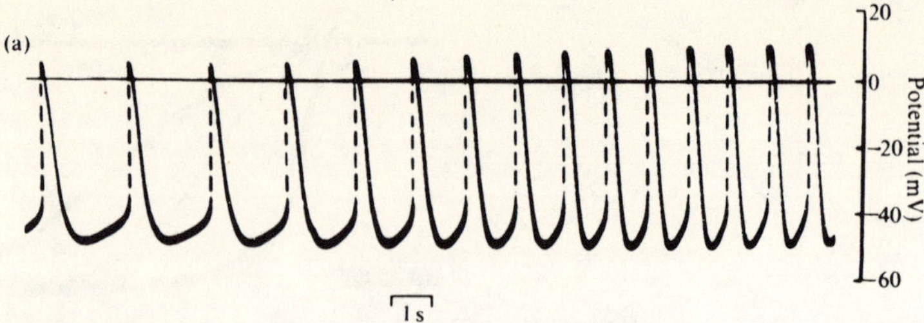

Figure 5-3
Membrane potential in frog sinus venosus. The sympathetic nerve was stimulated during the break in the baseline. (From O. F. Hutter and W. Trautwein, *J. Gen. Physiol.* 39:715, 1956.)

terminates the plateau. The effect of heart rate on P_{K^+} also contributes, as will be explained.

How do adrenergic mediators exert their effects? Recent evidence indicates they alter the kinetics of Ca^{++} channels as well as the number of channels that are functional. The channels are thought to possess a cyclic adenosine monophosphate– (cyclic AMP-) dependent protein kinase. Epinephrine and norepinephrine are known to stimulate formation of cyclic AMP from ATP. In the presence of the cyclic nucleotide, the kinase phosphorylates the cell membrane. The resulting change in conformation is thought to allow the Ca^{++} channels to become functional. This attractive hypothesis accounts for the fact that intracellular injection of cyclic AMP reproduces qualitatively all the effects of adrenergic mediators on the action potential and tension.

Effect of Frequency

At a normal heart rate of 70 beats per minute the action potential lasts about 300 ms. At 200 beats per minute the whole cycle lasts only 300 ms! Obviously, the action potential must shorten to preserve diastolic filling time. To understand the mechanism, recall that the plateau depends on a delicate balance of small conductances and is terminated by an increase in the ratio $P_{K^+}/(P_{Na^+} + P_{Ca^{++}})$. P_{K^+} takes 100 to 300 ms to recover from activation after each action potential. At high heart rates, P_{K^+} remains partly activated, and I_{si} does not fully recover from inactivation. Consequently, a smaller change is required to alter the ratio of ion permeabilities in favor of repolarization. Tachycardia also enhances tension, even though end-diastolic volume and hence fiber length decrease. The positive inotropic effect of tachycardia reflects the total time over many cycles during which the heart is depolarized beyond the threshold potential for activation of Ca^{++} influx. This loads the SR, raises the concentration of ionized Ca^{++} during systole, and recruits additional crossbridges.

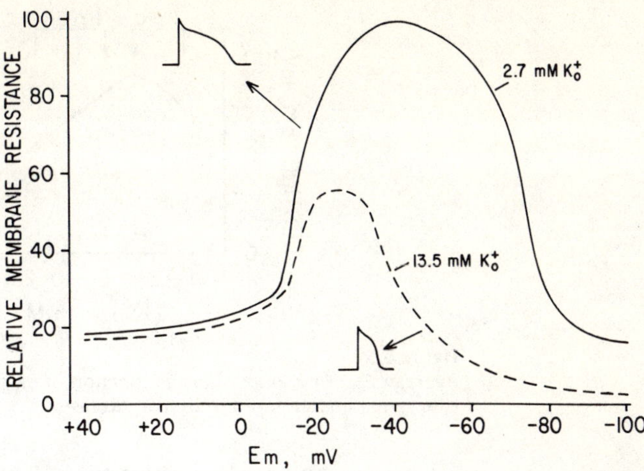

Figure 5-4
$[K^+]_o$ influences the transmembrane resistance (reciprocal of conductance) in Purkinje fibers, particularly at voltages characteristic of the action potential plateau. (Modified from E. E. Carmeliet, *Circulation* 24:499, 1961. By permission of the American Heart Association, Inc.)

Interaction of K^+, Ca^{++}, and Na^+

About a century ago Ringer discovered that cardiac contractility depends on the relative proportions of K^+, Ca^{++}, and Na^+ in the bathing medium. The positive inotropic effect of Ca^{++} is opposed by K^+. This antagonism is due to greater outward g_{K^+} (low transmembrane resistance) in the presence of high $[K^+]_o$; see Figure 5-4. Outward g_{K^+} shortens the action potential, so less time is available for Ca^{++} entry. The longer action potential produced by low $[K^+]_o$ has the reverse effect. The antagonism between $Na^+{}_o$ and $Ca^{++}{}_o$ is a direct consequence of the mechanism and stoichiometry of the Na^+-Ca^{++} exchange mechanism, explained in Chapter 4.

Clinical Application

Effect of Extracellular K^+

The normal plasma $[K^+]$ in humans ranges from 3.3 to 4.9 mEq per liter. Concentrations less than 1.5 mEq per liter or greater than 12 mEq per liter are generally fatal. Hyper- and hypokalemia are common complications of various metabolic, circulatory, and renal disorders, and release of K^+ from injured cells as in coronary artery occlusion can cause high local concentrations of extracellular K^+. Electrocardiographic changes in hyperkalemia are shown in Problem 1, pages 288–290.

Hyperkalemia

The most important effect of raising $[K^+]_o$ is depolarization. Refer to Figure 3-5, p. 33, and notice that only 10 percent of Na^+ channels are available at

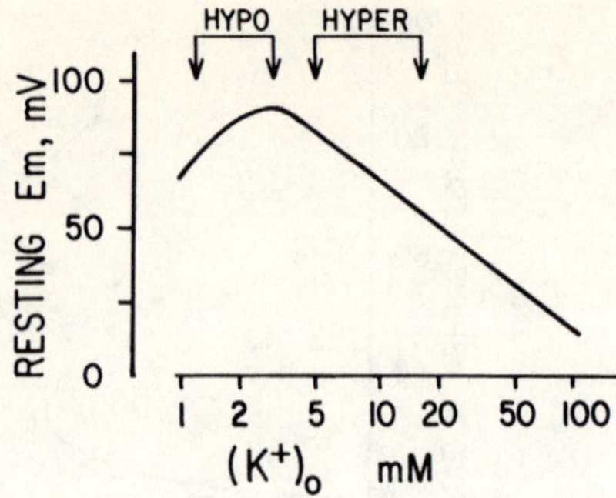

Figure 5-5
Average E_m in Purkinje fibers as function of extracellular $[K^+]$. Arrows indicate range encountered in human disease.

potentials positive to −60 mV. Figures 3-5 and 5-5 demonstrate why concentrations greater than 8 mM are so dangerous: About one-third the available Na^+ channels are inactivated at 8 mM. Inactivation of Na^+ channels decreases the magnitude and rate of rise of the action potential and thereby slows conduction. Excitability decreases markedly, again because of inactivation, and contributes to failure of the action potential to propagate.

One would think that hyperkalemia would decrease outward I_{K^+}, prolong the action potential, and thereby promote contraction. In fact precisely the reverse occurs, because $[K^+]_o$ greatly decreases transmembrane resistance (increases conductance). Notice in Figure 5-4 that resistance is lower than normal at all potentials in the presence of hyperkalemia, and that this effect is greatest in the plateau range. Tracer studies demonstrate that this low transmembrane resistance is due to higher g_{K^+}. The phenomenon is due to the inward rectifying properties of the K^+ channels. Exactly how $[K^+]_o$ alters the rectifying properties of its own channels is not known.

Greater g_{K^+} in hyperkalemia opposes pacemaker potentials and tends to block conduction at the AV node. Premature contractions caused by local differences in E_m and conduction velocity are common. Moreover, slow conduction and short refractory period favor reentry, and depolarization per se often initiates automaticity. It is hardly surprising that death in hyperkalemia is generally due to ventricular fibrillation.

Hypokalemia

Note in Figure 5-5 that depolarization may occur with low as well as high $[K^+]_o$. In hypokalemia, depolarization is accompanied by a large decrease in

g_{K^+}, which allows the ever-present inward Na^+ leak to lower E_m. The duration of the action potential is increased, as expected with low g_{K^+}. In addition, the Na^+ pump (Na^+-K^+ ATPase) becomes limited by K^+. All the effects attributable to depolarization per se are as described for hyperkalemia, including a strong tendency to ventricular fibrillation.

Calcium Channel Antagonists

Drugs that block voltage-dependent Ca^{++} channels in heart and vascular smooth muscle have proved effective in treatment of cardiac arrhythmias and ischemic heart disease. They are also useful in management of some forms of hypertension, presumably because Ca^{++} channels are largely responsible for action potentials in vascular smooth muscle. The blockers are thought to interact with the Ca^{++} channel when it is in the inactivated state. Consequently, the degree of block depends, in part, on E_m. This behavior permits considerable therapeutic specificity. For example, cells depolarized by ischemic injury may have slowly propagating Ca^{++}-dependent action potentials. These potentials can cause active arrhythmias, as explained in Chapter 3. The ischemic cells are preferentially affected by the blockers because they are partly depolarized. Since the Ca^{++} channel blockers have little effect at normal E_m, they do not impair I_{si} and tension development in nonischemic portions of the myocardium.

Recently chemical modification of a Ca^{++} channel antagonist produced a drug that increases Ca^{++} currents. This drug appears to prolong the "open time" of the channel. Since this effect is also highly voltage-dependent, the drug has promise as a positive inotropic agent with specificity for abnormal cells. Development of Ca^{++} channel modifiers well illustrates the fruitful interaction of basic and applied research.

Ischemia, pH

The intracellular pH of normal working myocardium is near 7.0. pH falls 0.2 to 0.4 pH units within 5 minutes after the onset of ischemia but changes very little with hypoxia in the presence of normal blood flow. The principal sources of retained H^+ are carbonic, phosphoric, and lactic acids. Intracellular acidosis suppresses I_{si} with little change in outward currents. The resulting decrease in duration of ventricular action potentials contributes to the development of arrhythmias, decreases intracellular Ca^{++} stores, and is partly responsible for a large fall in tension development.

References

1. Bean, B. P. Nitrendipine block of cardiac calcium channels: High affinity binding to the inactivated state. *Proc. Natl. Acad. Sci. U.S.A.* 81:6388, 1984.

2. Carmeliet, E. E. Repolarization and frequency in cardiac cells. *J. Physiol.* (Paris) 73:903, 1977.

*3. Noble, D. *The Initiation of the Heart Beat.* New York, London: Oxford University Press, 1979. Pp. 85–130.

4. Reuter, H. Localization of β adrenergic receptors, and effects of noradrenaline and cyclic nucleotides on action potentials, ionic currents and tension in mammalian cardiac muscle. *J. Physiol.* (Lond.) 242:429, 1974.

5. Schwartz, A., and Triggle, D. J. Cellular action of calcium channel blocking drugs. *Annu. Rev. Med.* 35:325, 1984.

*6. Tsien, R. W., and Siegelbaum, S. Excitable Tissues: The Heart. In T. E. Andreoli, J. F. Hoffman, and D. D. Fanestil (eds.), *Physiology of Membrane Disorders.* New York: Plenum, 1978.

7. Yatani, A., and Goto, M. The effect of extracellular low pH on the plateau current in isolated single rat ventricular cells — a voltage clamp study. *Jpn. J. Physiol.* 33:403, 1983.

6 : The Electrocardiogram

This is not a chapter on applied electrocardiography. The objective, rather, is to explain how the electrocardiogram (ECG) arises, and how the basic electrophysiology already considered relates to its interpretation. Information on the sequence of ventricular depolarization, lead systems, normal standards, and configurations in clinical entities can be found in the references.

Genesis of the ECG

Thus far we have been concerned with intracellular action potentials, whereas the ECG is a recording of potentials in *extracellular* fluid. Extracellular potentials are caused by the local circuit currents that accompany a propagating action potential; refer again to Figure 3-4. The current flowing in each of the four limbs of the circuit in Figure 3-4 is the same. Inflow of depolarizing current (limb 1) is described by

$$-I_{Na^+} \cong C_m \frac{dV}{dt} \max.$$

It follows that current flow in the extracellular fluid (limb 4) is proportional to the rate of change of voltage — that is, the rate of change of the action potential. This means that extracellular currents are small when the action potential changes slowly and large when the action potential changes rapidly. Thus the plateau of the action potential generates very small extracellular currents and produces negligible change in potentials recorded extracellularly. Since the plateau is very long, *depolarization and repolarization are separated by an interval of nearly constant potential in external recordings. Consequently, depolarization and repolarization can be recognized as discrete events.* This is the central idea that must be grasped to interpret the ECG.

The relation between the action potential and extracellular recordings is illustrated in Figure 6-1. Ignore the dashed lines for the moment. Extracellular recordings of voltages from a single fiber or a small bundle are called *electrograms*. Phases 0 and 1 of the intracellular action potential generate a biphasic spike in the electrogram. Phase 2 of the action potential changes too slowly to produce detectable extracellular voltages, and a stable baseline is recorded in the electrogram. During phase 3 the

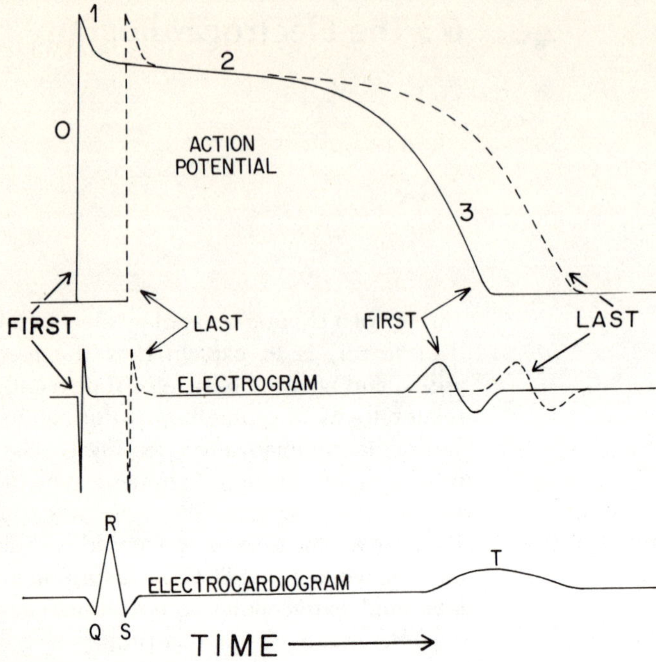

Figure 6-1
Schematic showing how the ventricular action potential and its time derivative are related to the ECG. Potentials caused by the first and last fibers to be excited are shown by solid and dashed lines, respectively. The electrogram and ECG are drawn about 10 times their proper size, relative to the action potential.

action potential changes more slowly than in phases 0 and 1, but more rapidly than in phase 2, resulting in a small, broad deflection in the electrogram.

If two fiber bundles are placed in the same conducting medium, local current will enter and leave each bundle independently of the other. The electrical field produced by the whole heart is therefore a representation of the temporal and spatial summation of electrograms. Depolarization and repolarization can be identified in the ECG of the whole heart because of fast conduction in the Purkinje net, which allows summation of the depolarization phase of all electrograms well before the repolarization deflection begins at any location. The result is two summations representing depolarization and repolarization separated by an isoelectric interval.

The summation of electrograms is shown schematically in Figure 6-1 by the solid and dashed lines, representing respectively the first and last ventricular fibers to be excited by the Purkinje net. The ECG deflections corresponding to depolarization and repolarization are called the QRS complex and T wave, respectively.[1] QRS and T are empirical wave forms. They bear no relation to the magnitude, shape, duration, or even polarity of an electrogram recorded from a single cell. The interval between Q and T is exaggerated in Figure 6-1. Separation of the two deflections varies with the duration of the action potential plateau and with the degree of synchronization imposed by the Purkinje fibers. When the action potential is short, conduction velocity in Purkinje fibers is slow, or both, the Q–T interval is short or absent. The sinusoidal ECG in severe hyperkalemia is a good example; see Figure P-1E and F, page 289.

The QRS complex is typically 1 to 2 mV; phase 0 of a ventricular action potential is almost 50-fold larger. The magnitude of the ECG, like its shape, is empirical because it is affected by the resistance of all tissues between the heart and the recording electrodes on the skin. Furthermore, the ECG represents only a small fraction of the electrical activity of the cardiac fibers because of cancellation of electrical forces acting in various directions. Coronary occlusion well illustrates the influence of cancellation. Destruction of a sufficiently large mass of tissue creates an electrical imbalance detectable as a change in shape of the ECG. If, however, a second occlusion is so located that the fresh damage eliminates the imbalance, the shape of the ECG returns to normal! In fact, if the heart were a perfect sphere and all fibers were excited simultaneously, no ECG would be detected at all. It is helpful to think of the ECG as a *nonuniformity detector.*

Nonuniformities in both the heart and its surroundings contribute to the normal ECG. The heart is asymmetrically placed in a highly nonuniform volume conductor. The resistivities of lungs and body wall, for example, differ. The two ventricles are of different size and, from the electrical point of view, are open at the base. Most important, not all fibers are excited instantaneously. Excitation proceeds from endocardium to epicardium, and the apex and septum are depolarized about 30 ms before the base.

In summary, the ECG represents the spatial and temporal summation of electrograms. Its shape and magnitude are empirical and depend on nonuniformities in the heart's electrical field. Depolarization and repolarization are identifiable as separate events because of the long plateau of the action potential and fast conduction in the Purkinje net.

[1] Einthoven, who first recorded the ECG, chose to name the deflections beginning with the letter *P,* for the atrial wave. Arbitrariness has been an unfortunate characteristic of electrocardiography ever since.

The Concept of an Equivalent Dipole

The voltage distribution around an active fiber resembles that produced in a volume conductor by a *dipole,* defined as a point source and sink for current. Battery terminals, for example, constitute a dipole. This concept is applied to a muscle strip in Figure 6-2. The region ahead of the advancing depolarization is a source, and the depolarized region is a sink, for current. The complex distribution of potentials in the volume conductor is replaced by a single equivalent dipole moving toward or away from an electrode. According to convention, an approaching depolarization (positive head of the dipole) produces an upward deflection, and approaching repolarization (negative head) causes a downward deflection. The dipole constitutes a vector, since it has both magnitude and direction. The dipoles for all the constituent fiber bundles can be resolved by vector addition into a single equivalent electrical vector, which represents the activity of the whole heart at a particular instant. The dipole changes its magnitude and the orientation of its axis in three dimensions throughout systole. The mean electrical vector is a convenient way of describing the complex distributions of po-

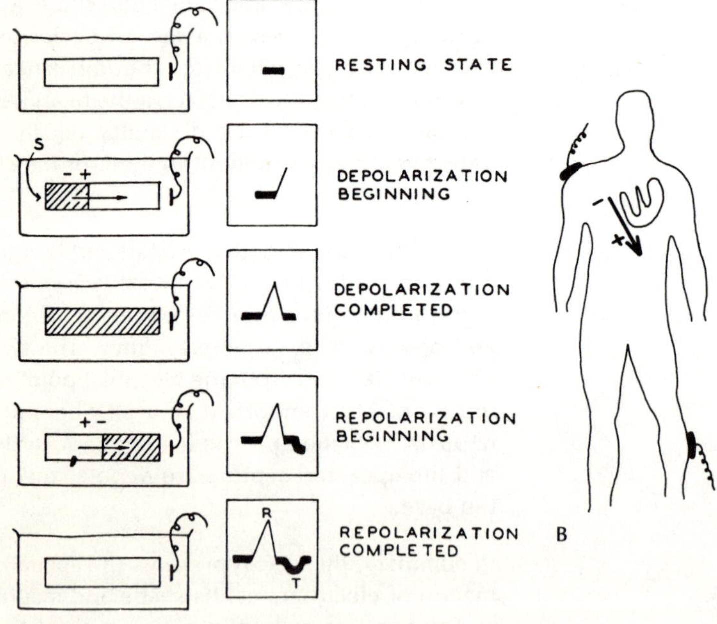

Figure 6-2
A. Tracings registered by an extracellular electrode during approach of a dipole. Shaded area is depolarized (outside is negative). (Reproduced with permission from B. S. Lipman, E. Massie, and R. E. Kleiger, *Clinical Scalar Electrocardiography* [6th ed.]. Copyright © 1972 by Year Book Medical Publishers, Inc., Chicago.) B. Representation of a mean instantaneous electrical vector for the whole heart.

tentials during excitation. The vector in Figure 6-2 would produce a negative deflection at the right arm and a positive deflection at the left leg. Thus the size, contour, and sign of the recording depend on the position of the electrode, which is, of course, arbitrary.

The Normal ECG

The Atria

Examples of atrial action potentials are shown in Figure 5-2. Notice that the atrial action potentials do not exhibit a distinct plateau. Consequently, atrial depolarization and atrial repolarization do not produce separately identifiable voltages in the ECG. The atria are relatively small, and conduction is slow because there is no Purkinje net. The atrial wave in the ECG is therefore a rather long deflection of low amplitude.

Sequences and Intervals

An idealized ECG is shown in Figure 6-3; the numerals denote sequential events. Voltages generated by the SA node (*1* in Figure 6-3) are too small to be detected. This is true of the AV node and Purkinje fibers as well. *Nevertheless, these specialized tissues largely determine the form of the ECG* because they control the timing of electrical events. Excitation reaches the AV node over Purkinje-like fibers at *2*, long before the atria are fully depolarized. Though conduction time across the AV node cannot be determined exactly, the interval between the beginning of the P wave and the first deflection of the QRS complex is a useful approximation.

Slow spread of excitation in the atria at *3* gives rise to the P wave. At *4* excitation reaches the Purkinje system, and the first deflection of the QRS complex (*5*) signals beginning activation of the ventricle. The duration of QRS is determined by conduction

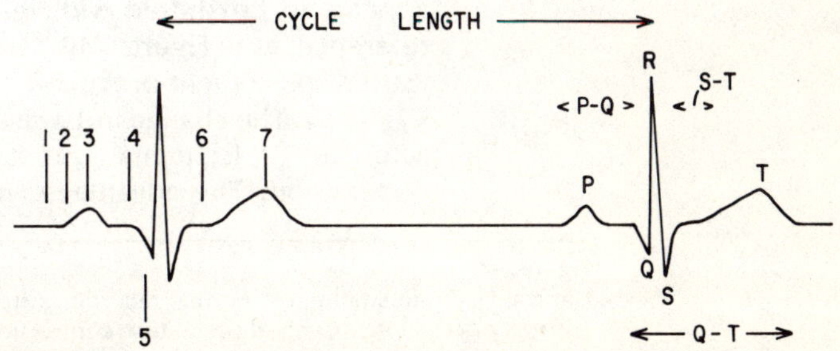

Figure 6-3
Schematic ECG showing the sequence of events (*left*) and waves and intervals (*right*). The numerals are explained in the text.

velocity in the Purkinje net. During the S–T interval (6), all ventricular cells are in the plateau phase of their action potentials. Consequently, there is little extracellular current flow, and the S–T segment is isoelectric, or nearly so. The S–T interval varies with intraventricular conduction time as well as with action potential duration. Phase 3 of the action potential is much slower than phase 0. Consequently, repolarization generates small local circuit currents that propagate slowly and give rise to the long, low-amplitude T wave. If the rate of repolarization increases, the T wave becomes tall and peaked. The time between the peak and the end of the T wave roughly corresponds to the relative refractory period. The duration of the various waves and intervals is given in Appendix 2.

The effects of hyperkalemia on the ECG are shown in Problem 1, pages 288–290. If you can reason out the mechanisms responsible for these ECG changes you have a satisfactory grasp of Chapters 2 through 6.

Clinical Application

The clinical ECG is recorded from a standard set of leads (electrode positions). Figure 6-4A illustrates typical normal wave forms for locations on the chest, progressing from right (V_1) to left (V_6). Television dramas firmly associate the ECG with ischemic heart disease. The basis for this application is the local circuit current that flows from normal cells to those depolarized by injury. If the potential in diastole is arbitrarily chosen as reference, an injury potential will displace that portion of the trace upward or downward. During systole, however, the surrounding normal cells will be depolarized also, so the potential difference and deflection of the base line disappear. The result is that the S–T segment appears to be shifted with respect to the diastolic reference, as in Figure 6-4B. The injury potential (upward displacement of the S–T segment) is evident at V_3 and V_4. The change in T-wave contour is also characteristic of ischemia, but its mechanism is not understood. The advantages of multiple electrode

Figure 6-4
Clinical ECGs illustrating (*A*) normal recordings from chest leads; (*B*) acute coronary occlusion; (*C*) atrial premature contractions; (*D*) atrial fibrillation; (*E*) interpolated ventricular premature contractions; (*F*) early ventricular premature contractions; (*G*) ventricular fibrillation; (*H*) complete AV block; and (*I*) 2:1 AV block. (From B. S. Lipman, E. Massie, and R. E. Kleiger, *Clinical Scalar Electrocardiography* [6th ed.]. Copyright © 1972 by Year Book Medical Publishers, Inc., Chicago.) Recordings reproduced with permission.

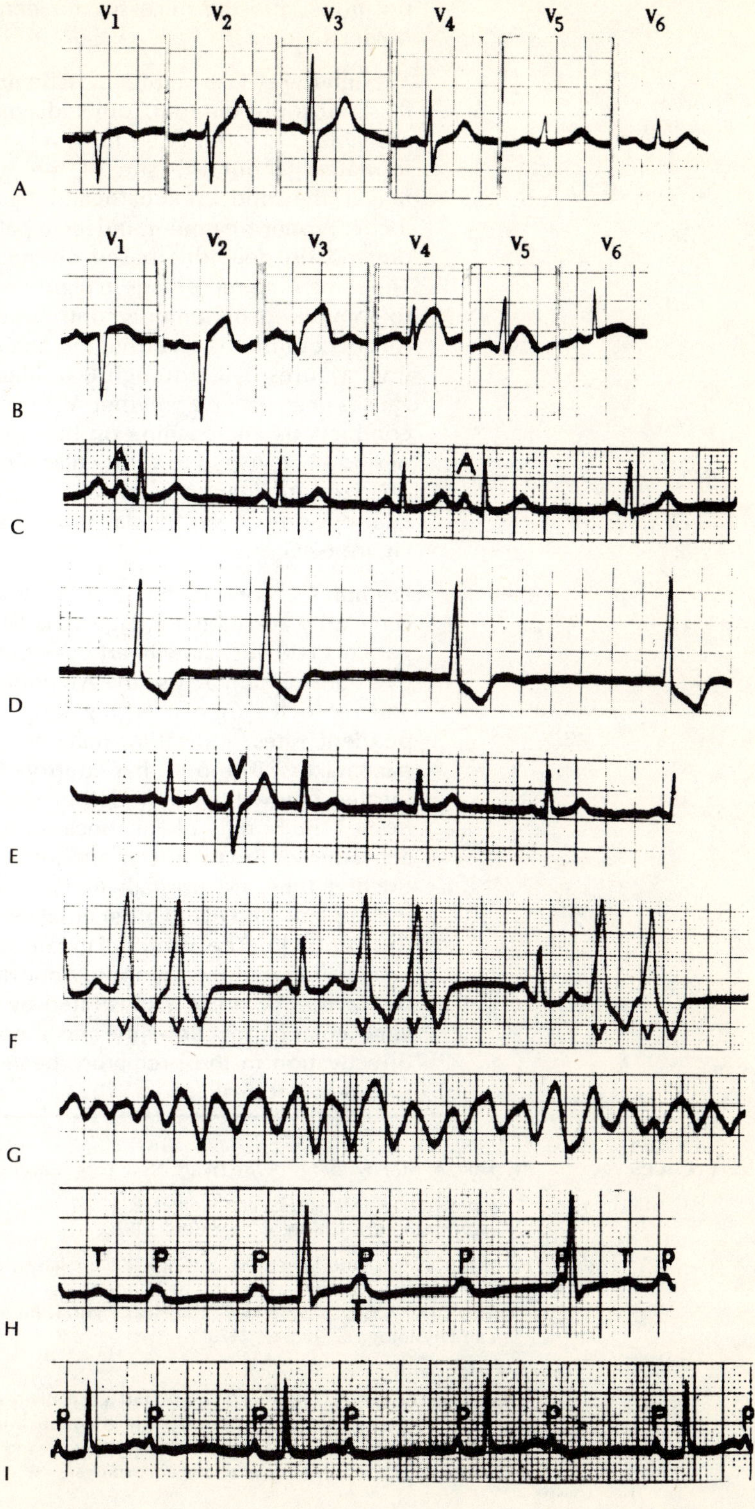
V1
V2
V3
V4
V5
V6
A
V1
V2
V3
V4
V5
V6
B
A
A
C
D
V
E
V
V
V
V
V
V
F
G
T
P
P
P
P
P
T
P
T
H
P
P
P
P
P
P
P
P
I

positions, and the necessity for empirical rules, is obvious.[2]

Though the ECG is helpful in ischemic heart disease it is not indispensable; other diagnostic tools are available. *Only* the ECG, however, can provide information about the site of the operative pacemaker, the conduction path, and the conduction velocity. Proper treatment, indeed a patient's life, may depend on decisions based on such information. The remaining recordings in Figure 6-4 were chosen to show the truly unique contribution of the ECG. All are continuous recordings at one electrode position. Figures 6-4C through 6-4F illustrate common causes of an irregular rhythm. Ventricular premature contractions encroaching on the relative refractory period (*F*) can lead to ventricular fibrillation, as emphasized in Chapter 3. An ECG recorded during a fatal episode of ventricular fibrillation is shown in Figure 6-4G.

Examples of conduction disorders that only the ECG can clarify are shown in Figures 6-4H and 6-4I. Both patients had very slow heart rates because of defective transmission across the AV node. In *H* the atria and ventricles are excited regularly but at two independent rates, indicating that they have different pacemakers. The one that controls the ventricle is located below the AV node but above the bifurcation of the bundle of His, because the sequence of activation of the ventricles and intraventricular conduction time are normal. In *I,* AV nodal block is incomplete, and every other atrial excitation reaches the ventricle. The ventricular rate is therefore exactly half that of the SA node. Abnormal conduction below the AV node is illustrated by the long intraventricular conduction time and abnormal sequence of activation in the premature beats shown in Figures 6-4E and 6-4F.

References

*1. Katz, A. M. *Physiology of the Heart.* New York: Raven, 1977. Pp. 257–362.

2. Lipman, B. S., Massie, E., and Kleiger, R. E. *Clinical Scalar Electrocardiography* (6th ed.). Chicago: Year Book, 1972.

3. Scher, A. M., and Spach, M. S. Cardiac Depolarization and Repolarization and the Electrocardiogram. In *Handbook of Physiology,* Section 2: The Cardiovascular System — The Heart, Vol. I. Bethesda, Md.: American Physiological Society, 1979.

[2]The clinical ECG is recorded at 25 mm/s and a sensitivity of 1 mV/cm. These standards do not allow identification of small conduction abnormalities in the ventricle and often obscure the low-voltage P and T waves. Existing amplifiers could produce more useful recordings.

II : Hemodynamics

7 : Pressure Gradients and Resistance to Blood Flow

Pressure is defined as force per unit area. The common units reflect the fact that pressure (P) within a fluid varies with depth below a free surface:

$$P = \gamma \times g \times h,$$

where γ is the density of the fluid (mass/unit volume), g is acceleration caused by gravity, and h is depth. Since g is a constant, pressure is given by specifying the fluid and the depth. Cardiovascular pressures are generally expressed in millimeters of mercury, or *torr*.[1] Pressure is the same in all directions at a given point, and when the fluid is at rest, pressure is the same at all points on a horizontal plane.

In addition to the gravitational potential energy just defined, an additional component of pressure exists in the vascular system as a result of the energy contributed by the heart. The height to which blood would rise in a vertical tube connected to a vessel would indicate the sum of the cardiac and gravitational components. The mean aortic pressure so measured is about 136 cm of blood, or 100 torr.

Pressure is often the only hemodynamic quantity available to a physician. However, in most instances, information about flow as well as pressure is required. Unfortunately, there is no direct relationship between arterial pressure at a particular point and blood flow. This is true because flow depends on the *difference* in pressure between an upstream and downstream site; see Figure 7-1. Pressure gradients along arteries are generally less than 1 percent of pressure at a point.

Pressure Gradients

The *causes* of pressure gradients in the circulation are

1. Hydrostatic columns
2. Transformations between kinetic and potential energy (Bernoulli's principle)

[1] Many journals, especially those published abroad, now insist on Système International (SI) units, based on the metric system. Pressure in SI is given as newton per square meter or Pascal (Pa). One kilopascal (kPa) = 7.5 mm Hg.

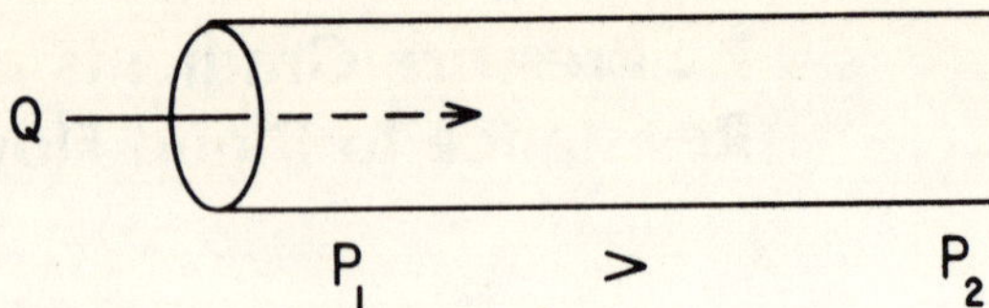

Figure 7-1
Flow (*Q*) is driven by a gradient in pressure (*P*).

3. Accelerations (Newton's second law)
4. Frictional losses (Poiseuille's law)

Cause 1 is important mainly in the venous system and is considered in Chapter 11. If the body is horizontal, cause 1 can be neglected. Causes 2 and 3 are of concern only in the largest arteries. The most important thing to remember about them is that the pressure gradients they produce are negligible under normal circumstances. Thus friction alone accounts for the large ΔP between arteries and veins. The potential energy in the large elastic arteries represents the major external work of the heart. This work is degraded to heat in friction as blood flows through the minute vessels. The friction occurs within the blood and not between the blood and the vessel wall.

Laminar Flow

The fundamental observations on the viscous properties of fluids were made by Newton. He measured the motion of various liquids in a barrel containing a centrally placed rotor. When the rotor turned, its motion was first transmitted to liquid close to it; the more remote portions moved later and more slowly. Thus the rotor created a *velocity gradient*. Newton correctly interpreted this gradient as the sliding of concentric layers of the liquid on one another. Flow of this type, with the liquid arranged in onionlike layers is called *laminar*.

Definition of Viscosity

The rate at which Newton's rotor transferred momentum to remote laminae depended on the liquid. He termed this property "defect of slipperiness"; we now call it *viscosity*. The laminae are of molecular dimensions, and viscosity denotes the tendency of molecules in adjacent laminae to interact. To gain an intuitive understanding, imagine a deck of cards on a table. If one pushes horizontally on the top card (applies a *shearing stress*), the cards slip over one another. The greater the shearing stress, the greater the distance the cards will move in an instant of time. The shearing stress is the horizontal pushing force divided by the area of the card. A force per unit area is a pressure. The velocity gradient (also called the *rate of shear*) in this analogy is the velocity of a card with respect to the one below it, divided by card thickness. Its dimensions are therefore cm/s per

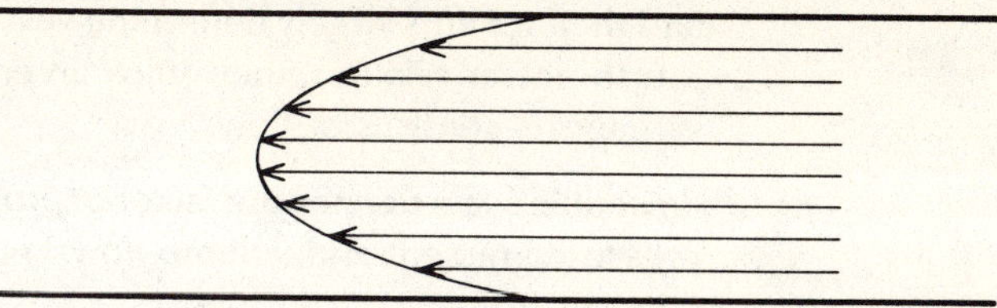

Figure 7-2
Rate of shear in steady laminar flow. Arrows indicate velocities of laminae at various radial positions.

cm, or s^{-1}. Viscosity (analogous to friction between the cards) is defined as the factor of proportionality relating shearing stress to rate of shear:

$$\eta = \frac{\tau}{dv/dr},$$

where η is viscosity, τ is shearing stress, v is velocity, and r is distance. If a shearing stress of 1 dyne produces a velocity gradient of 1 s^{-1}, a liquid has a viscosity of 1 poise. Water at room temperature has a viscosity of about 1 centipoise (10^{-2} poise). It is often convenient to express viscosity relative to that of water.

Laminae in a small vessel are represented as arrows in Figure 7-2. The lamina in contact with the vessel wall adheres to it and is at rest. The transmural velocity gradient (shear rate) is maximal at the wall and falls to zero at the center. There the fastest lamina moves at twice the average velocity. In steady flow the energy degraded to heat in friction between the laminae is balanced by the drop in potential energy along the tube, that is, the pressure gradient. This balance is expressed in Poiseuille's law, after the physicist (and physician) who obtained it by precise, direct measurements[2]:

$$Q = \Delta P \times \frac{r^4}{l} \times \frac{1}{\eta} \times \frac{\pi}{8},$$

where Q = volume flow (ml/min, for example), $\Delta P = P_1 - P_2$, r = tube radius, l = tube length, and η = viscosity. Notice the three terms: Flow depends on the pressure gradient, the geometry of the vessels, and the properties of blood. The numerical constants arise in the integrations.

Application to Circulation

The most striking feature of Poiseuille's law is that the flow varies as the *fourth power* of the radius. If the radius is halved (vasoconstriction), flow decreases 16-fold for the same ΔP. Most vascular smooth muscle fibers are oriented circumferentially,

[2]The derivation is given on pp. 21–23 of reference 6.

and their lengths largely determine vessel radius. Because of the fourth-power relation, they enjoy an enormous mechanical advantage as controls of flow.

Poiseuille's law defines the *factor of proportionality* between the pressure gradient and volume flow:

$$Q = \Delta P \times C,$$

where the hydraulic conductance, $C, = \frac{r^4 \pi}{l \eta 8}$. The reciprocal of the conductance, the resistance R, is more commonly used:

$$Q = \frac{\Delta P}{R},$$

where $R = \frac{l \eta 8}{r^4 \pi}$. This provides a practical means for determining whether vasoconstricton or vasodilation has occurred. This is true because l and η are generally constant in arterioles, the vessels in which resistance is greatest. For example, if we wish to know the resistance to flow through a human arm we measure arterial pressure, Pa, venous pressure, Pv, and flow:

$$R_{\text{Limb}} = \frac{Pa - Pv \text{ torr}}{\text{Q ml/min}} = \frac{100 - 2}{300} = 0.33.$$

The result is in peripheral resistance units (PRU). Similarly, the resistance of the entire systemic circulation (total peripheral resistance, or TPR) might be

$$TPR = \frac{Pa - P \text{ rt. atrium}}{\text{cardiac output}} = \frac{100 - 1}{5000} = 0.02 \text{ PRU}$$

The calculation of resistance as above is the first step in evaluating the vasomotor effect of any drug or stimulus.

If resistance is constant, a plot of ΔP versus Q yields a straight line; see Figure 7-3. The resistance ($\Delta P/Q$) is given by the slope. Note that resistance and hence the contractile state of the vascular muscles are the same at point 1 and at a higher pressure, point 2, since flow changes proportionately. Thus a rise in pressure does not necessarily indicate vasoconstriction. If resistance falls to a new, steady level, a new pressure-flow relation is obtained, indicating that vascular smooth muscle relaxed (Figure 7-3, line *b*). Intuitively, one might expect vasodilation to be accompanied by a fall in arterial pressure. Though this is often the case, pressure may actually rise despite vasodilation if flow increases sufficiently; see the shift from point 2 to point 3 in Figure 7-3. Clearly, one needs information about *both* pressure and flow to understand what is going on. This is particularly true since pressure is regulated within narrow limits, whereas flow

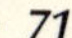

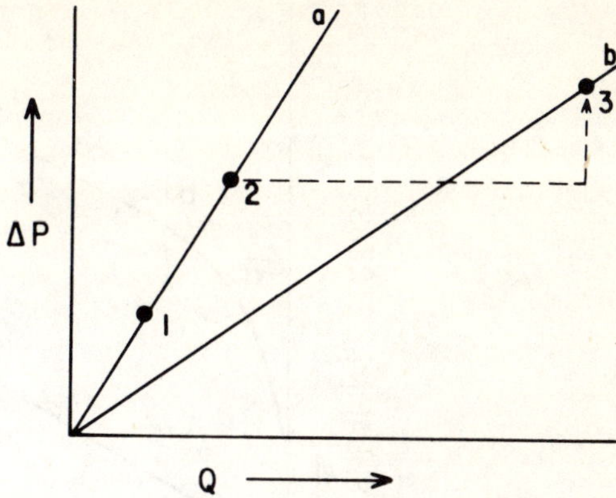

Figure 7-3
Lines denote pressure-flow relations at two resistances.

changes, often many-fold, to match transport to metabolism. Physicians carry blood pressure gauges, not flow meters, so they must always ask themselves how flow *might* have changed in order to interpret the measured pressures.

Poiseuille's law applies to steady, laminar flow in a single rigid tube. Blood flow in vessels, however, is pulsatile, and in very large vessels may not be laminar. Further complications arise when vessels are connected in networks. Finally, blood viscosity may vary with flow rate and vessel radius, as explained below. Nevertheless, Poiseuille's law remains an acceptable frame of reference if used with discretion.

Role of Viscosity

Though viscosity is a linear term in the Poiseuille relation, it can have a surprisingly large influence on flow in veins and, in certain pathological states, in arterioles as well. Thus far we have assumed that viscosity is a constant, independent of rate of shear. Fluids that behave this way are termed Newtonian. A plot of shear stress versus rate of shear for a Newtonian fluid in steady, laminar flow yields a straight line through the origin; see Figure 7-4, curve 1. The slope is, of course, the viscosity. Plasma is always a Newtonian fluid, even at very high protein concentration.

Solutions that contain suspended particles do not have a definite coefficient of viscosity. The *apparent* viscosity depends on the rate of shear, and hence volume flow, as in Figure 7-4, curve 2. The arrow indicates the *yield stress* that must be applied before flow will start from rest. Blood behaves as shown by curve 2 because it is a cell suspension. *The most important de-*

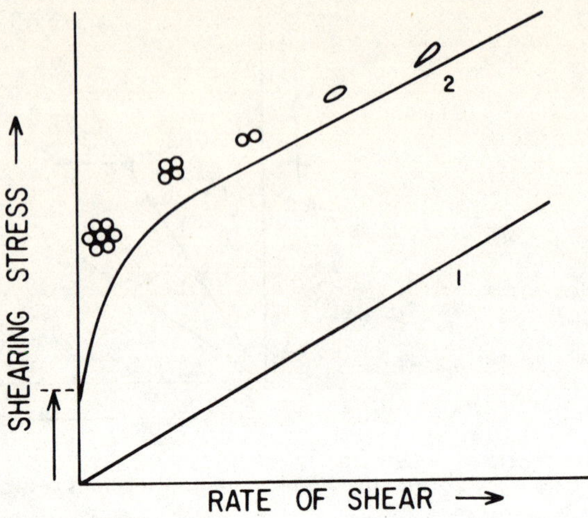

Figure 7-4
The ratio of shearing stress to rate of shear (slopes of curves) is the viscosity. Plasma viscosity is constant (*curve 1*), but blood viscosity is not (*curve 2*). Aggregated and disaggregated erythrocytes are shown above curve 2.

terminant of blood viscosity is the fractional concentration of erythrocytes. This is generally expressed as the hematocrit ratio:

$$\frac{\text{cell volume}}{\text{cell volume} + \text{plasma volume}}.$$

Effect of Hematocrit on Resistance

The hematocrit of shed blood ranges from 36 to 52 percent in normal human adults. Each curve in Figure 7-5 describes the viscosity-hematocrit relation at the indicated rate of shear. Shear rates in arterioles range from 20 to 200 s^{-1}; 1 to 10 s^{-1} is typical. The curves are not linear, despite the log scale of the ordinate, which indicates a greater than exponential rise in viscosity! At low shear, increasing the hematocrit from 40 to 60 percent would have about the same effect on resistance to flow as a 25 percent reduction in vessel radius, even though resistance varies as the fourth power of the radius.

Effect of Hematocrit on O_2 Offered

The product of flow and O_2 content per milliliter of blood is termed *O_2 offered.*[3] O_2 content depends in part on the hematocrit, which is regulated by a humoral system sensitive to the partial pressure of oxygen in arterial blood (PaO_2). If PaO_2 is chronically low, the rate of red cell production increases and the hematocrit rises. This allows each milliliter of blood to carry more oxygen and is an essential adaptation to residence at high altitude and to any disease that lowers PaO_2. The cost (increased viscosity and resistance to flow) is paid by the heart. People with

[3]This product has also been called *O_2 delivery*. However, O_2 is not delivered until it reaches the mitochondria.

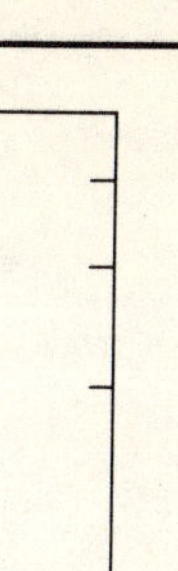

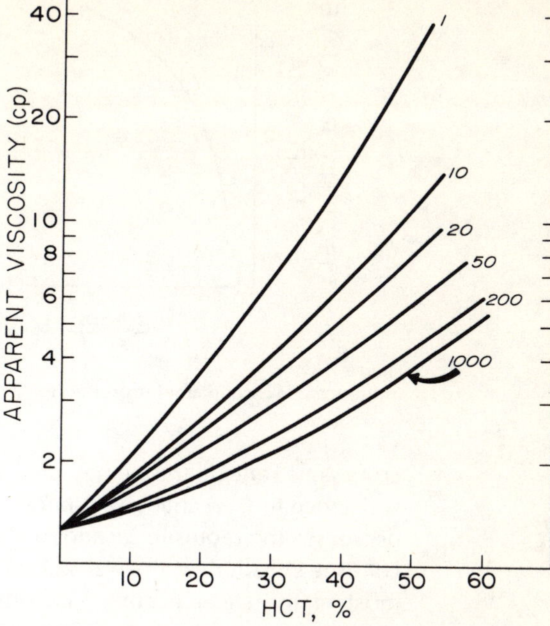

Figure 7-5
Apparent viscosity of blood in centipoise (logarithmic ordinate) as a function of hematocrit (*HCT*). Numbers adjacent to curves indicate shear rate in inverse seconds. (Modified from G. R. Cokelet, Hemodynamics. In P. C. Johnson [ed.], *Peripheral Circulation*. New York: Wiley, 1978.)

high hematocrits are precariously balanced because of the steep slopes of viscosity-hematocrit relations. A cardinal rule in physiology and medicine is that *if a little is good, more is not necessarily better.* The increase in hematocrit at high altitude is an example. Above 60 percent hematocrit, viscosity and resistance rise so steeply that flow decreases proportionately more than O_2 content increases, and O_2 offered falls. The therapeutic objective in this situation is to keep the cost–benefit ratio favorable.

Influence of Vessel Diameter

Fahraeus discovered that the hematocrit of *flowing* blood decreases progressively in tubes narrower than about 300 μm, even though the hematocrit of blood entering and exiting remains constant. The mechanism depends on the transmural velocity gradient (shear rate). The force balance on red cells directs them toward the center of a microvessel, leaving a cell-free plasma sheath near the wall. This sheath accounts for a major fraction of the volume in vessels that exhibit the Fahraeus effect. Laminae near the center move faster than those near the wall, so mean red cell velocity in microvessels exceeds plasma velocity. Mass balance is achieved by greater distances between red cells and hence lower (dynamic) hematocrit. Blood viscosity in mi-

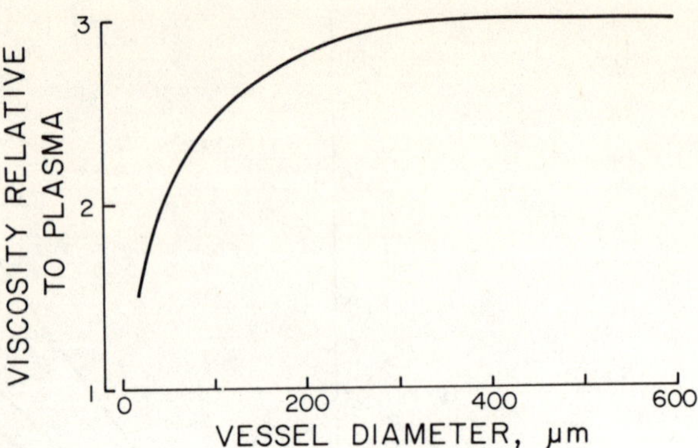

Figure 7-6
Influence of vessel diameter on the hematocrit of flowing blood.

crovessels reflects the hematocrit, as shown in Figure 7-6: The resistance to flow changes in parallel with viscosity. This greatly decreases the requisite ΔP and cardiac work. At the capillary the cell-free sheath near the wall acts as a lubricating layer in which most of the shear occurs. Viscosity in capillaries is therefore virtually identical to that of plasma.

How Red Cells Affect Viscosity

As is so often the case in physiology, to understand a complex system we first consider the properties of an individual cell (in this case the erythrocyte), and then the interactions among cells.

Mechanical Properties of Red Cells. A unique feature of an erythrocyte is its deformability. If freely suspended, an erythrocyte assumes a biconcave, discoid shape, indicative of the large excess of its surface area over its volume. The membrane is not distensible like a balloon. Instead, it is like a partly filled but unstretchable plastic bag. Since the membrane is flexible and the cell contents are fluid, the normal erythrocyte can assume many shapes if squeezed by simply shifting its volume about. Red cell deformability is essential because (1) it facilitates entry into capillaries and (2) it decreases the contribution of erythrocytes to blood viscosity.

The capillary, intuition to the contrary, is a rigid structure, and its diameter is generally *less* than that of the smallest erythrocyte. Consequently, erythrocytes fold into conical or teardrop shapes in capillaries, as shown in the photo on the cover of this book. Why did nature opt for deformable cells and small capillaries rather than small cells and large capillaries? The answer may be that transport is greatly facilitated by maximizing the

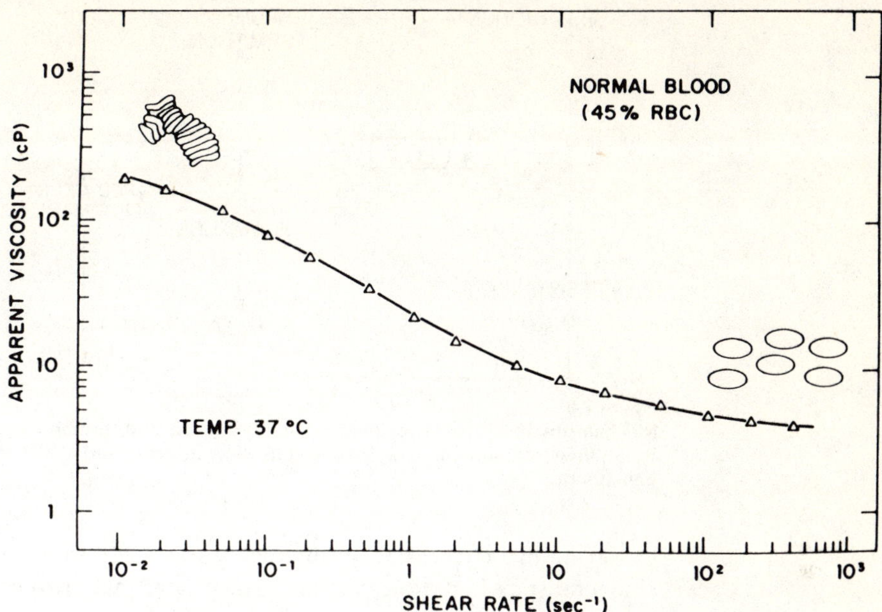

Figure 7-7
Quantitative relation between viscosity and shear rate for blood of normal hematocrit. Ranges necessitate log scales. (Data of S. Chien, S. Usami, and K. M. Jan, DHEW Publication No. [NIH] 76-1007, 1975, p. 277.)

number of capillaries per volume of tissue, as explained in Part III.

The principal problem created by narrow capillaries is that anything that decreases erythrocyte deformability increases resistance to blood flow. The cell shape with minimum ratio of surface area to volume is a sphere. A perfect sphere of constant surface area would not deform at all and could not survive the shearing stresses in circulation. Red cells become more spherical as they age, either in circulation or in a blood bank. Senescent red cells are filtered from circulation at narrow channels in the spleen that they cannot traverse.

Interactions of Red Cells. Blood viscosity is strongly influenced by interactions among red cells, as shown at upper left in Figure 7-7. The abscissa is directly proportional to flow and inversely proportional to radius. If blood is stationary, or flowing very slowly, erythrocytes form poker-chip-like aggregates called *rouleaux*. Protein, especially fibrinogen, greatly enhances cell-to-cell bonding. Rouleaux constitute an extra source of friction (viscosity) because part of the applied shearing stress is dissipated in deforming them or breaking them apart.

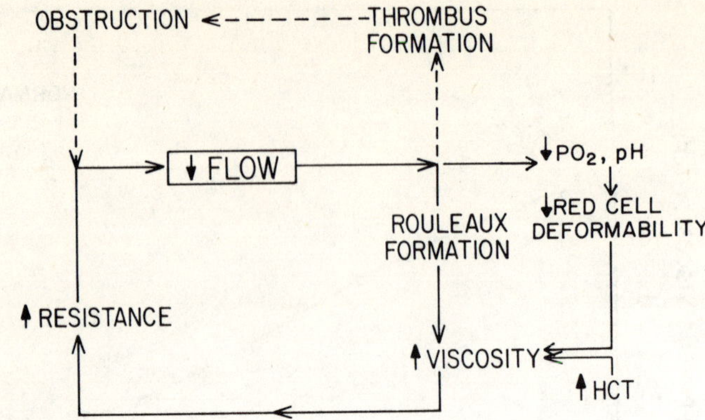

Figure 7-8
Mechanisms responsible for high resistance, stasis, and thrombosis when blood flow is abnormally low, arranged to show positive feedback. (*HCT* = hematocrit.)

Under normal circumstances the high velocity and small radius characteristic of arterioles result in shear rates that prevent formation of rouleaux. Since arterioles are chiefly responsible for vascular resistance, changes in resistance should be interpreted as indicative of vasoconstriction or vasodilation unless flow rate is abnormally low.

The situation in venules is quite different. Radius is large and red cell velocities are low, so rouleaux are generally present. *Viscosity rather than vessel geometry is the main determinant of resistance in the veins.* Consequently, the positive feedback loops shown in Figure 7-8 can be initiated by any factor that decreases venous flow sufficiently.

Rouleaux are virtually eliminated at shear rates greater than 20 s^{-1} at normal concentrations of plasma proteins. Nevertheless, viscosity falls between 20 and 500 s^{-1} because erythrocytes deform into elongated, streamlined shapes that offer less resistance to flow. At higher shear rates viscosity is constant.

Clinical Application

Many progressive, life-threatening illnesses involve positive feedback, or "vicious cycles." The system diagrammed in Figure 7-8 is a good example. It applies to common low flow states such as venous stasis and hemorrhagic shock, as well as to hyperviscosity syndromes. Coronary and cerebral thrombosis involve some of the same mechanisms.

For now enter the loop at "↑ viscosity." A dramatic example is sickle cell crisis, caused by a congenital defect in hemoglobin. When a sickle cell gives up more than a critical amount of O_2, it becomes a solid, elongated structure that is very rigid indeed. This increases resistance. The circulation functions at near-constant arterial pressure, so a rise in resistance decreases flow. Low flow increases the amount of O_2 that must be extracted from each red cell, because fewer red cells reach the tissue per unit time. This further increases the tendency for sickling. If flow is low enough, rouleaux formation begins and viscosity increases further. Thus the effects of sickle cell crisis (high O_2 extraction and rouleaux formation) promote the cause, that is, hyperviscosity. If shear rates fall low enough, platelet aggregation and thrombosis lead to irreversible injury.

The tendency for rouleaux formation increases with hematocrit and with the concentration of fibrinogen, which promotes cell-to-cell bonding. Fibrinogen may be produced in excess in certain malignancies. Hyperviscosity may be localized to sites of low blood flow. For example, rouleaux formation distal to an atherosclerotic plaque is an important initiating factor in thrombosis of coronary and cerebral arteries.

References

1. Burton, A. C. Role of geometry, size and shape in the microcirculation. *Fed. Proc.* 25:1753, 1966.
2. Caro, C. G., Pedley, T. J., Schroter, R. C., and Seed, W. A. *The Mechanics of the Circulation.* New York, London: Oxford University Press, 1978. Pp. 151–180, 385–407.
3. Chien, S., Usami, S., and Skalak, R. Blood Flow in Small Tubes. In E. M. Renkin and C. C. Michel (eds.), *Handbook of Physiology,* Section 2: The Cardiovascular System, Vol. IV. Microcirculation, Part 2. Bethesda, Md.: American Physiological Society, 1984.
4. Cokelet, G. R. Hemodynamics. In P. C. Johnson (ed.), *Peripheral Circulation.* New York: Wiley, 1978. Pp. 81–110.
5. Cokelet, G. R., Meiselman, H. J., and Brooks, D. E. *Erythrocyte Mechanics and Blood Flow.* New York: Liss, 1980.
*6. McDonald, D. A. *Blood Flow in Arteries.* Baltimore: Williams & Wilkins, 1974. Pp. 17–30, 41–45.
7. Schmid-Schönbein, G. W., Skalak, R., Usami, S., and Chien, S. Cell distribution in capillary networks. *Microvasc. Res.* 19:18, 1980.
8. Young, T. On the functions of the heart and arteries (The Croonian Lecture). *Philos. Trans. R. Soc. Lond.* 99:1, 1808.

8 : Pressure and Flow in Large Vessels

The heart is an intermittent pump; its output is zero for about two-thirds of each cycle. The large arteries store part of the stroke volume for release in diastole and store part of the heart's energy output as a rise in pressure. Release of this potential energy provides the driving force for diastolic flow.

Components of arterial pressure are identified in Figure 8-1. Note especially that pulsations are superimposed on a much larger steady pressure. A physician's blood pressure cuff allows an estimate of peak pressure in systole (P_s) and minimum pressure in diastole (P_D). The difference between these is called the *pulse pressure*. Mean pressure over the entire cycle ($\bar{P}a$) can be estimated as

$$\bar{P}a \cong P_D + \tfrac{1}{3}(P_s - P_D).$$

$\bar{P}a$ is the only arterial pressure of consequence for blood flow through an organ. Nevertheless, the increasing use of phasic pressure for diagnosis and patient monitoring necessitates thorough understanding of the origin and transmission of the pulse.

Determinants of Phasic Pressures

Arterial Compliance

Figure 8-2 shows an aortic segment attached to a syringe at one end and a pressure gauge at the other. A force applied to the plunger raises the pressure and displaces a certain volume, ΔV. The ratio $\Delta V/\Delta P$ is the distensibility, or *compliance*, of the segment. In young persons compliance is constant through about 150 torr and then decreases sharply. The nonlinearity is due to the presence of both elastic and collagen fibers in the wall. Elastic fibers are about 15 times more extensible. At small volumes only the elastic fibers are under tension; the collagen merely unfolds. At large volumes the collagen fibers are fully straightened, and as they take up the load the pressure rises steeply. The aorta is thus analogous to a soft rubber inner tube protected from blowout by a hard rubber casing. As with a tire, an aortic blowout occurs only if there is extensive local damage. Deterioration of elastic fibers accounts for the low arterial com-

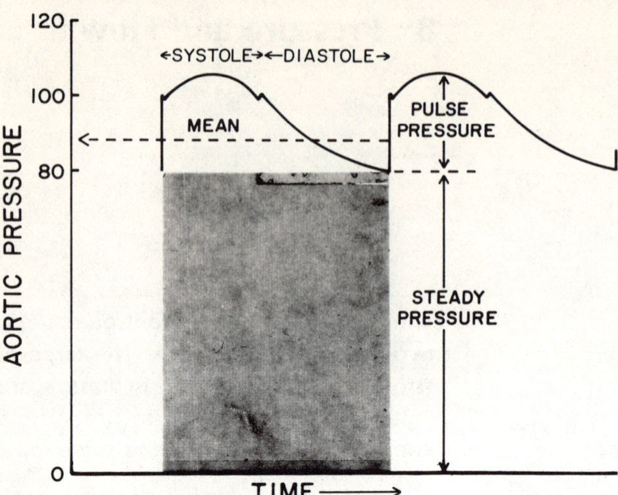

Figure 8-1
Components of phasic arterial pressure.

pliance and large pulse pressures characteristic of the elderly. Compliance changes so slowly, however, that it can be considered constant on the time scale of physiological adjustments.

Arterial Inflow Versus Outflow

The increase in arterial pressure during systole reflects the difference between the instantaneous rate of inflow from the ventricle and the rate of outflow through the minute vessels. The rate of inflow depends on stroke volume, ventricular contractility, and afterload. The rate of *outflow depends solely on the total peripheral resistance* (*TPR*). Heart rate affects pulse pressure through changes in stroke volume and by changing the time available for outflow from the aorta through the peripheral resistance. Though the importance of each determinant of phasic pressure is seldom known, much can be deduced from qualitative thinking about their interrelations.

Transmission of the Pressure Pulse

The Pulse Wave

Volume does not increase in all arteries simultaneously, because of the inertia of the long blood columns. The stroke volume accumulates first in the most proximal vessels. The resulting increment in pressure forces blood into adjacent sections, and so on. Thus, the pressure pulse travels as *a wave of distension* toward the periphery. This wave is very long — on the

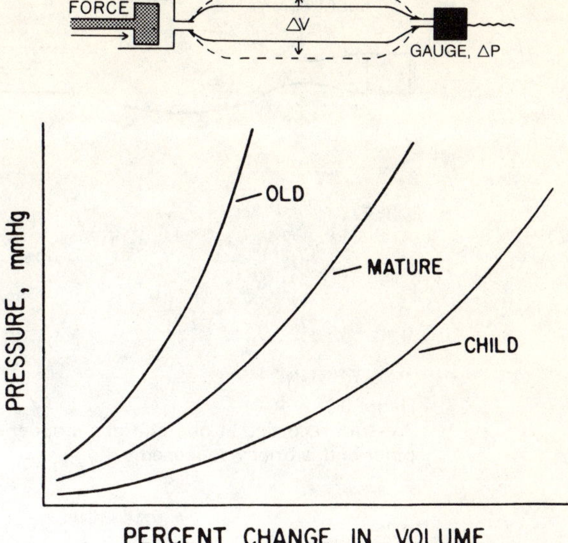

Figure 8-2
Distensibility curves for human aortas.

order of several meters. The rate at which it propagates is chiefly determined by vascular compliance. The "stiffer" the vessels the faster the propagation. In young adults the pulse wave velocity is about 5 m per second; velocity may double with advancing age.

The velocity of the pressure pulse is about 10 times the mean velocity of blood flow in the large arteries. To clarify the difference between the pulse wave and the movement of blood, consider a bicycle inner tube stoppered at both ends, so that flow along the tube is impossible; see Figure 8-3. If one end is tapped or briefly squeezed, the volume so displaced distends the adjacent section, and raises the pressure there. This in turn distends more peripheral sites, and a wave of distension and pressure propagates to the opposite end. There it encounters an infinite resistance (the stopper). Since the total volume is constant, the volume increment at the distal end comes from the proximal end. There the pressure is less than the steady-state value. The difference in pressure between the ends causes the pulse wave *reflected* from the distal resistance to propagate backward. Reflection from the proximal end then occurs, and so on. A pressure gauge at either end records a sinusoidal oscillation. Note that it is heavily damped in transmission. The vascular system behaves in similar fashion.

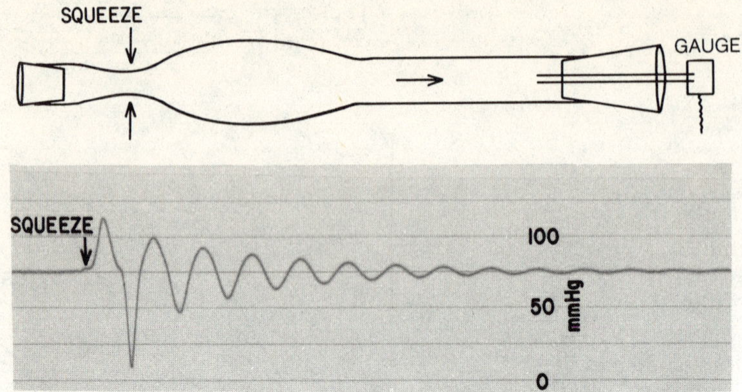

Figure 8-3
Pressure recorded at one end of a stoppered bicycle inner tube when the other end is briefly squeezed.

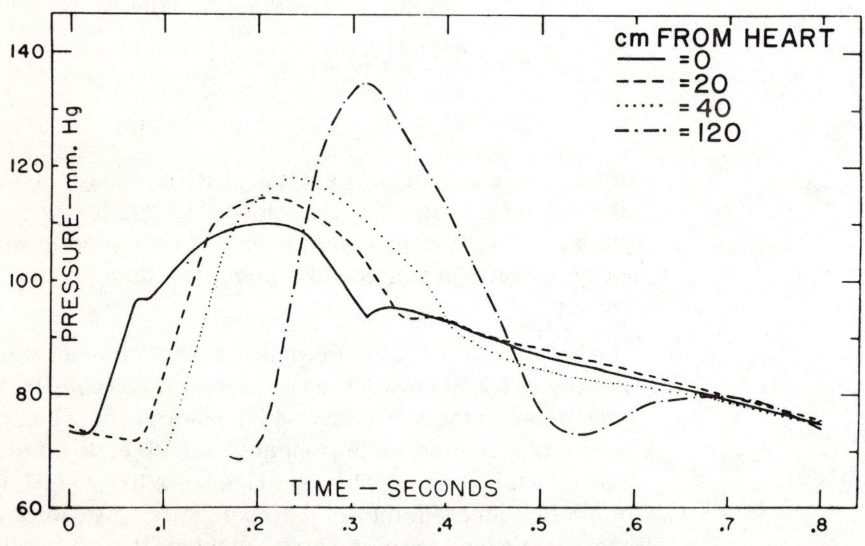

Figure 8-4
Superimposed recordings of arterial pressure at various distances from the aortic valve. The peripheral pulses are delayed, peaked, and damped. (From J. W. Remington and E. H. Wood, *J. Appl. Physiol.* 9:433, 1956.)

Change in Pulse Contour

Pulses recorded at various distances from the aortic valve are superimposed in Figure 8-4; note that the steady component of pressure is not shown. The central pulse is progressively damped in transmission. Damping affects high-frequency components to the greatest extent, so the rapid initial rise and oscillations caused by valve closure are obliterated in the peripheral pulses. Consequently, *only central pulses can be used to assess aortic valve function or to time the application of cardiac assistance devices* that act during diastole. Moreover, the recording apparatus itself must be properly damped. A small air bubble in the catheter or pressure gauge can make a central pulse look like a peripheral one. Physicians must keep these technical matters in mind when interpreting data collected in intensive care units.

Pulse contour is altered by wave reflection as well as damping. The body behaves as though composed of one reflection site above the diaphragm and another below. The reflected wave is largest near the reflection sites and is obliterated by damping before it reaches the aortic root. The reflected pulse sums with, or cancels, the antegrade pulse. This is responsible for the peaking of the peripheral pulse shown in Figure 8-4 and for the subsequent pressure oscillations. Students are often disturbed by the fact that peak pressure in the peripheral pulse exceeds that in the central one. Notice, however, that central pressure exceeds peripheral pressure earlier in time. Mean pressure — the determinant organ flow — is indeed slightly higher at the central site. In summary, peripheral pulses are delayed, damped, and peaked and are hardly more useful than a recording of mean pressure.

Mean Pressure in Arteries

Figure 8-5 shows pulses recorded simultaneously in the ascending aorta and in a small, unnamed artery in the dog's leg. Both vagi were stimulated in order to arrest the heart. With pulsation eliminated, the upstream pressure is only 2 torr greater than the downstream pressure. This can also be demonstrated by electri-

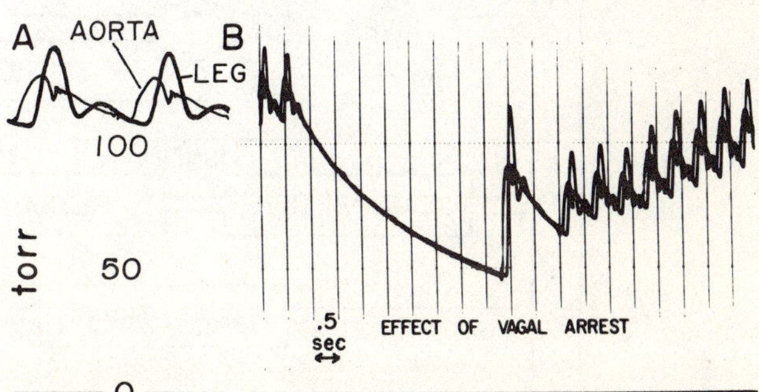

Figure 8-5
Phasic pressures in ascending aorta and a small leg artery; distance between catheter tips was 30 cm. When pulsation is eliminated by cardiac arrest the mean pressures are almost the same at the upstream and downstream sites.

cally damping the pulsations. The experiment proves that the ΔP caused by viscous resistance is negligible between the aorta and the smallest peripheral arteries. This is of the utmost importance, for it tells us that *the mean pressure available to drive blood through all the organs is the same*. The reason resistive losses in large vessels are so small is given in Chapter 10.

Organ Resistances in Parallel

Since the organs share a common pressure, they may be considered lumped resistances in parallel, as shown in Figure 8-6. The total conductance through the systemic circulation is equal to

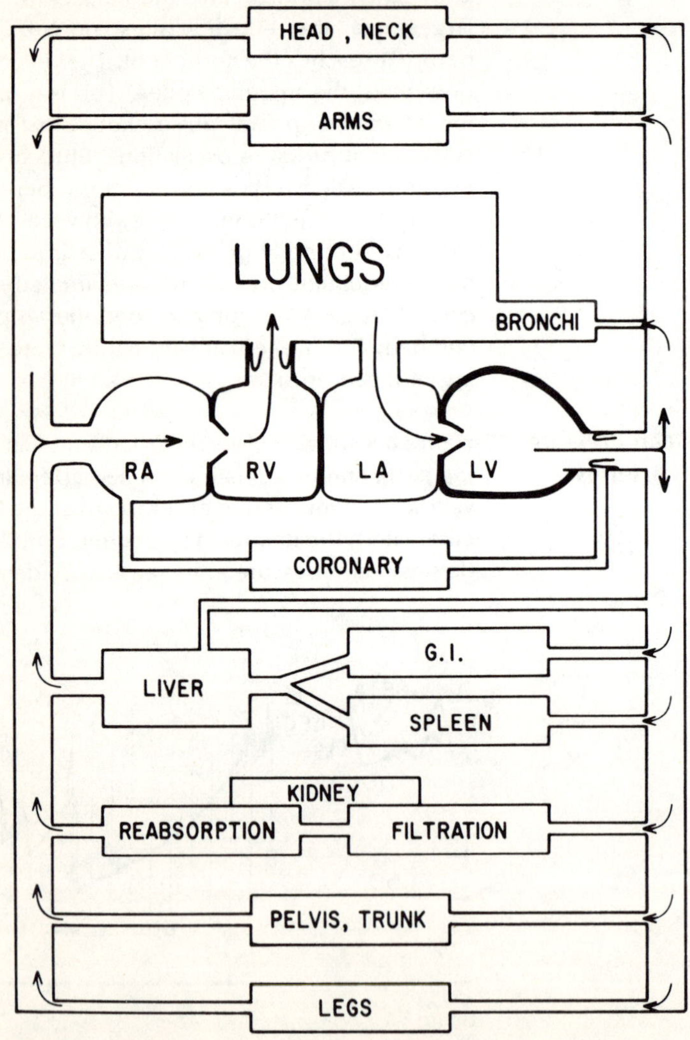

Figure 8-6
Schematic illustrating parallel connection of systemic organs. The two ventricles (*RV, LV*) are connected in series. (*RA* = right atrium; *LA* = left atrium; *G.I.* = gastrointestinal tract.)

the sum of the individual organ conductances:

$$1/TPR = 1/R_{\text{kidney}} + 1/R_{\text{legs}} + 1/R_{\text{brain}} + 1/R_{\text{etc.}}.$$

This arrangement has several very important consequences:

1. Each organ can control its own flow by changing its conductance.
2. The cardiac output can therefore be redistributed to meet changing requirements.
3. Redistributions generally have little effect on mean arterial pressure.

The contribution of flow redistribution to adaptation to stress is developed in Chapter 13.

The most important exception to the general rule is the pulmonary circulation, which is in series with the systemic. Other exceptions include the liver, which is in series with the mesenteric circuit and in parallel with other organs. The kidney can be regarded as a glomerular organ for filtration in series with a tubular organ for reabsorption.

Pressure-Flow Relations in Larger Arteries

Gradients Caused by Acceleration

The velocity of blood, and hence its kinetic energy, changes throughout the cardiac cycle, but the pressure gradients required to produce these accelerations are negligibly small except at the aortic valve. Pressure-flow relations at the valve are shown in Figure 8-7. Note first that the *difference* between left ventricular pressure and aortic pressure (lower panel) is only a small fraction of total pressure at the valve. The difference is positive and maximal as blood is accelerated from rest to peak velocity, and then reverses (aortic pressure > ventricular) during the last two-thirds of systole. This reverse ΔP decelerates the blood; note the decline in forward velocity. Because the blood has momentum, ejection continues in late systole despite the reverse ΔP. The phenomenon demonstrates that flow is determined by the gradient in total energy, kinetic as well as potential. A positive ΔP across the aortic valve throughout systole is diagnostic of obstructive disease. The *factor of safety* built into the aortic valve is so large that major resistive losses do not develop, even at very high cardiac output, until the cross-sectional area of the valve is less than half normal. This accounts, in part, for the long latent period before the appearance of symptoms in aortic stenosis.

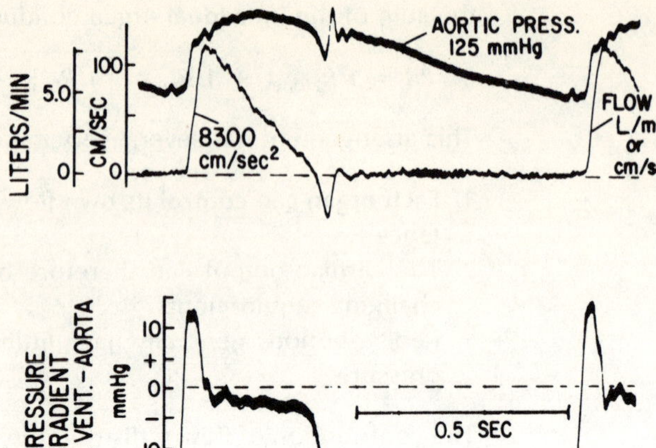

Figure 8-7
The pressure gradient from left ventricle to aorta (*lower panel*) is shown for correlation with aortic pressure and flow. Since the cross-sectional area of the aorta was held constant, flow could be expressed in cm/sec or L/min. The maximum acceleration (dv/dt) was 8300 cm/s^2 (Modified from M. P. Spencer and F. C. Greiss, *Circ. Res.* 10:274, 1962. By permission of the American Heart Association, Inc.)

Pressure Gradients Caused by Energy Transformations

The total energy (E) expressed per unit volume of flowing blood is

$$E = \gamma g h + P + \tfrac{1}{2} \gamma v^2,$$

where v is blood velocity. The first term represents energy of position and can be neglected if the system is horizontal. P denotes potential energy of pressure, and the last term represents kinetic energy. If frictional losses are nil (as they are in large vessels), the law of conservation of energy tells us that an increase in v must be accompanied by a corresponding decrease in P. Energy redistributions occur at sites of abnormal narrowing, or *stenosis*. Since the same volume flows through the normal and stenotic portions of a vessel, the velocity and kinetic energy must be higher in the stenosis. The pressure tending to distend the stenotic segment is correspondingly lower, so stenosis tends to progress.

In resting horizontal persons, about 97 percent of total energy is potential. Even when the cardiac output is greatly increased, less than 20 percent of the heart's external work is used to impart momentum to the blood. This accounts for the fact that diseases that increase cardiac output are much better tolerated than those that raise arterial pressure.

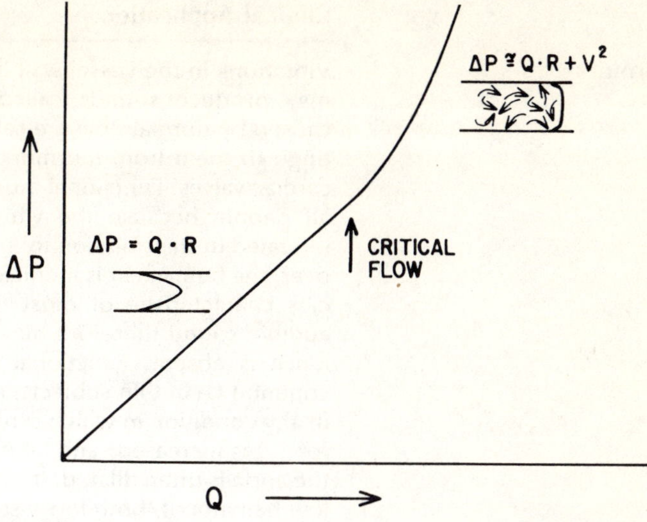

Figure 8-8
Linear slope indicates range of laminar flow. Nonlinearity is due to development of turbulence.

Turbulence and Its Significance

The basic assumption in the derivation of Poiseuille's law is that flow be laminar. Above a critical flow rate, however, the laminae break down into eddies that move randomly in all directions. Such flow is said to be *turbulent*; see Figure 8-8. The kinetic energy of the eddies is dissipated as heat. Consequently, additional pressure (potential energy) must be applied to achieve the same flow. This extra pressure varies as the square of the velocity.

The tendency to turbulence is given by the Reynolds number, *Re*:

$$Re = \frac{v D \gamma}{\eta},$$

where v = linear velocity, D = diameter, γ = density, and η = viscosity. *Re* is dimensionless because it is a ratio of inertial forces to cohesive forces. The former tend to disrupt the laminae, the latter to maintain them.

The *Re* at which turbulence begins is about 1000 in vivo. In normal human beings, peak systolic velocity in the thoracic aorta is 50 to 300 cm/per second at rest, and aortic diameter is 2.5 to 4.0 cm. Blood has a density of 1 and viscosity of 0.04 poise at normal hematocrit and high shear rate. *Re* for these conditions varies from about 3000 to 30,000, so flow in the thoracic aorta is turbulent during most of systole. Systolic flow is also turbulent in the pulmonary artery.

Clinical Application

Murmurs

Vibrations in the vessel wall induced by turbulence may produce sounds called *murmurs.* Murmurs caused by normal flow are called *functional,* to distinguish them from murmurs caused by disease of cardiac valves. Functional murmurs are not heard in all people because the vibrations are greatly attenuated in transmission to the body surface. Moreover, the human ear is inefficient at the low frequencies characteristic of most murmurs. Absence of audible sound therefore may not mean that turbulence is absent. Functional systolic murmurs are common (1) in thin subjects, especially children; (2) in any condition in which cardiac output (and therefore v) is increased; and (3) in the elderly, in whom the aorta is often dilated. In anemia accompanied by low hematocrit, both low viscosity and high cardiac output contribute to functional murmurs. Conversely, functional murmurs are seldom heard in people with abnormally high hematocrits, in whom viscosity may be twice normal. Indeed, hyperviscosity may "mask" a murmur that is not functional! Beyond the aorta, velocity and diameter decrease markedly, and turbulence seldom occurs. Velocities during diastole are too low to permit turbulence. Diastolic murmurs are never functional and are only partly due to turbulence.

Effect of High Flow on the Vessel Wall

Recall from Chapter 7 that shear stress increases with flow velocity and is greatest near the wall. If the shear stress, or viscous drag, is high enough, the intima is deformed, and its permeability to lipids and macromolecules is increased. Thus high flow velocities contribute to the prevalence of atherosclerosis in large vessels. Deformation of the vasa vasorum, the vessels that nourish the arterial wall, may also contribute to atherogenesis.

Indirect Measurement of Arterial Pressure

Blood pressure in humans is generally measured by means of a *sphygmomanometer.* This device consists of an inflatable cuff, which is wrapped around an arm or leg. The cuff is inflated to a pressure sufficient to occlude the underlying artery. The pressure in the cuff is measured as the cuff is slowly deflated. When cuff pressure falls just below peak blood pressure, a high-velocity jet enters the distal, unoccluded artery. The resulting turbulence and abrupt distension cause audible vibrations. This cuff pressure is taken to represent peak systolic pressure. As the cuff is deflated further, the vibrations (called Korotkoff sounds) increase in intensity, then become muffled, and finally disappear. Disappearance of sound is well correlated with minimum diastolic pressure. The pressures corresponding to appearance and disappearance of the Korotkoff sounds are termed systolic and diastolic, respectively, by clinicians.

References

1. Bruns, D. L. A general theory of the cause of murmurs in the cardiovascular system. *Am. J. Med.* 27:360, 1959.

*2. Caro, C. G., Pedley, T. J., Schroter, R. C., and Seed, W. A. *The Mechanics of the Circulation*. New York, London: Oxford University Press, 1978. Chap. 12.

3. Dobrin, P. B. Vascular Mechanics. In J. T. Shepherd and F. M. Abboud (eds.), *Handbook of Physiology,* Section 2: The Cardiovascular System, Vol. III. Peripheral Circulation and Organ Blood Flow, Part 1. Bethesda, Md.: American Physiological Society, 1983.

4. Heistad, D. D., Markus, M. L., Larsen, G. E., and Armstrong, M. L. Role of vasa vasorum in nourishment of the aortic wall. *Am. J. Physiol.* 240:H781, 1981.

5. McDonald, D. A. *Blood Flow in Arteries*. Baltimore: Williams & Wilkins, 1974. Pp. 238–255, 309–315, 389–398.

6. Simon, A. C., Safar, M. E., Levenson, J. A., London, G. M., Levy, B. I., and Chou, N. P. An evaluation of large arteries' compliance in man. *Am. J. Physiol.* 237:H550, 1979.

9 : Integrated Events of the Cardiac Cycle

This brief chapter contains no concepts but many essential facts about how events are related in time. These facts are used in every physical examination; they must be mastered for permanent retention.

Phases of the Cycle and Valve Positions

The cardiac cycle is divided into four phases, according to what is going on in the ventricles. During *isovolumic contraction,* ventricular pressure rises above atrial pressure but does not yet reach arterial pressure (pulmonary or aortic). The atrioventricular (AV) valves (mitral and tricuspid) are closed, and the semilunar valves (aortic and pulmonary) are closed. When aortic pressure is exceeded, the *ejection* phase begins; the AV valves remain closed, but the semilunar valves open. When ejection ceases, the aortic and pulmonary valves close, and ventricular pressures fall toward atrial pressures. During this phase of *isovolumic relaxation* all valves are again closed. When the ventricular pressures drop below atrial pressures, the AV valves open, and ventricular *filling* begins; aortic and pulmonary valves, of course, remain closed. The phases of the cycle are identified at the top of Figure 9-1. You will find it necessary to keep referring to this schematic as you study. Read this chapter once to identify the variables and events. Then reread with attention to the causal and temporal relations between pressures (lower half of the figure) and flows (upper half).

Events during Systole

Isovolumic Contraction

Systole occupies about one-third of the cycle at normal heart rates. Electrical systole begins with the first component of the ventricular complex (QRS). Mechanical systole begins about 0.02 to 0.04 second later. The first rise in ventricular pressure tenses the AV valves, which, at normal heart rates, are almost coapted at the end of diastole. The AV valves are held in place by the chordae tendineae, but the leaflets bulge into the atria. This bulge produces a small rise in atrial pressure. Sudden tensing of the AV valves produces the main components of the first heart sound. Ventricular contraction before ejection begins is

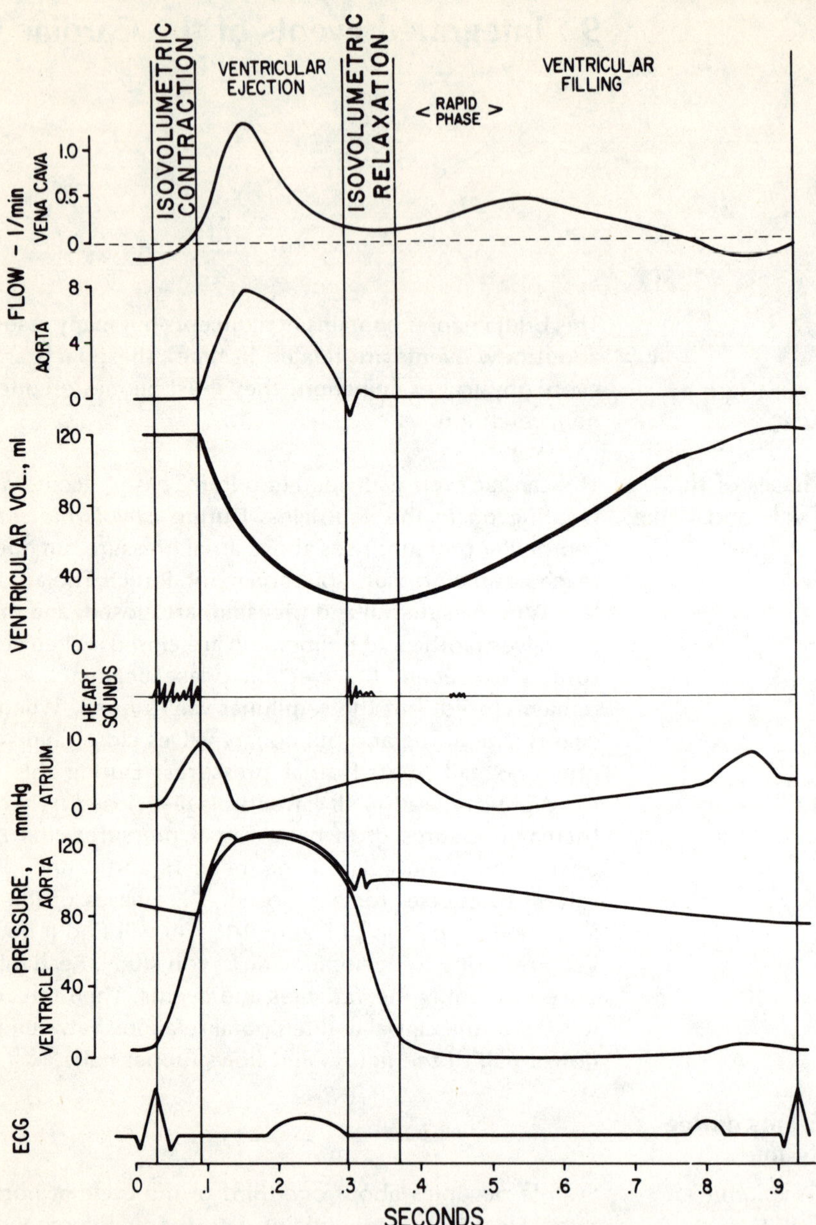

Figure 9-1
Summary of simultaneous events of cardiac cycle. Atrial and ventricular pressures are not drawn to the same scale.

isovolumic but not isometric, because the ventricle shortens from base to apex. This shape change creates a strain within the wall that squeezes and narrows the intramural coronary vessels. The duration of isovolumic contraction is 0.06 to 0.08 second.

Ejection

Shortly after the ventricle is fully depolarized (ventricular complex of ECG is completed), ventricular pressure exceeds aortic pressure, and ejection begins. The principal decrease in ventricular volume and peak rate of flow in the aorta occur early in systole. The eddy currents created in the sinuses of Valsalva by the high-velocity stream prevent the valve cusps from blocking the orifices of the coronary arteries. Note especially that the ventricle does not empty completely. The decrease in ventricular volume relative to end-diastolic volume is called the *ejection fraction*. It amounts to 0.6 to 0.8 in healthy hearts.

Outflow from the atria is prevented by high intraventricular pressure that holds the AV valves shut. Nevertheless, ejection strongly influences atrial pressure and flow in the great veins. As ventricular fibers shorten, they pull the base of the heart toward the apex. This stretches the atria and increases their capacity. The resulting fall in atrial pressure produces a brisk increase in vena caval flow. Atrial filling is responsible for the slow rise in atrial pressure and decreased flow rate in the venae cavae during the latter part of systole.

Events during Diastole

Isovolumic Relaxation

Ventricular pressure falls rapidly as active tension decays. Release of potential energy stored in elastic fibers during systole helps to expand the ventricles and accelerates the pressure drop. The large pressure gradient that develops between aorta and ventricle drives a small back-flow that slams the aortic valve shut; refer to Figure 8-7, p. 86. The abrupt tensing of the semilunar valve leaflets gives rise to the second heart sound and to a sharp oscillation in aortic pressure called the dicrotic notch. This latter and the second heart sound are usually well correlated with the end of the T wave of the ECG. Pulmonary valve closure contributes to the second heart sound. Meanwhile, venous return continues to expand the atria, so atrial pressure increases further. The duration of isovolumic relaxation is 0.06 to 0.10 second at normal heart rates.

Ventricular Filling

About 0.04 second after ventricular pressure drops below atrial pressure the AV valves open. Blood dammed up in the atria during systole rushes into the ventricles. This *rapid filling phase* lasts about 0.1 second. Ventricular wall tension continues to fall during this time. Consequently, ventricular pressure remains slightly below atrial pressure, despite the large initial increment in ventricular volume. A low-frequency, low-intensity vibration accompanies rapid ventricular filling and in thin individuals (especially children) is audible as a third heart sound. The rate of filling slows as atrial and ventricular pressures approach equilibrium. Flows in the venae cavae and pulmonary veins decrease in late diastole as rising pressure dissipates the gradient for venous return. At slow heart rates, filling practically ceases before atrial contraction begins.

Electrical activation of the atria (P wave of ECG) is followed within 0.02 second by a rise in atrial and ventricular pressures that lasts about 0.1 second. At slow heart rates this adds little additional volume to the ventricles, because the resistance to retrograde flow back into the great veins is less than resistance to forward flow if the ventricles are nearly full. (Note that caval flow goes below the baseline.) At rapid heart rates, however, passive filling is incomplete, and atrial contraction becomes essential. This is why atrial fibrillation has such a deleterious effect on cardiac output when the ventricular rate is high. Atrial contraction is important for filling even at slow heart rates if inflow to the ventricle is impeded by mitral or tricuspid valve stenosis. Under normal circumstances, the most important effect of atrial contraction is to produce a quick stretch of the ventricular muscle fibers. The increment in fiber length permits the ventricles to develop greater tension in the subsequent systole. It is convenient to think of the atria as *booster pumps* for the ventricles. This mechanical function depends on the AV node, which delays ventricular systole until after atrial contraction is completed.

When the atrial fibers relax, atrial pressure falls, and the leaflets of the AV valves float into close proximity. The time for this prepositioning is again provided by the AV nodal delay. With the valves already almost closed, the rise in ventricular pressure in early systole causes virtually no reflux of blood into the atria.

We have finally completed one cardiac cycle and are back to isovolumic contraction. The only way to feel secure about all this is to work your way through a few more cycles on your own.

10 : Microcirculation: Sites of Resistance and Exchange

The minute vessels control peripheral resistance, the distribution of flow, the surface area for blood-tissue exchange, and the capacity of blood reservoirs. Each of these functions depends on a category of vessels with common anatomical characteristics.

Intraorgan Resistances in Series

Vascular categories are traversed seriatim, so they can be regarded as lumped resistances in series; see Figure 10-1. Except for the capillaries, they are shown as variable resistances, to indicate control by nerves and vasoactive substances. The pressure drop attributable to each vessel category is shown in Figure 10-2 for the mesenteric vascular bed. The ΔP indicates the contribution to total resistance.

Small Arteries

Branches of the main artery to an organ serve a *distributive* function, as for example the interlobar, arcuate, and interlobular arteries of the kidney. The smallest distributing arteries are about 200 μm in diameter. The regional distribution of flow can be controlled by varying the appropriate resistances. For example, the ratio of cortical to medullary flow in kidney and the ratio of subepicardial to subendocardial flow in the ventricles may change under various circumstances. Distributing vessels are interconnected in a repetitive, arcadelike pattern, called the *macromesh*. The pressure drop across the macromesh is generally small. If a distributing vessel becomes occluded, local metabolites decrease resistance to flow through interconnections, and flow proceeds around the obstruction. This *collateral circulation* is of particular importance in the heart and other organs of high O_2 consumption.

Arterioles

Precapillary vessels 20 to 200 μm in diameter have a thick, continuous smooth-muscle coat and are classed as true arterioles. They are connected in *repetitive* arcades to form the *micromesh*. The large ΔP across these arterioles identifies them as the principal sites of resistance; note Figure 10-2. *Arterioles therefore control total flow through an organ.* Arteriolar resistance also influences hydrostatic pressure in the capillaries. This pres-

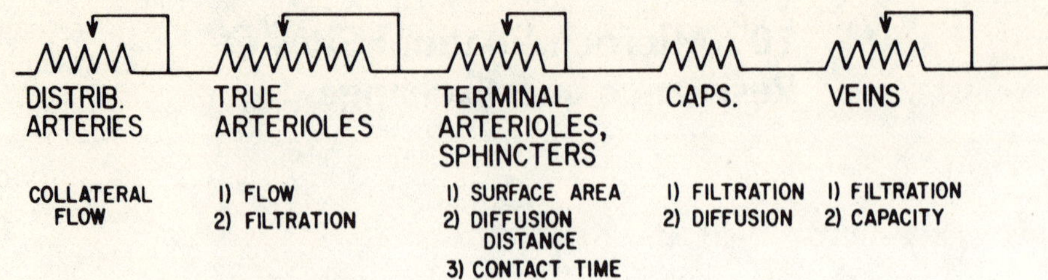

Figure 10-1
Schematic showing intraorgan resistances in series.

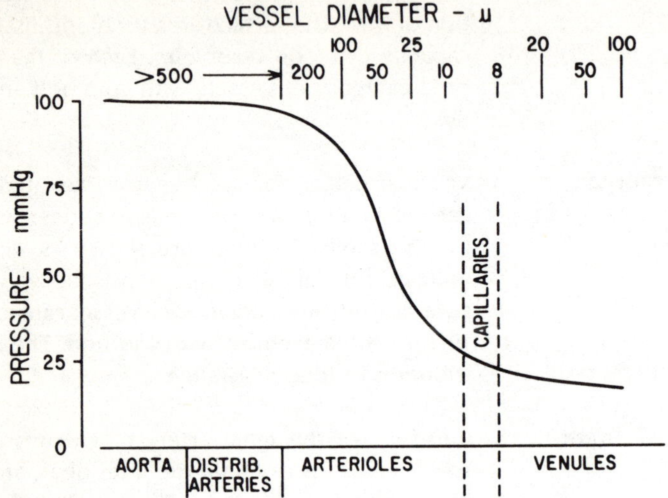

Figure 10-2
Distribution of pressures in mesenteric circulation. (Based on data of R. W. Gore, *Circ. Res.* 34:581, 1974. By permission of the American Heart Association, Inc.).

sure largely determines the rate of filtration (or reabsorption) of interstitial fluid, as explained in Chapter 14. Constriction seldom fully occludes the arteriolar lumen. Arteriolar constriction and dilation often occur in rhythmic cycles. Each vessel cycles independently of its neighbor, so only very small regions of tissue are deprived of flow at a particular time. Though each arteriole obeys Poiseuille's law, the change in resistance across the entire network is less than that predicted by the fourth-power rule.

Terminal Arterioles and Precapillary Sphincters

Arterioles smaller than about 20 μm have a discontinuous smooth-muscle coat and are classified as terminal arterioles. Each controls inflow to a sheaf of 5 to 25 capillaries. The sheaves overlap like courses of brick. The terminal arteriole and its capillary sheaf constitute a *microvascular unit* for blood-tissue exchange. In some organs a ring of smooth muscle at the entrance to an individual capillary allows finer control of capillary function. Terminal arterioles and precapillary sphincters tend to respond more vigorously than true arterioles to tissue metabolites. Since the lumen is very small, constriction of terminal arterioles tends to block entry of red cells into the capillaries beyond. The ΔP across terminal arterioles is small, however, so these vessels are not major controls of resistance and total flow through an organ. The principal function of terminal arterioles is to produce appropriate changes in the number of actively perfused capillaries. Thus flow and capillary density should be regarded as semi-independent variables, controlled by distinct smooth-muscle effectors. Active capillary control is superimposed on passive, hemodynamic factors that influence passage of erythrocytes and granulocytes through branching networks.

Capillaries

The capillary is the principal site of exchange between blood and tissue. When metabolic rate is low, as in resting skeletal muscle, most capillaries are not actively perfused. Additional capillaries and intercapillary anastomoses are *recruited* when the metabolic rate increases, as in exercise. Capillary density sets the surface area for transcapillary exchange and also determines the distances substances must move by diffusion between blood and tissue. Finally, capillary density influences flow velocity in capillaries, and hence the time available for transcapillary exchange. Capillary function in blood-tissue transport is considered further in Chapter 16.

Venules

The principal function of venules is to contain about 80 percent of the blood volume. Venules are also important in filtration, because venous pressure affects capillary pressure. Though the pressure drop in veins is small, it is not always a small fraction of the total pressure drop across an organ. If the arterioles are fully dilated, as in heavy exercise, venous resistance becomes an important determinant of flow.

Role of Network Geometry

The length and diameter of an individual vessel decrease progressively with branching. However, the total length, total cross-sectional area, and total capacity of vessels within an organ increase with branching. These geometrical changes are different for each vessel category.

Friction in laminar flow depends largely on the surface area of the laminae, which increases with each branching. Therefore, the pressure drop per unit length varies directly with the number of vessels. This explains why the ΔP along the aorta and major arteries is so small; there simply are not enough of such vessels to cause an appreciable pressure drop. Vessel number cannot be the only determinant of ΔP, however, for there are far more capillaries than arterioles, but the ΔP is small in capillaries and large in arterioles. The additional factor to be taken into account is the effect of branching on flow velocity.

Recall from Chapter 7 that friction depends on the rate of shear, and hence on velocity. (If you have ever burned your hands sliding down a rope, you know this by experience.)

$$\underset{\text{cm/s}}{\text{Velocity}} = \underset{\text{cm}^3\text{/s}}{\text{volume flow}} / \underset{\text{cm}^2}{\text{cross-sectional area}}$$

Cross-sectional area increases at each branching, so velocity and pressure-drop per unit length of vessel fall progressively from aorta to capillary. From Poiseuille's law one can show that the ΔP in the branches exceeds that in the parent vessel by

$$\frac{N A^2_p l_b}{A^2_b l_p},$$

where N = number of branches, A = cross-sectional area, l = vessel length, p = parent vessel, and b = branches. The increment in A with branching varies from 1.2 in certain arterioles to about 6 at the capillaries. In the true arterioles the proportional increase in N is greater than the proportional increment in A, so ΔP per unit length is large. Moreover, arterioles are quite long (500–10,000 μm) so the total ΔP is large. In contrast, ΔP is very small in capillaries because their huge aggregate cross-sectional area results in very low linear velocities. Since capillaries are 100 to 3000 μm long, the time required for transit is on the order of 1 second. This is sufficient time for exchange of diffusible substances between blood and tissue. Metabolites can diffuse across arterioles and venules. Nevertheless, capillaries play the dominant role in transport largely because transit time in other vessels is too brief (<100 ms).

The small ΔP in postcapillary vessels reflects the fact that the cross-sectional area after each venous confluence is three to six times greater than the cross-sectional area of the concomitant arteries. Large cross-sectional area also explains why veins contain about 80 percent of the blood volume. Velocities, transit times, and volume flow at various locations in a loop of cat mesentery are shown in Figure 10-3. Relating these data to the pressure changes in Figure 10-2 will be helpful.

Relation of Capillary Structure to Function

Capillaries behave like a filter with pores of molecular dimensions. The pores are large enough to permit *hydrodynamic flow* of an ultrafiltrate of plasma. Normal function of skin, muscle, and most of the viscera requires that the volume filtered be small and that protein be retained within the vascular compart-

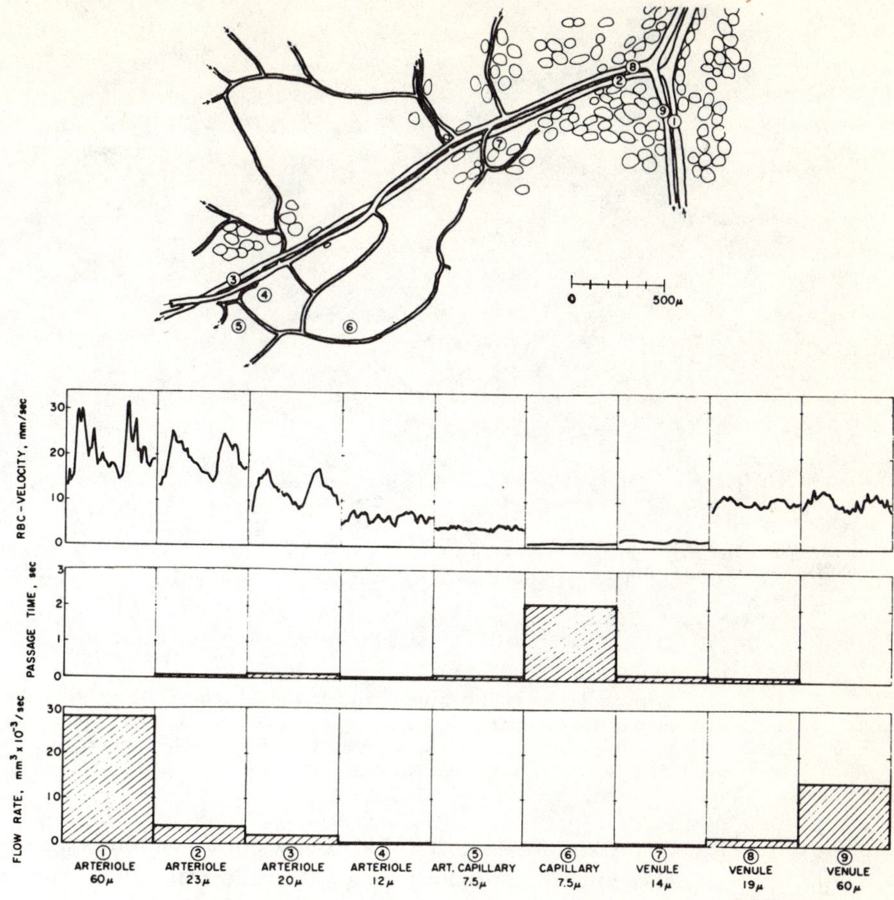

Figure 10-3
Red cell velocities, transit times, and flow rates in a vascular loop of cat mesentery. Width of each panel corresponds to 625 msec. (From P. Gaehtgens, H. J. Meiselman, and H. Wayland, *Microvasc. Res.* 2:151, 1970.)

ment. The same pores permit diffusion of water-soluble molecules between capillaries and tissue. The pores are formed by the cleft where two endothelial cells overlap. The one shown in Figure 10-4 is about 0.5 μm long and 6 to 10 nm wide over most of its length. At the point labelled *TJ* (tight junction), the slit narrows to 4.0 to 4.5 nm. In this region the two cells are held together by a hydrated mesh of fine filaments, rather like a wet felt gasket. The effect is to restrict egress of plasma protein.

Physiologists have estimated the size and abundance of aqueous pores by determining the rate at which molecules of known dimensions diffuse across the capillary. Data for cat hind limb are shown in Table 10-1. In the last column, permeability is expressed in terms of flux per unit concentration difference per weight of limb. If the capillary were no barrier, capillary perme-

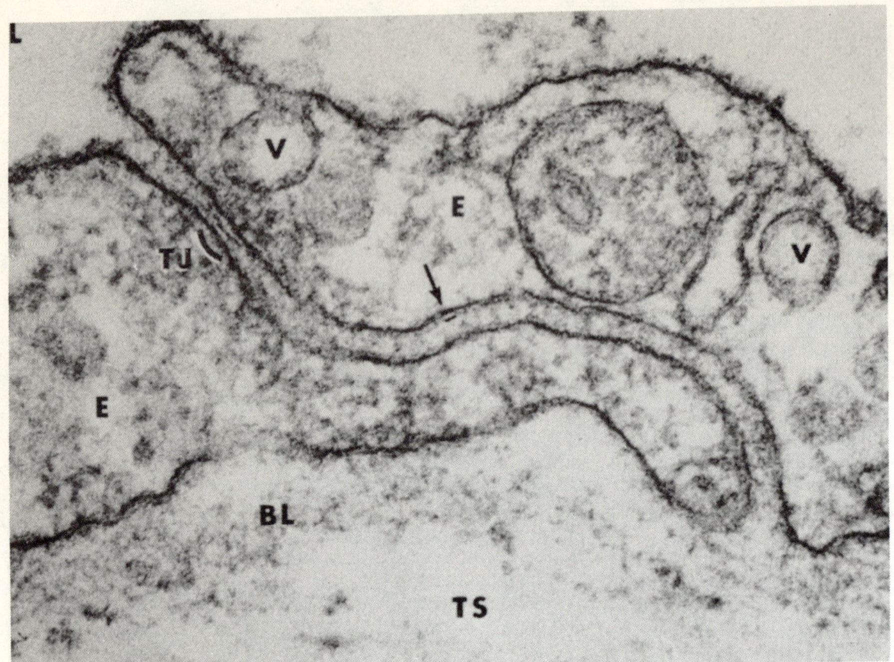

Figure 10-4
Arrow indicates cleft between two endothelial cells (*E*) bounded by the lumen (*L*) on one side and the tissue space (*TS*) and basement lamina (*BL*) on the other. Cells contain large vesicles (*V*). Parenthesis indicates tight junction (*TJ*). (From J. H. Luft, *Fed. Proc.* 25:1780, 1966.)

ability and the free diffusion coefficient for various substances should change proportionally with molecular size. In fact, permeability changes much more. The theory of restricted diffusion indicates that the capillaries in 100 grams of cat muscle behave like an artificial membrane 7000 square centimeters in area and 0.5 μm thick, containing 5×10^{12} aqueous pores 8 nm in diameter. Though such pores would occupy only 0.15 percent of membrane area they are sufficient to account for known rates of diffusion of water-soluble substances.

Brain capillaries are an exception. Their slit pores are completely occluded at the tight junction and are very impermeable to water-soluble molecules. At the opposite extreme, glomerular capillaries are roughly 200 times more permeable to water than are muscle capillaries but much *less* permeable to protein. This suggests a high density of small pores but no large ones. Micrographs of glomerular ultrastructure can be found in reference 11. Notice in Table 10-1 that albumin's permeability is small but not zero, even though its equivalent diameter is considerably greater than that of the tight junction. This behavior is best explained by diffusion through a few very large pores. The larg-

Table 10-1
Comparison of Permeabilities of Cat Limb Capillaries with Free Diffusion Coefficients, for Molecules of Increasing Size

Substance	Molecular Weight (daltons)	Approximate Molecular Diameter (nm)	Free Diffusion Coefficient ($cm^2/s \times 10^{-5}$)	Permeability $\frac{cm^3/s}{100\ g}$
Water	18	0.30	3.2	3.7
Urea	60	0.52	1.95	1.83
Glucose	180	0.74	0.91	0.64
Sucrose	342	0.96	0.74	0.35
Raffinose	504	1.14	0.56	0.24
Inulin	5,500	2.8	0.23	0.036
Myoglobin	16,500	3.8	0.15	0.005
Serum albumin	69,000	7.2	0.085	<0.001

Source: Modified from data of E. M. Landis and J. R. Pappenheimer. In W. F. Hamilton and P. Dow (eds.), *Handbook of Physiology*. Section 2, Circulation. Bethesda, Md.: American Physiological Society, 1963. Vol. 2, p. 961.

est of these are found in liver, spleen, and bone marrow, where protein and even intact cells may enter and exit the blood stream.

Thus far we have considered the capillary as an inert barrier. In fact, it is capable of transporting certain large molecules by engulfing them on the luminal (or antiluminal) side and releasing them on the other. Though some of the apparent permeability to very large molecules may be accounted for in this way, the amount of water so transported is negligible. Endothelium is, in fact, very metabolically active and plays a major role in certain endocrine regulations and in control of vascular smooth muscle.

Capillary Distensibility

The capillary is a rather rigid structure, despite its fragile appearance. It can withstand up to 100 torr without rupture. How can an endothelial tube with little connective tissue support have such mechanical properties? The answer lies in its extremely small size and the law of Laplace; see Figure 10-5.

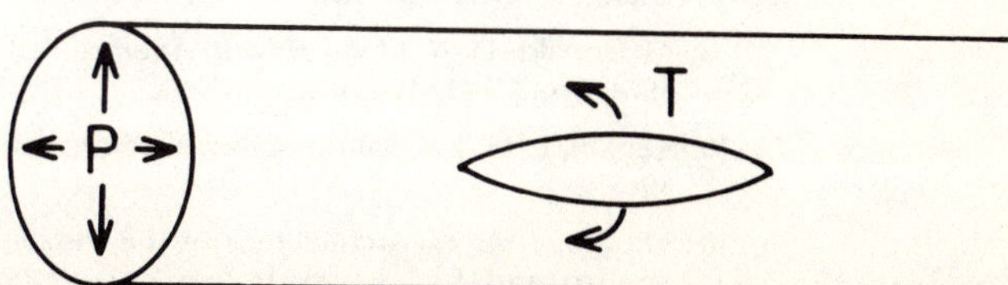

Figure 10-5
Law of Laplace as applied to a capillary. Edges of a longitudinal slit are pulled apart by the circumferential tension (*T*) in the wall.

For a cylinder

$T = r \times \Delta P$

where r = radius, ΔP = transmural pressure, and T is the circumferential tension in the wall that resists the pressure. If capillary radius and transmural pressure are 2 μm and 25 torr, respectively, wall tension is 7 mg per centimeter. Tension in the wall of the aorta is about 50,000 times greater.

Clinical Application

Microvascular geometry was long regarded as a dead, clinically irrelevant subject. It now appears that genetic hypertension in the rat is due, in part, to a decrease in the number of arterioles and to other structural changes in the microcirculation. The relative contributions of vessel geometry, blood viscosity, cardiac output, and active vasoconstriction to various hypertensive states are currently under intensive study throughout the world.

References

1. Engelson, E. T., Skalak, T. C., and Schmid-Schönbein, G. W. The microvasculature in skeletal muscle: 1. The arteriolar network in rat spinotrapezius muscle. *Microvasc. Res.* 30:29, 1985.

2. Fung, Y.-C. Stochastic flow in capillary blood vessels. *Microvasc. Res.* 5:34, 1973.

3. Granger, H. J., Meininger, G. A., Borders, J. L., Morff, R. J., and Goodman, A. H. Microcirculation of Skeletal Muscle. In M. A. Mortillaro (ed.), *The Physiology and Pharmacology of the Microcirculation*, Vol. 2. New York: Academic, 1984.

4. Honig, C. R., Odoroff, C. L., and Frierson, J. L. Active and passive capillary control in red muscle at rest and in exercise. *Am. J. Physiol.* 243:H196, 1982.

5. Hutchins, P. M., and Darnell, A. E. Observation of a decreased number of small arterioles in spontaneously hypertensive rats. *Circ. Res.* 34[Suppl. 1]:161, 1974.

6. Lund, N., Damon, D. N., and Duling, B. R. Capillary grouping in hamster tibialis anterior muscle: Flow patterns and physiological significance. *Int. J. Microcirc. Clin. Exp.* 5:359, 1987.

7. Mayrovitz, H. N., Wiedeman, M. P., and Noordergraff, A. Microvascular hemodynamic variations accompanying microvessel dimensional changes. *Microvasc. Res.* 10:322, 1975.

8. McDonald, D. A. *Blood Flow in Arteries*. Baltimore: Williams & Wilkins, 1974. Pp. 37–41, 46–54.

*9. Renkin, E. M. Regulation of the microcirculation. *Microvasc. Res.* 30:251, 1985.

10. Rhodin, J. A. G. Architecture of the Vessel Wall. In D. F. Bohr, A. P. Somlyo, and H. V. Sparks, Jr. (eds.), *Handbook of Physiology*, Section 2: The Cardiovascular System — Vol. II. Vascular Smooth Muscle. Bethesda, Md.: American Physiological Society, 1980.

11. Valtin, H. *Renal Function: Mechanism Preserving Fluid and Solute Balance in Health*. Boston: Little, Brown and Co., 1973. Chap. 10.

11 : Gravity and Venous Return

Harvey was the first to show that venous return to the heart must equal arterial outflow in the steady state. In human beings, seated or standing, long hydrostatic columns raise transmural pressure in dependent arteries and veins. Since veins are very distensible, blood tends to pool below heart level. Nature circumvents the effect of gravity on venous return by use of "sump pumps" and by neural control of flow and distensibility. In addition, reservoirs are provided to buffer transient discrepancies between cardiac inflow and outflow. Figure 11-1 is an overview of the material in this chapter and the next.

Venous Capacity and Distensibility

The venous wall contains collagen but few elastic fibers, so it is very noncompliant. On the other hand, an empty or partly filled vein is very distensible, because its capacity is large and the collagen fibers are not stressed until the vein is completely full. Thus veins are like large, noncompliant plastic bags, not small, compliant balloons. (All this should sound familiar; we used the same ideas to describe the pressure-volume relation for the relaxed heart.) Because of their enormous capacity and distensibility, veins contain about 80 percent of the total blood volume.

An empty vein has a flat profile, and its pressure is virtually zero; see Figure 11-2. As a vein fills, pressure remains almost constant until the venous cross section is circular. At that point addition of more volume creates tension in the wall, and pressure rises sharply. Veins can tolerate high pressure without blowout, because collagen, the principal component of the wall, is extremely strong. This permits use of vein segments for arterial grafts.

The long, flat slope of the volume-pressure relation explains why venous hemodynamics is so difficult to study. We often want to know how *volume* and its distribution change, but volume must be inferred from pressure. These inferences are imprecise because trivial pressure changes often correspond to large changes in volume.

Venous distensibility, capacity, and pressure can be varied by smooth-muscle fibers; compare curves *A* and *B* in Figure 11-2.

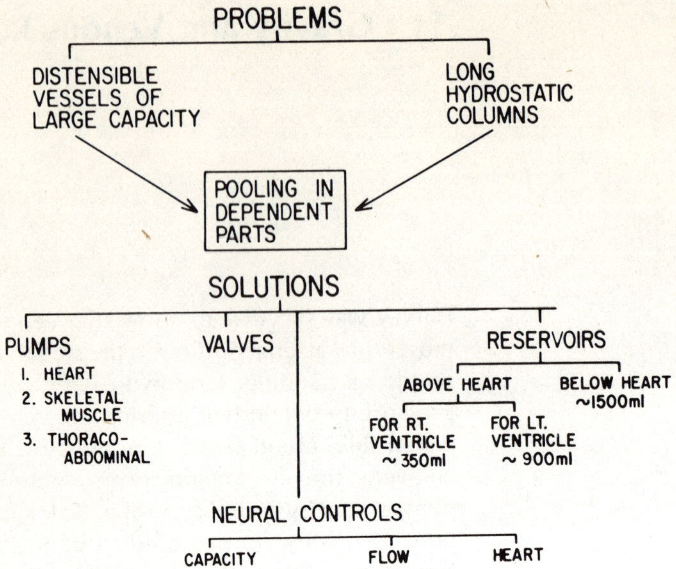

Figure 11-1
Overview of physiology of venous return.

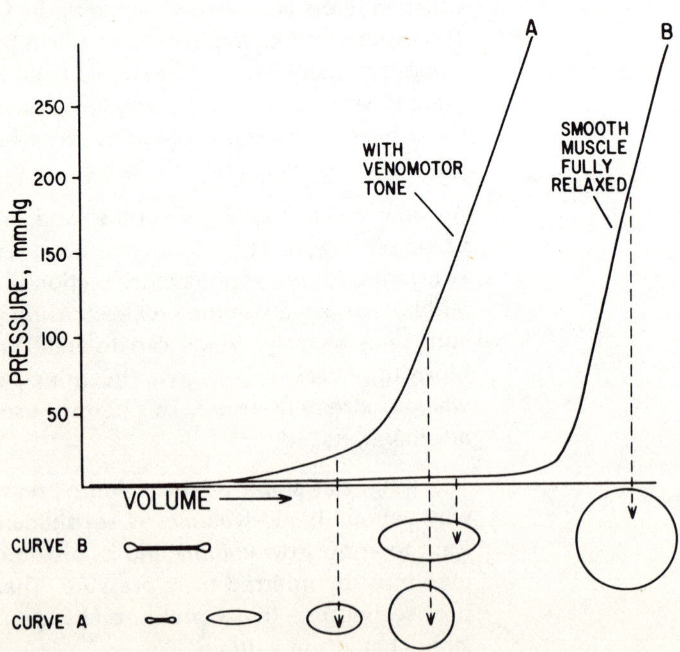

Figure 11-2
Effect of venomotor tone on dimensions and pressure-volume relations for an isolated systemic vein.

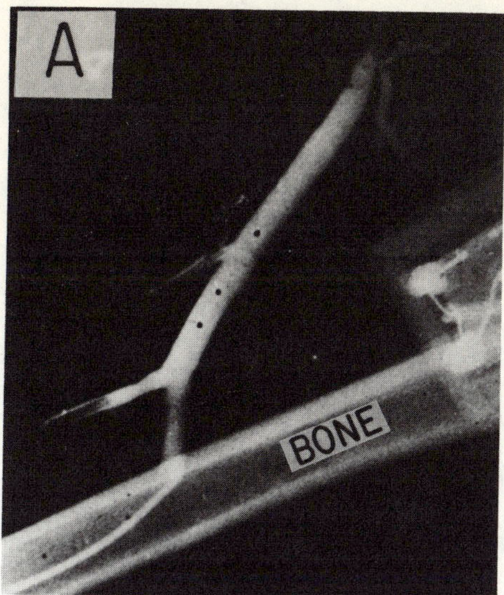

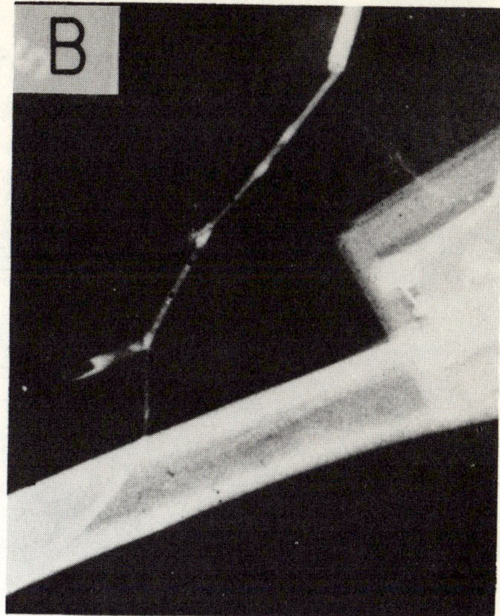

Figure 11-3
Venoconstriction in dog leg vein induced by a norepinephrine infusion. (From unpublished data of Dr. Thomas W. Morris, University of Rochester, Rochester, N.Y.)

The muscles are partly contracted under normal circumstances. This contractile activity, called *venomotor tone,* largely determines vein compliance at low volumes. In effect, venomotor tone converts a large, noncompliant bag into a smaller one. Ability to vary venous capacity is essential for adaptation to gravitational stress and changes in blood volume.

Venoconstriction in situ is illustrated in Figure 11-3. Both ends of a vein in a dog hind limb were cannulated, and the vein was perfused with a substance opaque to x-rays. Pressure in the vein was maintained constant at 40 torr. The smooth muscle contraction induced by norepinephrine almost completely occluded the lumen. Equally dramatic vasoconstriction can be induced by reflex or psychic stimulation of sympathetic nerves. Selective venoconstriction is a major factor in controlling distribution of the blood volume.

Hydrostatic Columns

Venous pressure falls to zero close to the heart, so the veins in the neck are normally collapsed. Collapse does not materially affect resistance to flow. In contrast, hydrostatic columns below the heart impede venous return. The concepts are illustrated in Figure 11-4. In *A*, a large reservoir delivers flow to a horizontal and vertical U tube. If both arms of the U are of unequal length, the increment in potential energy (γgh) from the top to the bottom of the proximal arm is exactly equal to the decrement in potential energy from bottom to top of the distal arm. As long as

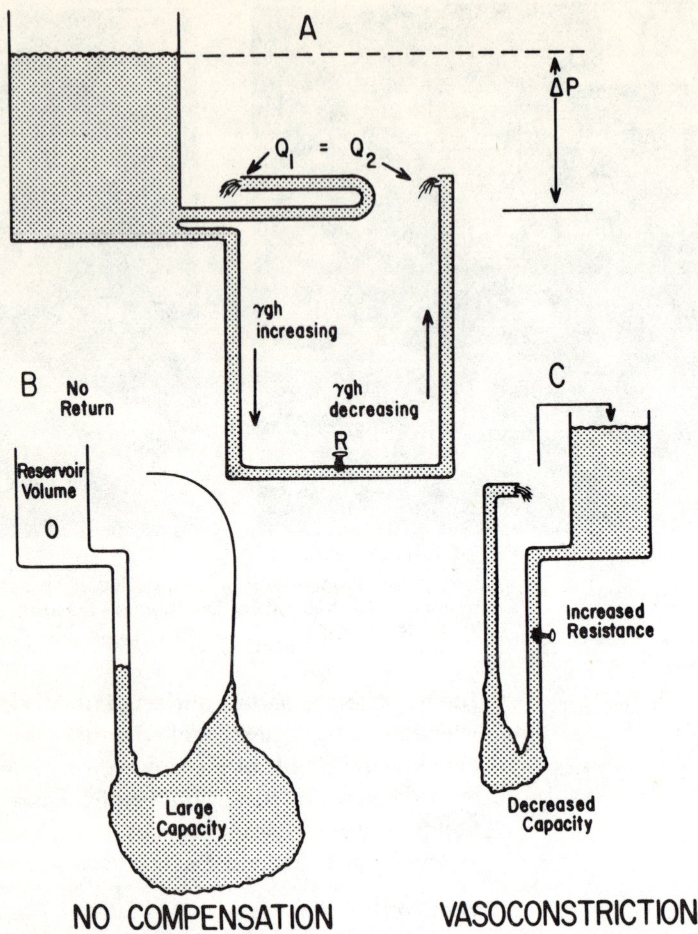

Figure 11-4
The effect of shifting rigid and distensible systems from a horizontal to a vertical position. See text for explanation.

there is free communication between the two arms the presence of a resistance (*R*) at the bottom makes no difference. Since the gravitational component balances out, flow is not affected by shifting the U tube from the horizontal to the vertical position. When we stand, the long arterial and venous columns between heart and foot are analogous to the system in Figure 11-4, *from the standpoint of energetics*. Consequently, there is no need for an extra energy source to drive venous blood upward. Sump pumps are nonetheless essential to control pressure and capacity.

Role of Venous Distensibility

Despite the previous paragraph, gravity seriously impedes venous return: Cardiac output transiently decreases about 30 percent immediately after rising. The essential difference between the circulation and the system in Figure 11-4A is that the veins (analogous to the distal arm of the U) are very distensible. Moreover, the capacity of veins below the heart exceeds the volume of the reservoir above the heart. Figure 11-4B illustrates the situation without compensating adjustments. Blood entering dependent parts accumulates in the venous capacity. The difference between venous return (from parts above the heart) and cardiac output is drawn from reservoirs. As the reservoirs are depleted, cardiac output falls progressively. It would not fall to zero, however, because loss of consciousness (fainting) would occur first. Fainting is adaptive in that it restores the horizontal position.

More practical adaptations are shown in Figure 11-4C. The initial deleterious effects of the upright position (decreased arterial pressure and central blood volume) stimulate mechanoreceptors that induce reflex venous and arteriolar constriction.[1] Venoconstriction limits depletion of the central reservoirs by decreasing the capacity of veins below the heart. Once this smaller capacity is filled, it strongly resists distention, and the system becomes identical to that in Figure 11-4A. However, venoconstriction takes 2 to 3 minutes to develop, during which time the thoracic reservoirs continue to be depleted. The function of arteriolar constriction is to decrease the rate of pooling during this time by decreasing flow to the dependent parts.

Clinical Application

Confinement to bed is the physician's most frequent prescription. Unfortunately, prolonged recumbency profoundly impairs reflex compensations for gravitational stress. The power (and limitations) of these reflexes can be demonstrated with a human centrifuge. A person sits at the end of a long rotor; the gravitational field is adjusted by varying the rate of rotation. Hydrostatic pressure (γgh) varies directly with g. At 5 g, venous pressure at the foot is about 300 torr when the person is seated. Since arterial pressure increases by the same amount, venous return would continue if pooling could be avoided. Arteriolar and venous constriction are remarkably effective in defending venous return, provided sufficient time is allowed. If the centrifuge accelerates slowly, well-conditioned subjects tolerate about 5 g for prolonged periods. An antigravity suit (a rigid garment that applies counterpressure to the veins) increases this tolerance only slightly.

[1] Virtually all physiological effects are themselves stimuli in that they initiate reflex compensations.

Apart from their power, the most striking feature of venomotor reflexes is their *lability*. A slight cold, a sleepless night, several days of bed rest, or even one martini can reduce tolerance to less than 2 *g*. Prolonged bed rest is especially debilitating, for it decreases blood volume as well as venomotor tone. The giddiness (low cerebral blood flow) on arising after a long illness is familiar to all. Surgeons recognize how rapidly one becomes deconditioned and generally have their patients walking about on the first postoperative day.

Venous Pressure Recumbent and Upright

Thus far we have been mainly concerned with venous flow. However, pressure per se has important physiological effects. Central venous pressure determines the end-diastolic length of ventricular muscle fibers, and hence active tension. Peripheral venous pressure approximates end-capillary pressure and thereby influences the rate at which fluid is filtered through the capillary into the intercellular spaces.

The reference level for venous pressure is the right atrium, located at about the fourth intercostal space at the sternum. Right atrial pressure fluctuates slightly above or below atmospheric pressure. Venous pressures are often measured with water rather than mercury manometers. In the horizontal position pressure in the smallest peripheral veins is 15 to 20 cm H_2O (11–15 mm Hg). Pressure in large arm veins should be less than 12 cm of water; it does not reflect central venous pressure because of valves at the thoracic inlet.

The effect of standing on pressure in a vein of the foot is shown in Figure 11-5A. The subject was instructed to relax the muscles of the catheterized foot and to bear all his weight on the opposite leg. Pressure rose from 10 mm Hg recumbent to 87 mm Hg (118 cm blood) as the leg veins gradually filled from below. The vertical distance between the foot and right atrium was about 120 cm, indicating that an uninterrupted hydrostatic column existed. If venous pressure had remained at 87 mm Hg, fluid would have been filtered at about 1 ml per minute, and in 2 hours the foot would have been about twice its normal size! Such swelling is called *edema*.

The principal mechanism for decreasing hydrostatic pressure — and hence the rate of edema formation — is muscle contraction, as in walking. In Figure 11-5B rhythmic walking in place lowered venous pressure to 17 mm Hg, only 7 mm Hg higher than when the subject was recumbent. In the sitting position, with legs dangling passively, venous pressure rose to 60 mm Hg, roughly

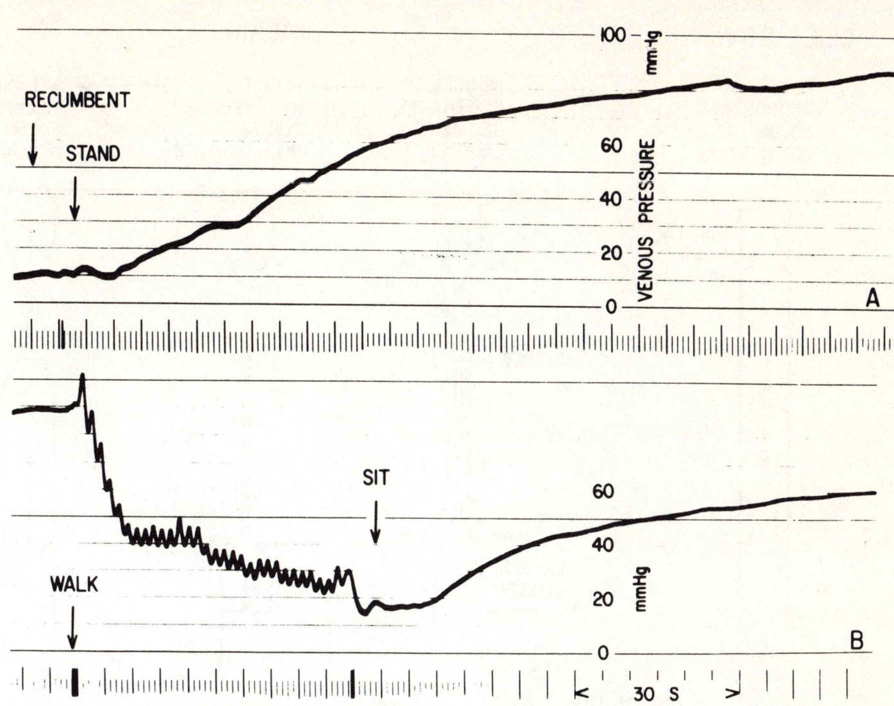

Figure 11-5
Effect of the muscle venous pump on venous pressure at the ankle.

two-thirds the maximum pressure observed upright. This should be borne in mind when one is caring for people confined to bed and chair by stroke or other chronic illness.

The Muscle Venous Pump

The mechanism by which muscle contraction shortens hydrostatic columns and lowers venous pressure is shown in Figure 11-6. Veins are provided with numerous valves, which, during quiet standing, are held open by the flow of blood. During walking, veins are compressed by the contracting muscles, and a segment of the vein is emptied. Because of the valves, blood flows only in the upward direction. When the muscle relaxes, the proximal valve closes, and a segment of empty vein interrupts the hydrostatic column. This segment fills from below, but if the next step occurs soon enough, the column remains interrupted, and distal venous pressure remains low. The cycle shown in Figure 11-6 is referred to as the *muscle venous pump.* The functions of this pump (and the thoracoabdominal pump yet to be considered) are (1) to decrease capillary filtration pressure and edema formation; (2) to decrease pooling on arising, before vasomotor adjustments are fully developed; and to (3) accelerate venous return, especially during running. The crucial

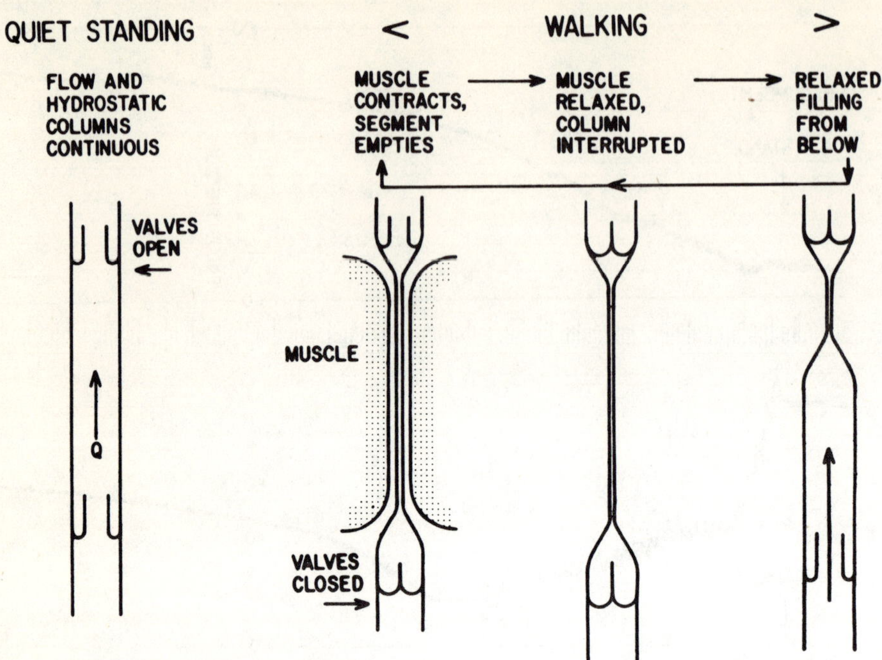

Figure 11-6
Mechanism of muscle venous pump.

role of the muscle venous pump is revealed if a runner stands quietly after a race. With maximum vasodilation and high cardiac output, the thoracic blood volume is dangerously depleted in seconds. To avoid fainting runners must continue mild exercise for several minutes.

Clinical Application

Varicose Veins and Venous Thrombosis

Proper function of the venous pumps depends on the integrity of venous valves. The valves may be congenitally defective, and any condition that impedes venous return (i.e., pregnancy) can make them incompetent. Incompetence creates a long hydrostatic column that distends distal segments, causing lower valves to leak, which distends more segments, and so on.[2] Dilated venous segments are called *varices*. The associated venous hypertension causes edema and initiates arteriolar constriction. The resulting decrease in flow may be severe enough to cause ulceration. Low flow also increases the risk of venous thrombosis: Recall the pathophysiology of low flow states outlined in Figure 7-8.

[2]Notice that this is another example of disease as positive feedback.

Blood flow in immobile limbs tends to be low even without varices, and arteriolar constriction decreases it even further if the limbs are dependent. Failure to recognize these effects of position is responsible for what has been termed "nursing home thrombosis," "travel thrombosis," and so on. Venous thrombosis is a potentially fatal illness that can be prevented by simply moving the feet.

The Thoraco-abdominal Pump

The vertical distance between the diaphragm and the first venous valve in the thigh is about 20 cm. The intra-abdominal veins are not distended by this column because they are perfectly counterpressurized by the viscera. (The specific gravity of the viscera is about the same as that of blood.)

The heart and thoracic veins lie in the virtual space between the visceral and parietal pleura. During normal quiet breathing, intrapleural pressure varies from 3 to 7 mm Hg *below* atmospheric pressure. A collapsible tube is distended as much by a decrease in pressure outside as by an equal rise in pressure inside. Consequently, the transmural pressure tending to fill the thoracic veins is the sum of venous and thoracic pressures. Negative intrathoracic pressure contributes to venous return by, in effect, applying suction to the top of the hydrostatic column.

During inspiration the chest expands and the diaphragm descends. This lowers intrathoracic pressure (more negative), raises abdominal pressure, and increases the total ΔP for venous return. The effect of abdominal pressure in emptying splanchnic veins is identical in principle to the action of the muscles on leg veins. During expiration, pleural pressure rises and abdominal pressure falls, so the abdominal veins refill and thoracic inflow decreases. Since venous return falls if breathing stops, inspiration facilitates venous return more than expiration impedes it.

Together, the contractile properties of the veins and auxiliary pumps permit us to spend more than half our lives standing or seated. However, the effectiveness of these adaptations depends on the blood volume and its distribution, as described in the next chapter.

References

1. Roth, C. F. Venous System: Physiology of the Capacitance Vessels. In J. T. Shepherd and F. M. Abboud (eds.), *Handbook of Physiology*, Section 2: The Cardiovascular System — Vol. III. Peripheral Circulation and Organ Blood Flow, Part 1. Bethesda, Md.: American Physiological Society, 1983.

*2. Shepherd, J. T., and Vanhoutte, P. M. *Veins and Their Control.* Philadelphia: Saunders, 1975. Pp. 190–195, 210–232.

12 : Blood Volume and Its Distribution

Total Blood Volume

The volume of blood in the body is easily measured in a laboratory or clinic. A known amount of a substance that cannot leave the circulation is injected intravenously. A commonly used indicator is a radioactive substance covalently bound to protein. After thorough mixing, a venous sample is drawn and the concentration of indicator is measured.

$$\text{Blood volume} = \frac{\text{amount injected}}{\text{concentration}}.$$

Plasma and erythrocyte volumes can be determined if the hematocrit is known. The hematocrit of blood in a large vein or artery is about 10 percent higher than the mean for all vessels because of the Fahraeus effect discussed in Chapter 7. Consequently

$$\text{plasma volume} = \text{blood volume } [1 - (0.9 \text{ Hct})].$$

Between 4 and 90 years of age, total blood volume averages 77 ml per kilogram of lean body weight in both sexes. Thus, a 70-kg person has about 5.4 liters of blood. The constancy of blood volume is even more remarkable when measured in a particular individual over many years. The neuroendocrine system that regulates blood volume is considered in Chapter 25.

The ideal value or *set point* for blood volume regulation can be altered by prolonged exposure to certain stimuli. For example, with three weeks of bed rest or of weightlessness in space, blood volume decreases by up to 20 percent. This volume loss contributes to postural hypotension and fainting. On the other hand, the increase in blood volume (up to 25 percent) after physical training or residence in a hot climate improves tolerance to gravitational stress. Such stress is termed *orthostatic*.

In the absence of hemorrhage, dehydration, and heart failure, blood volume regulation is so precise that only the *distribution* of volume affects cardiovascular responses to acute stress. Volume distribution is not regulated and is affected by position, vasomotor tone, exercise, temperature, and various drugs and diseases.

Intrathoracic Blood Volume

It is convenient to consider volume distribution in functional rather than strictly anatomical terms. The body may be regarded as two interconnected reservoirs, one within the thorax, the other outside it. The intrathoracic reservoir accounts for about half the distensibility of the venous system.

The thoracic blood volume can be estimated by indicator dilution if the time course of change of concentration is recorded. The procedure is considered in Chapter 13, p. 126. Table 12-1 gives values for human adults. The total intrathoracic blood volume comprises a reservoir for the left heart (about 900 ml) and a reservoir for the right heart (roughly 350 ml). About 75 percent of the blood in the left ventricular reservoir is contained in pulmonary capillaries and venules.

A reservoir can be regarded as *reserve of capacity,* or a *reserve of volume*. The large capacity of the intrathoracic reservoirs protects the ventricles from excessive stretch and the lungs from high capillary pressure and edema. The thoracic reservoir fills in the supine position (because of gravity), during water immersion (counterpressure), and during cold exposure (venoconstriction). Thoracic reservoirs are depleted during orthostatic stress, hemorrhage, and dehydration. The pressure changes that accompany these volume shifts are very small: A 1000-ml hemorrhage depletes the thoracic reservoirs by about 500 ml but decreases central venous pressure only 2 to 3 torr. The change in myocardial fiber length, however, is large and would cause a correspondingly large change in ventricular performance. Fortunately, we are provided with volume as well as pressure detectors with which to initiate reflex compensation, as explained in Chapter 25.

Table 12-1
Average Values for Thoracic Blood Volume and Its Components in Humans

Location	Estimated Volume (L)	% Total Blood Volume[a]
Total intrathoracic	1.13–1.51	21–28
Left heart and pulmonary vessels[b]	0.80–1.10	15–20
Right heart and venae cavae	0.32–0.43	6–8

[a] If 100% = 5.4 L.
[b] If left ventricular diastolic volume = 150 ml.

Effect of Respiration on Thoracic Reservoirs and Cardiac Output

The values shown in Table 12-1 are means with respect to time. In fact, thoracic blood volume varies roughly ± 250 ml during normal quiet breathing. This variation is due to oppositely directed, cyclical changes in the output of the two ventricles.

Inspiration distends the pulmonary venules by increasing their transmural pressure (outside more negative). This increase in reservoir capacity decreases left ventricular filling and stroke volume, as shown in Figure 12-1. In contrast, the thoracoabdominal pump increases systemic return during inspiration, so the output of the right ventricle rises and adds more volume to the pulmonary veins. The reverse changes occur during expiration,

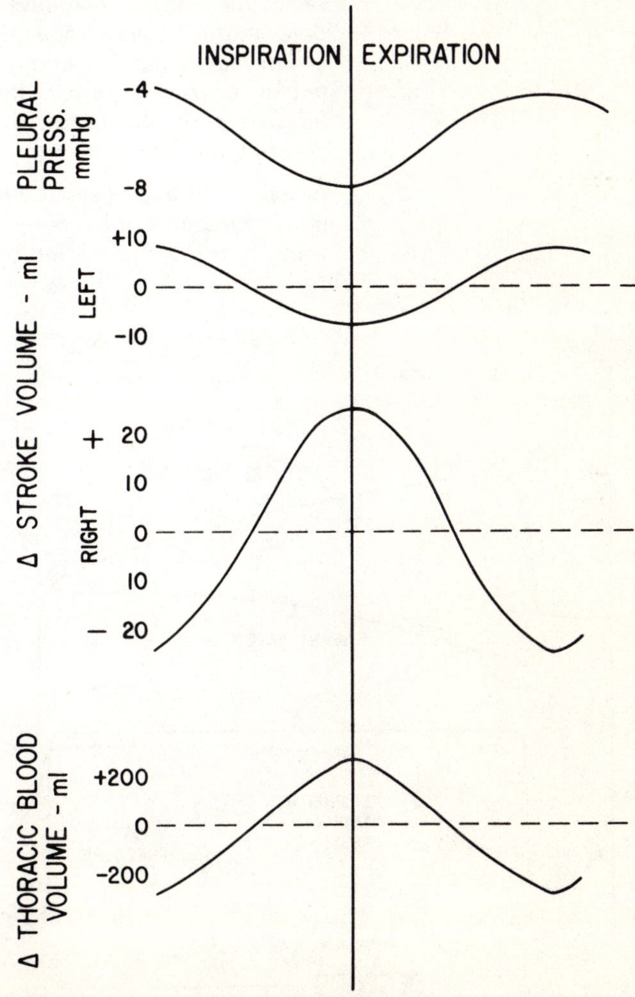

Figure 12-1
Respiratory variation in thoracic blood volume and concomitant changes in the stroke volumes of the two ventricles.

so the output of the two chambers is identical over a complete respiratory cycle. Notice that the right ventricular output changes ± 25 percent. The larger volume of the pulmonary reservoir makes the left ventricle far less dependent on moment-to-moment changes in venous return; its output varies only ± 5 percent during a respiratory cycle. Total thoracic blood volume (bottom panel of Figure 12-1) varies with the algebraic difference between right and left ventricular outputs.

Clinical Application

The Valsalva Maneuver

Straining against a closed glottis raises intrathoracic pressure and impedes venous return. This act, called the Valsalva maneuver, accompanies lifting, defecation, sustained coughing, and parturition. It can be hazardous, especially in people with hypertension or coronary artery disease. Its circulatory effects are generally divided into four stages, as indicated by the numbers at the top of Figure 12-2.

In *stage 1,* thoracic pressure rises sharply. It is transmitted directly to the arteries, but not the peripheral veins, which are protected by venous valves.

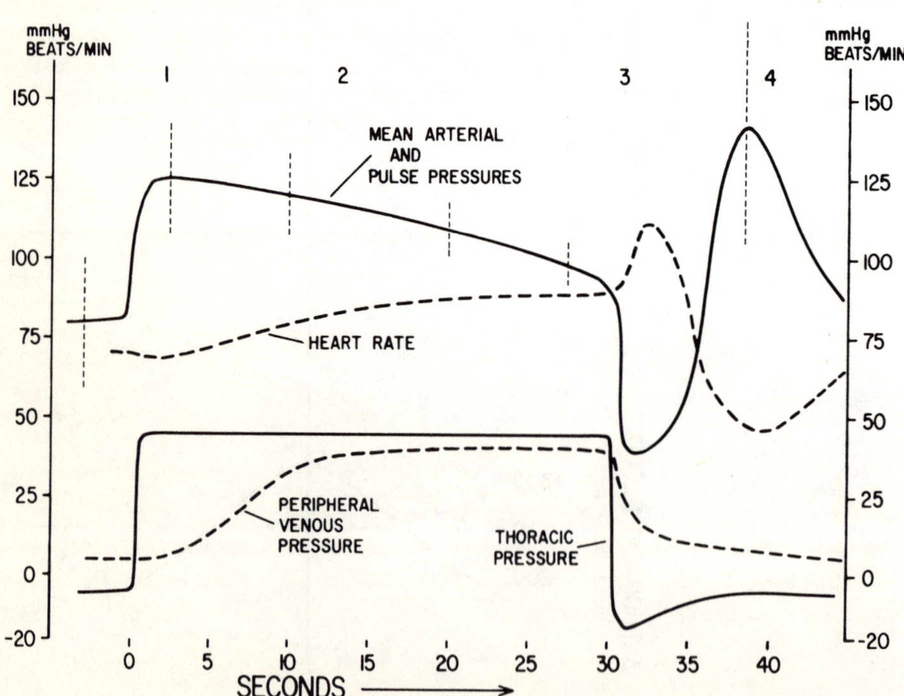

Figure 12-2
Time course of pressures during four stages of the Valsalva maneuver. Dashed vertical lines denote pulse pressure.

In *stage 2*, high thoracic pressure obstructs venous return, so peripheral venous pressure rises. Output of both ventricles is drawn from thoracic reservoirs. As these are depleted, ventricular filing pressure and stroke volume decline; note the large decrease in pulse pressure indicated by the vertical dashed lines in Figure 12-2. Sensors that detect arterial pressure (baroreceptors) initiate reflexly mediated tachycardia, vasoconstriction, and increased ventricular contractility. These reflex changes minimize decreases in cardiac output and mean arterial pressure.

In *stage 3*, the subject suddenly relaxes and then inspires deeply after the long breath hold. As blood dammed up in the veins surges into the chest, peripheral venous pressure falls, and right ventricular stroke volume increases enormously. The capacity of the pulmonary veins increases because of the deep inspiration, so venous outflow into the left ventricle and left ventricular stroke volume decrease. The drop in systemic arterial pressure reflects the fall in intrathoracic pressure and drop in left ventricular output. Baroreceptors are stimulated even more intensely and initiate further increases in heart rate, contractility, and peripheral resistance.

In *stage 4*, the right ventricle rapidly fills the pulmonary veins, and left ventricular output increases abruptly. Since the peripheral resistance is high (from stage 3) mean arterial pressure and pulse pressure rise sharply. The hypertensive overshoot in stage 4 can be large, particularly in hypertensive persons. Baroreceptor reflexes and the Starling relationship eventually restore the circulation to normal. The intense sympathetic discharge in stage 3 and vagal slowing of the heart in stage 4 can initiate conduction disorders and active arrhythmias, particularly if the myocardium is nonhomogeneous. Death from ventricular fibrillation after straining at stool is not uncommon in patients with arteriosclerotic disease.

The Extrathoracic Reservoirs

The principal extrathoracic reservoir for orthostatic responses is the venous system of the legs. (Recall that the splanchnic veins are perfectly counterpressurized.) The *mean* distending pressure over the length of the legs is approximately 60 torr. At that pressure in a standing subject about 500 ml of blood would accumulate in one leg at room temperature, and 800 ml or more in a hot environment. Most of this volume comes from the thoracic reservoirs. Sitting is almost as stressful. At 35 torr, the mean distending pressure seated, the volume pooled in the legs is about 70 percent of that observed when standing. Most of the volume consists of whole blood and accumulates in the first few minutes, but a slow further increase continues for several hours. The slow component is due to transcapillary filtration (edema) and can decrease the total blood volume by up to 15 percent.

Intrathoracic Blood Volume, Cardiac Output, and Orthostatic Stresses

Intrathoracic blood volume sets ventricular filling pressure and fiber length. It is therefore one of the major determinants of cardiac output. Nevertheless, cardiac output is constant over a wide range of thoracic blood volumes; see Figure 12-3. This constancy reflects the fact that cardiac output is a regulated variable. During an orthostatic stress, or hemorrhage, sympathetic nerves shift the ventricle to a more advantageous function curve. This defends the stroke volume against the fall in thoracic blood volume and ventricular end-diastolic pressure. At the same time, reciprocal changes in sympathetic and vagal tone to the SA node increase heart rate. The increase in heart rate affords a simple, bedside estimate of the fall in stroke volume and blood volume, if the relationships in Figure 12-3 are kept in

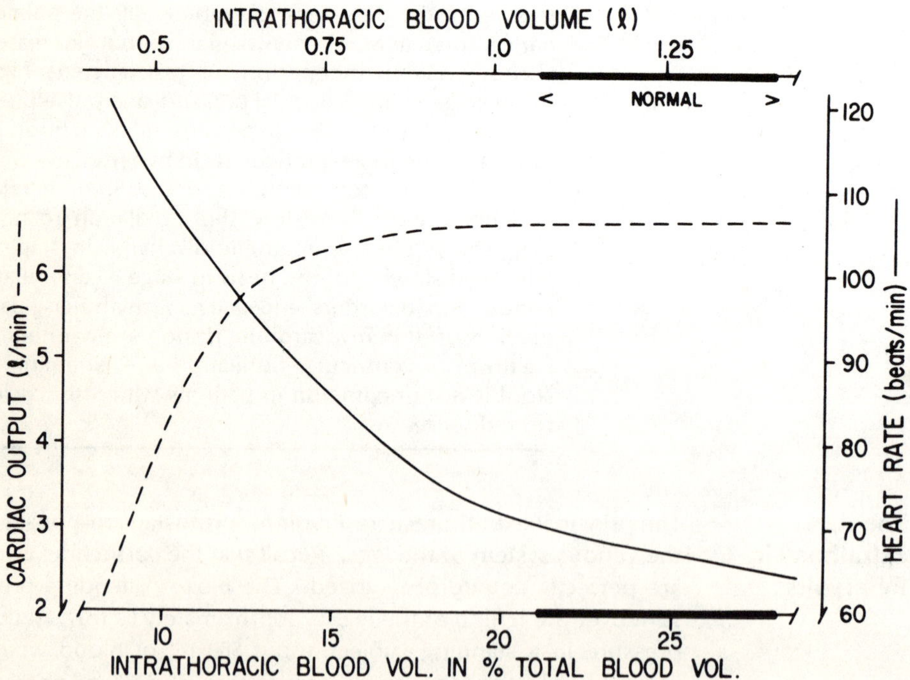

Figure 12-3
Intrathoracic blood volume as a determinant of heart rate and cardiac output in normal persons.

mind. The compensations just described, and arteriolar constriction in the legs, occur within a few heart beats. Venoconstriction develops more slowly, however, so despite reflex compensations and auxiliary venous pumps, 200 to 400 ml of blood leaves the thorax on arising. As shown in Figure 12-3, this greatly depletes the volume reserve for defense of cardiac output. Since the volume reserve is so fully engaged in the upright position under normal circumstances, it is easy to understand why postural hypotension and fainting are so common if total blood volume falls or compensations are impaired.

Clinical Application

Orthopnea

Redistributions of volume into and out of the thorax have been studied with a device like a child's teeterboard; see Figure 12-4. If the iliac crest is at the fulcrum, the thoracic reservoir lies on one side and the legs on the other. The arms fall about equally on both sides. Measurements on legless people indicate that the splanchnic bed can be ignored. Volume shifts between thorax and legs cause headward or footward torque (force × distance from fulcrum).

A centroid of volume can be determined for the chest and another for the legs. Knowing the torque and the distance of these centroids from the fulcrum, one can calculate the shift in volume. Some 200 to 400 ml moves out of the thorax on arising in the morning and returns to the thorax within 30 minutes after reclining. In normal persons the pulmonary veins can take up much more than 400 ml with little rise in venous pressure or change in lung compliance. However, if the heart is operating on a depressed Starling curve the pulmonary veins are nearly full. Under these conditions a small increment in volume, as in recumbency, causes a large increase in lung pulmonary venous pressure and decrease in compliance. The lungs become more difficult to inflate and deflate, and the patient experiences shortness of breath, or *dyspnea*. Dyspnea initiated by orthostatic volume shifts is called *or-*

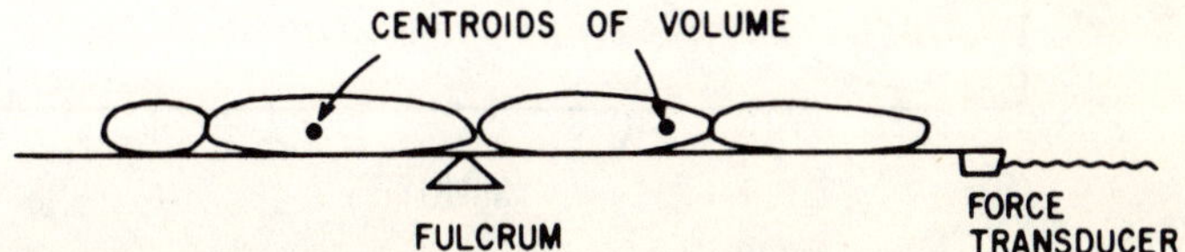

Figure 12-4
Teeterboard method for detecting change in distribution of volume between intrathoracic and extrathoracic reservoirs.

thopnea. Sitting or standing generally produces prompt relief.

Nongravitational Volume Shifts

Major volume redistributions can occur in recumbent persons; an example is shown in Figure 12-5. A normal subject was studied on the teeterboard after orthostatic volume shifts were over and the baseline was stable. Intravenous norepinephrine induced arteriolar and venoconstriction. There is very little smooth muscle in pulmonary veins, so vasoactive drugs change systemic, but not pulmonary, venous capacity. In the experiment shown, about 200 ml accumulated in the thorax in 15 minutes without inducing symptoms. However, in a patient with a depressed ventricle and nearly full thoracic reservoirs, norepinephrine can precipitate orthopnea, or even pulmonary edema. Norepinephrine need not be infused; more often it is released endogenously in response to pain or fright.

Treatment of acute pulmonary edema requires that cardiac output briefly exceed venous return. To this end contractility can be enhanced with a positive inotropic agent, positive airway pressure can be applied to impede venous return, or volume can be trapped in the legs by use of tourniquets or a venodilator drug.

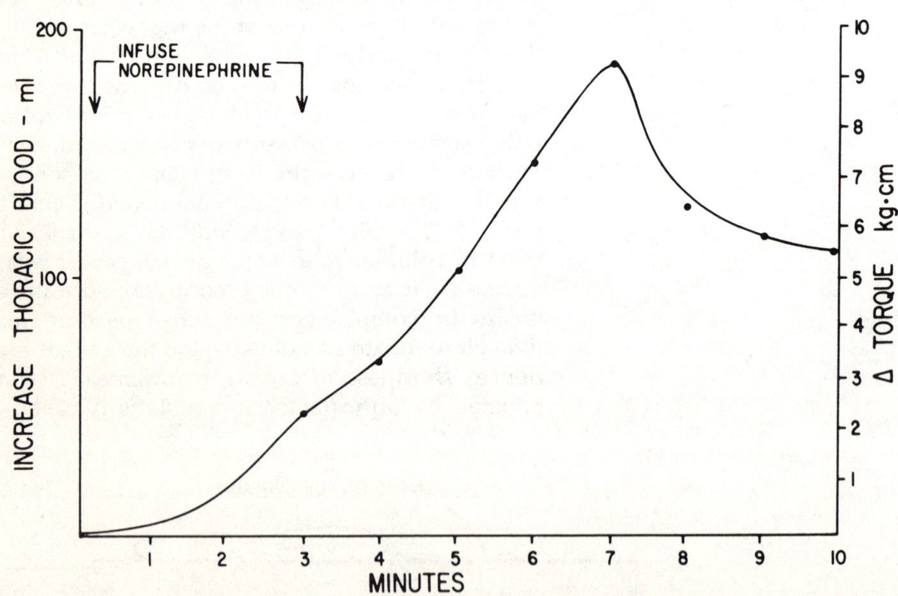

Figure 12-5
Effect of an intravenous infusion of norepinephrine to redistribute blood into the thorax. (Unpublished data based on the teeterboard method, courtesy Dr. S. M. Tenney, Dartmouth Medical School.)

Gross venodilation in a normal person can dangerously deplete the thoracic reservoirs. This situation occurs in people given autonomic blocking drugs or spinal anesthesia. (The latter blocks autonomic as well as somatic nerves to the legs.) Such patients may have low cardiac output and hypotension unless the foot of the bed is elevated to promote venous return.

Techniques used to monitor volume distribution are not generally available; in all likelihood you will be limited to measurements of peripheral venous pressure. You must therefore rely on your "book learning" in thinking about the role of the veins in clinical problems.

References

*1. Blomqvist, C. G., and Stone, H. L. Cardiovascular Adjustments to Gravitational Stress. In J. T. Shepherd and F. M. Abboud (eds.), *Handbook of Physiology*, Section 2. The Cardiovascular System — Vol. III, Peripheral Circulation and Organ Blood Flow, Part 2. Bethesda, Md.: American Physiological Society, 1983.

2. Cassidy, S. S., and Mitchell, J. H. Effects of positive and negative pressure breathing on right and left ventricular preload and afterload. *Fed. Proc.* 40:2178, 1981.

3. Engel, G. L. *Fainting*. Springfield, Ill.: Thomas, 1962. Pp. 6–33.

4. Fenn, W. O., Otis, A. B., Rahn, H., Chadwick, L. E., and Hegnaur, A. H. Displacement of blood from the lungs by positive pressure breathing. *Am. J. Physiol.* 151:258, 1947. (This describes the teeterboard technique.)

5. Rothe, C. F. Reflex control of veins and vascular capacitance. *Physiol. Rev.* 63:1281, 1983.

6. Rowell, L. B. *Human Circulation Regulation During Physical Stress*. New York, London: Oxford University Press, 1986.

13 : Cardiac Output and Regional Blood Flow

Blood flow and phasic pressure recordings are monitored routinely in medical and surgical intensive care units and operating rooms. Such information is invaluable, but only if properly collected and interpreted. The *responsibility* for this cannot be delegated to the technicians who run the apparatus!

Methods of Evaluating Flow and Metabolism

The Fick Principle

Suppose a substance is consumed (or produced) at a steady rate x. The Fick principle states that x is equal to the difference between the rate of delivery and the rate of removal. If the substance enters and leaves only via the blood,

$$x = \dot{Q}a\ Ca - \dot{Q}v\ Cv,$$

where $\dot{Q}a$ = rate of arterial flow, $\dot{Q}v$ = rate of venous flow, Ca = arterial concentration of the substance, and Cv = venous concentration.

If $\dot{Q}a = \dot{Q}v = \dot{Q}$,

$$x = \dot{Q}\,[Ca - Cv], \text{ or}$$

$$\dot{Q} = \frac{x}{Ca - Cv}.$$

In practice, the substance of interest is usually O_2, and x is the volume of O_2 consumed per minute ($\dot{V}O_2$). CO_2, foreign gases, and radioactive substances have also been used. Note that either flow or rate of metabolism can be so determined.

Cardiac Output Using the Fick Principle

The venous O_2 content (CvO_2) differs markedly in samples drawn from various organs. If we wish to know the total cardiac output, we must have a thoroughly mixed sample derived from all the organs to obtain the mean CvO_2. This is done by inserting a catheter into a peripheral vein and advancing it through the right heart into the pulmonary artery. CaO_2 and CvO_2 are estimated from the concentration of hemoglobin (Hb) and the percent saturation of Hb with O_2. Dissolved O_2 is less than 2 percent of the total when the subject is breathing room air and is often neglected. It must be measured if the subject is breathing O_2 at high partial pressure (PO_2). The following is a sample calculation:

O_2 capacity of blood = [Hb] (g/L) × 1.39 ml O_2/g Hb.
Dissolved O_2 = 0.029 ml/L per mm Hg PO_2.
Combined O_2 (HbO_2) = O_2 capacity × % saturation of Hb.
O_2 content = dissolved O_2 + combined O_2.
Assume [Hb] = 150 g/L.
Assume the saturation of Hb in arterial blood (SaO_2) = 94%.
Then HbO_2 = (150 g/L × 1.39 ml/g) × 0.94 = 196 ml/L.
Assume arterial partial pressure (PaO_2) = 95 mm Hg.
Then Dissolved O_2 = 0.029 ml/L per mm Hg × 95 mm Hg = 2.8 ml/L.
Arterial O_2 content = 196 ml/L + 2.8 ml/L = 198.8 ml/L.*

In similar fashion, the O_2 content of mixed venous blood ($C\bar{v}O_2$) was found to be 149 ml per liter. Then the O_2 *extraction* (*E*) is $CaO_2 - C\bar{v}O_2$ = 0.05 liters per liter.

Assume $\dot{V}O_2$ = 0.25 L/min.

$$\text{Cardiac output (C.O.)} = \frac{0.25\ \text{L/min}}{0.05\ \text{L/L}} = 5.0\ \text{L/min.}$$

The only assumption is that a steady state exists throughout the measurement. Simpler methods have supplanted the above calculation, except for quantitative evaluation of congenital cardiac defects in patients in whom the systemic and pulmonary flows are different.

The Fick Principle for Regional Flow

The Fick principle can be used to determine organ blood flow if a known rate of consumption or uptake can be created by administering a test substance. To measure coronary or cerebral flow, the subject breathes an appropriate mixture of O_2 with nitrous oxide or krypton. These inert gases diffuse from the blood so readily that the rate of accumulation in tissue is limited solely by blood flow. To measure the accumulation, arterial and venous samples are withdrawn simultaneously, and the time courses of concentration are plotted; see Figure 13-1. The area between the arterial and venous concentration curves is the arteriovenous difference during the time required for complete equilibration. The numerator in the Fick equation (the amount of inert gas dissolved in the organ) cannot be measured directly.

*O_2 content is commonly expressed as ml/dl, or as vol %.

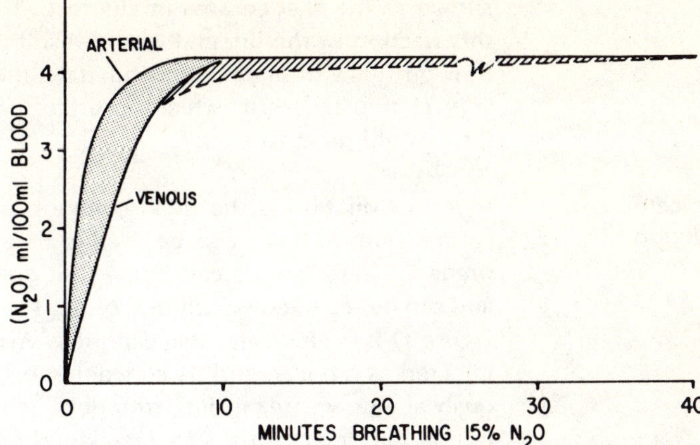

Figure 13-1
Time courses of equilibration of arterial and coronary or cerebral venous blood with N_2O. See text for explanation of stippled and shaded areas.

It is estimated by multiplying the venous concentration at equilibrium by the ratio of tissue concentration to blood concentration. This ratio, called the partition coefficient, is assumed to be a constant for a particular gas and tissue. For example, the partition coefficient for nitrous oxide and myocardium determined in vitro is about 1.1. Since the weight of the organ is not known, the tissue concentration is multiplied by 100 to express the flow in milliliters per minute per 100 g of organ. The modified Fick equation is

$$\dot{Q} = \frac{CvN_2O \times Pc \times 100}{\int_{t_0}^{t_{eq}} (a - v)dt},$$

where

CvN_2O = content of N_2O in venous blood at equilibrium.
Pc = partition coefficient.
$a - v$ = arteriovenous difference for N_2O.
t_0 = time zero.
t_{eq} = time at which tissue reaches equilibrium with venous blood.

In practice, the tissue is assumed to be at equilibrium at an arbitrary time (10 min in the case of N_2O). The normal integral is the stippled area in Figure 13-1.

The principal assumption in the inert gas method is that the *entire* organ has come into equilibrium with venous blood. In disease, however, poorly perfused regions may not reach equilibrium at the usual time. Uptake by poorly perfused regions is shown as the shaded area in Figure 13-1. Inability to measure this fraction of the integral would result in an overestimate of flow per 100 g of organ. Unfortunately, this error is large in the very circumstances in which accurate measurement of organ flow would be most useful.

Indicator Dilution Techniques

Indicator dilution is the most common method of measuring cardiac output. It can also be used to determine flow to certain organs. It requires a steady state, but only for a few seconds, and can be repeated rapidly and often. The principle is shown in Figure 13-2. An indicator that cannot leave the vascular system is injected as a bolus, and its concentration is recorded continuously at a downstream site. After delay in transit the concentration at the detector rises to a peak and follows an exponential decay. Then

$$\frac{\text{amount injected}}{\frac{\text{amount}}{\text{vol}} \times \text{time}} = \frac{\text{vol}}{\text{time}},$$

or flow, where amount/vol is the mean concentration between the appearance time (*Ta* in Figure 13-2) and the disappearance time (*Td*).

Dilution curves obtained with indocyanine green in an anesthetized dog are shown in Figure 13-3. These curves differ from Figure 13-2 in that the dye reappeared at the withdrawal site before *Td,* because of recirculation. In order to obtain the required integral, one can use the fact that the dye disappears exponentially. If the curve before recirculation is plotted semilogarithmically, the initial linear downslope extrapolated to zero concentration approximates *Td*. Cardiac output computers perform this operation automatically. A less precise but gener-

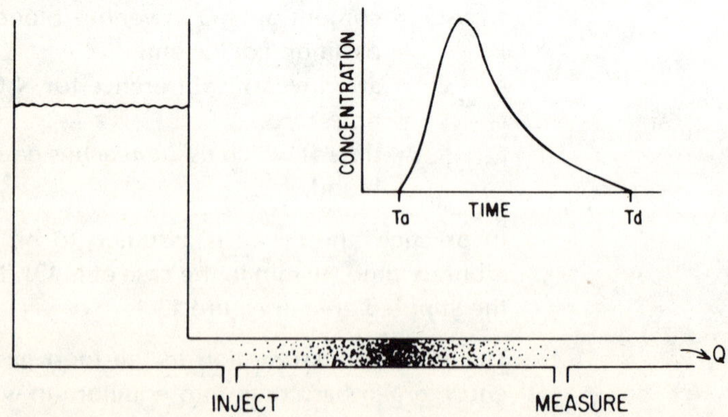

Figure 13-2
Principle of flow measurement by indicator dilution.

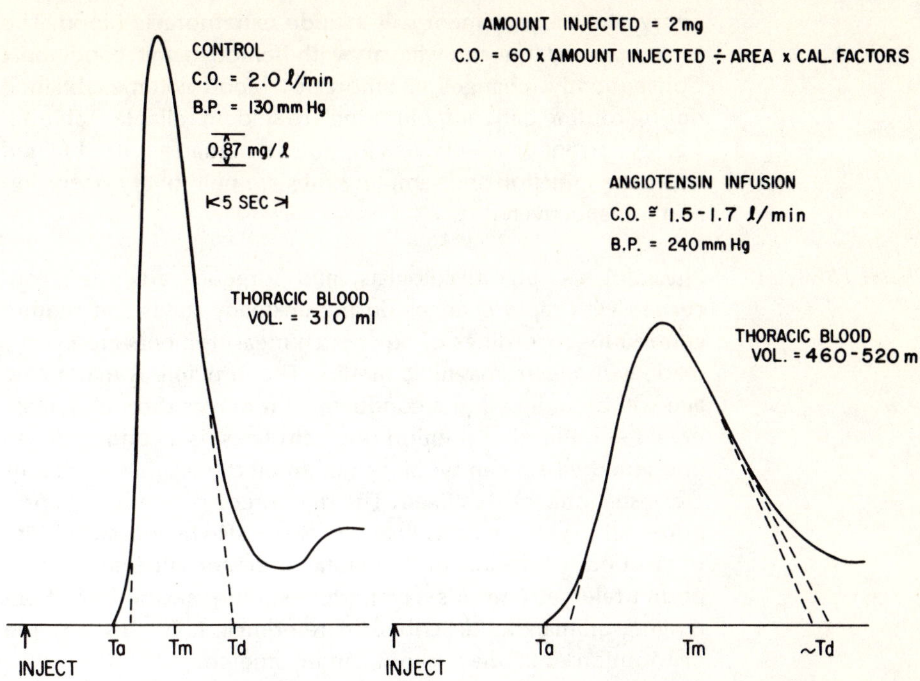

Figure 13-3
Dilution curves recorded in a 20-kg dog using indocyanine green as the indicator. The injection catheter was in the pulmonary artery; the sampling catheter, in the ascending aorta.

ally satisfactory method is to extrapolate the steepest slopes of the original curve to the abscissa and to the point where they intersect. The result is a triangle, whose area = ½(*Td* − *Ta*) × height, as in Figure 13-3. Recirculation introduces negligible error except when the cardiac output is low. The curve labelled *angiotensin infusion* in Figure 13-3 illustrates how acute cardiac failure caused by high outflow resistance increases the error of estimation.

Recently, heat has become the most commonly used indicator of cardiac output. The injectate, a bolus of saline at known temperature, returns to body temperature before it reappears at the sampling site. This eliminates the recirculation problem.

Estimating Thoracic Blood Volume

The indicator dilution curve provides *volume* as well as flow data: vol/*t* × *t* = vol. If vol/*t* is cardiac output, and *t* is the mean time required for the indicator to reach the detector (*Tm*), we obtain the thoracic blood volume discussed in Chapter 12. The calculated thoracic blood volume is strongly dependent on injection and sampling sites. If the indicator is injected into an arm vein or even the right atrium and is sampled from a peripheral artery, the measurement will include extrathoracic blood. The error may be large and will vary with hemodynamic conditions. Consequently, changes in "thoracic" blood volume obtained during routine patient monitoring are seldom reliable. Table 12-1 gives current best estimates for normal human adults obtained when the injection and sampling sites are pulmonary artery and aorta, respectively.

Phasic Flow

Physiologists, pharmacologists, and surgeons are often concerned with rapid changes during unsteady states and require continuous recordings of flow. Such measurements are usually made with electromagnetic meters. The principle is that a voltage will be induced in a conductor if it moves through a magnetic field. Blood, a solution of electrolytes, is a conductor. An unopened vessel can be placed in an electromagnet so that its cross-sectional area is fixed. The measured voltage is then proportional to volume flow. Phasic flow can also be measured with ultrasound. Ultrasonic probes suitable for chronic implantation permit telemetry from several arteries in unanesthetized, free-ranging animals as described in reference 4. In this way the distribution of cardiac output can be studied.

Normal Cardiac Output at Rest

Cardiac output at rest varies with body size and shape. It is therefore customary to divide the output by body surface area. The normalized output is called the *cardiac index* (L/min per m^2). A formula for estimating surface area is included in Appendix 2. Cardiac index is the same for both sexes. It is highest in children and decreases by about one-third between 20 and 75 years of age, as shown in Figure 13-4.

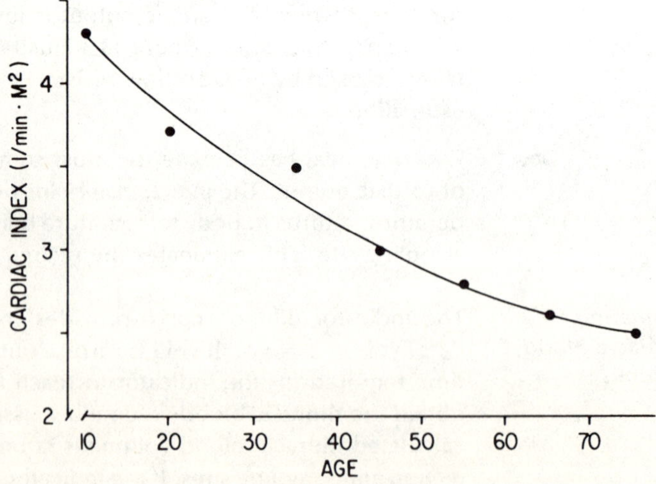

Figure 13-4
Effect of age on cardiac index at rest in a thermoneutral environment.

Absence of exercise is not necessarily the same as absence of stress. Standing, emotional tension, pregnancy, hot humid environments, hypoxemia, and many illnesses increase the resting cardiac output. The extent of such increases is so idiosyncratic and so dependent on age and acclimatization that no quantitative statement can be made, except that the changes can be large. For example, environmental temperatures about 40°C accompanied by high relative humidity can increase "resting" cardiac output threefold in an unacclimatized individual. The ability of such a person to work, or respond to another stress, is limited by the extent that the *reserve of cardiac output* is already engaged.

The Cardiac Output Reserve

Contributions of Heart Rate and Stroke Volume

Stroke volume is nearly maximal when one is recumbent and decreases by about a third when one sits or stands, because of the changes in volume distribution and preload discussed in Chapter 12. The fall in stroke volume is compensated for by increased heart rate, so the *expansion factors* for stroke volume and heart rate depend on position.

Average changes in heart rate and stroke volume in young adults working erect are shown in Figure 13-5. The reserve of stroke volume is fully utilized with very light work. In contrast,

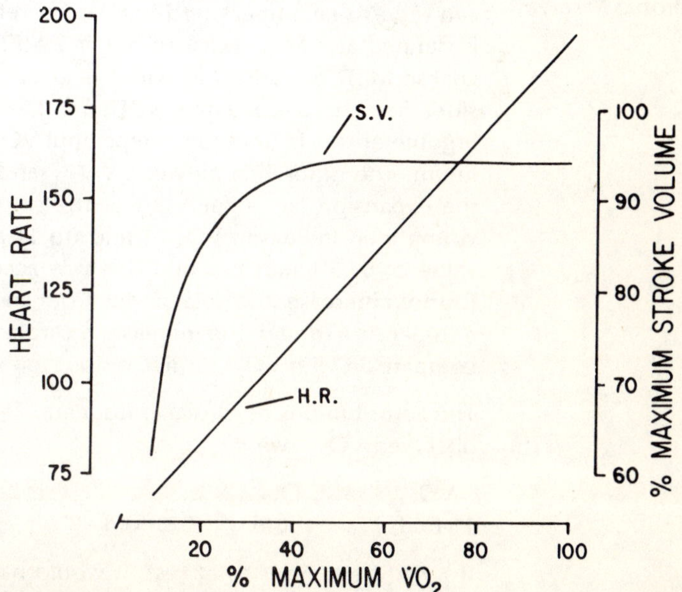

Figure 13-5
Components of the cardiac output reserve as functions of aerobic capacity. (*S.V.* = stroke volume; *H.R.* = heart rate.)

heart rate increases linearly with work and $\dot{V}O_2$. This linear relation is so reliable it can be used to predict the aerobic capacity or maximum $\dot{V}O_2$ ($\dot{V}O_{2_{max}}$). Age, sex, and body size must be taken into account.

In certain cardiac arrhythmias, heart rate may exceed 160 beats per minute at rest. Under these abnormal conditions, filling is limited by diastolic time, and cardiac output falls. This does not happen during normal exercise because (1) sympathetic nerves shorten systole and increase contractility, as explained in chapters 1 and 5, and (2) the thoracic blood volume is maintained by the thoracoabdominal and muscle venous pumps.

Resting heart rates of about 40 beats per minute are observed in well-conditioned athletes. Such people have physiological cardiac hypertrophy that allows stroke volumes much greater than predicted for age and body size. This enables them to work at lower heart rates that demand less O_2 consumption by the myocardium. Since their maximal heart rates approach 200 beats per minute, their maximal cardiac outputs approach 35 liters per minute. Use of exercise training to lower heart rate and improve cardiac efficiency is described in reference 1.

Relation between Cardiac Output and Aerobic Reserve

Cardiac output is adjusted to allow work to be done aerobically; see Figure 13-6. The lower abscissa expresses $\dot{V}O_2$ relative to $\dot{V}O_2$ at rest. Since resting $\dot{V}O_2$ is about the same for everyone, it can serve as an unmeasured standard of reference. Resting $\dot{V}O_2$ is defined as 1 MET, twice resting is 2 MET, and so on. The O_2 cost in MET for various activities is given in Appendix 4. Consider first the upper curve in Figure 13-6. Work on a bicycle ergometer was increased in steps until $\dot{V}O_2$ approached a maximum. The difference between $\dot{V}O_{2_{max}}$ and $\dot{V}O_2$ at rest defines the expansion factor for $\dot{V}O_2$, or the *aerobic reserve*. Trained young men increased $\dot{V}O_2$ 11-fold (to 11 MET), from an initial value of 0.18 L/min per m^2. This was accompanied by only a fourfold increase in cardiac index from an initial value of 3.5 L/min per m^2. Though the increase in cardiac output was small in comparison with $\dot{V}O_2$, cardiac output too was nearly maximal.

The contributions of cardiac output and O_2 extraction (E) to the observed $\dot{V}O_{2_{max}}$ were

$$\dot{V}O_{2_{max}} = C.O._{max} \times E.$$
$$\text{11-fold} \uparrow = \text{4-fold} \times \text{2.75-fold}$$

If E had been 5 vol % at rest, it would have been 13.75 vol % during maximal effort. In a few superathletes $\dot{V}O_2$ and cardiac output can (briefly) increase 20-fold and 6-fold, respectively.

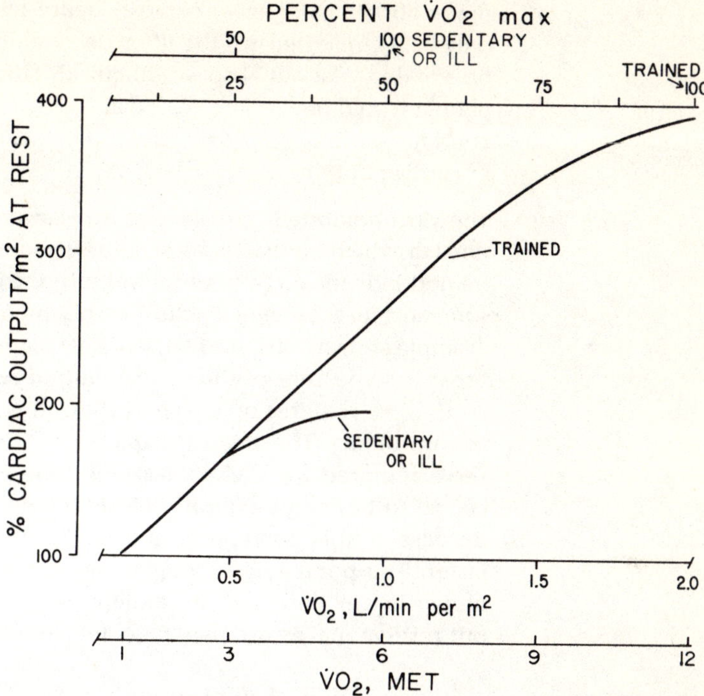

Figure 13-6
Relation between aerobic capacity and cardiac output in trained young athletes and in deconditioned subjects whose $\dot{V}O_{2_{max}}$ is half as great. Lower abscissa units are multiples of the $\dot{V}O_2$ at rest (1 MET).

$\dot{V}O_{2_{max}}$ is useful for defining potential expansion factors, but such heavy work can be sustained for only 2 to 5 minutes. Even the most strenuous manual labor (sugar cane cutting, lumbering) is done at less than 50 percent of $\dot{V}O_{2_{max}}$. Notice in Figure 13-6 that in trained subjects increases in $\dot{V}O_2$ were accompanied by *proportional* increases in cardiac output through 60 to 70 percent of $\dot{V}O_{2_{max}}$. Since aerobic capacity was large, less than 25 percent of the cardiac output reserve was utilized for routine work in these trained individuals. The remainder, and anaerobic metabolism, are used only for brief bursts of intense activity. In nature (and in crossing a New York City street), such bursts are essential for survival.

Illness and Deconditioning

In developed countries many people are sedentary and deconditioned. Surprisingly, all these people have about the same $\dot{V}O_2$ and cardiac output at rest and at low work rates as do trained athletes. Let us assume for illustrative purposes that the expansion factors for cardiac output and $\dot{V}O_2$ in an ill or deconditioned person are half those for trained subjects; notice the upper abscissa and lower curve in Figure 13-6. Then at a $\dot{V}O_2$ of only 0.75 L/min per m^2, the ill or deconditioned person would be working "flat out" and would quickly fatigue. Young, trained people would be hardly stressed at 0.75 L/min per m^2 and could continue for long periods because of their still untapped reserve of cardiac output.

The deconditioned person is at a disadvantage even at work rates at which cardiac output is the same as in a young, well-trained individual. This is true because the deconditioned person must use a *larger fraction* of his or her reserves. In the example shown in Figure 13-6, work at half the ill person's $\dot{V}O_{2_{max}}$ "costs" 80 percent of the cardiac output reserve, whereas the same work requires only 40 percent of the reserve of a trained young subject. The larger the fraction of the cardiac output reserve required for a given task the more strenuous it is *perceived* to be, and the more quickly the person senses fatigue. Because of this perception, old or deconditioned people tire faster. The popularity of jogging and other conditioning techniques is well deserved: Expanding $\dot{V}O_{2_{max}}$ and the cardiac output reserve makes ordinary tasks feel less tiring.

Clinical Application

Physicians must weigh the costs of bed rest against its benefits. Recall from Chapter 12 that prolonged bed rest impairs compensation for orthostatic stress and decreases total blood volume. It also affects cardiac function and exercise tolerance. The effect of 20 days in bed on 5 young men is shown in Figure 13-7. Two were physically trained beforehand (upper curves), and three were sedentary. After bed rest, heart rate was higher and O_2 extraction larger at all work rates. Since maximum heart rate was unchanged, the fall in maximum cardiac output was due to reduced stroke volume. All 5 subjects then began intensive physical training. The increase in aerobic capacity was larger in the previously sedentary individuals. These men doubled their $\dot{V}O_{2_{max}}$ relative to the value at the end of bed rest.

Inappropriate fatigue is one of the cardinal manifestations of disease. Its mechanism is precisely the reverse of physical training, that is, $\dot{V}O_{2_{max}}$ is progressively decreased. Ordinary tasks then demand a larger fraction of the (reduced) aerobic capacity and therefore are perceived to be more tiring. Fatigue and the aerobic reserve can be evaluated in MET by use of Appendix 4. Such semiquantitative thinking is an essential component of history taking

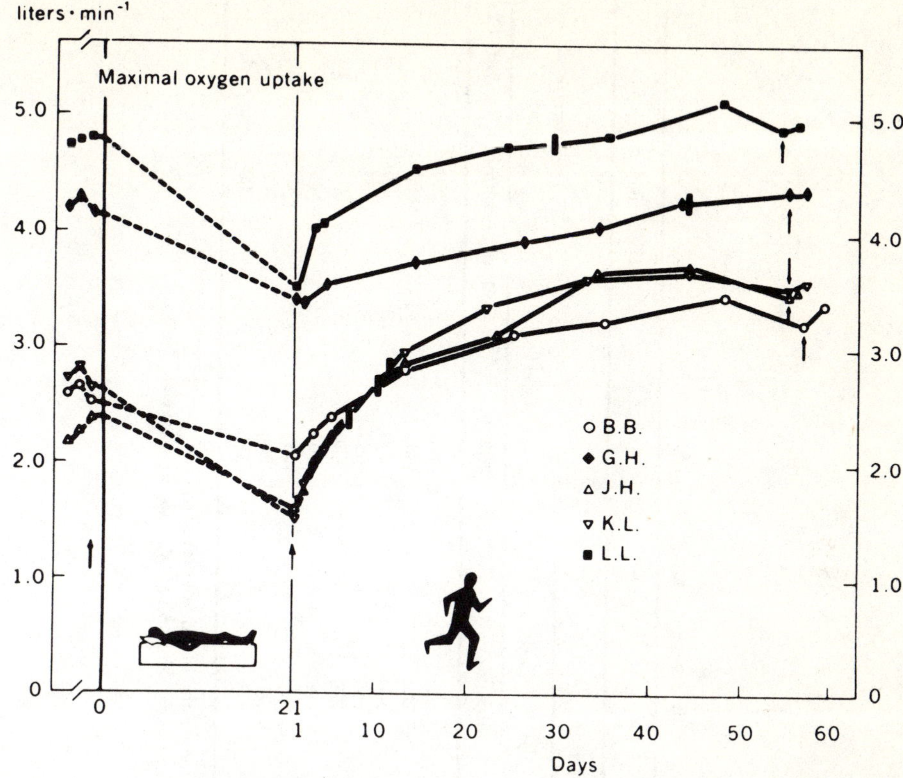

Figure 13-7
Changes in $\dot{V}O_{2_{max}}$ measured on a treadmill before and after bed rest and at various times during training. (From B. Saltin, G. Blomqvist, J. H. Mitchell, R. L. Johnson, Jr., K. Wildenthal, and C. B. Chapman, *Circulation* 38[Suppl. 7]:1, 1968. By permission of the American Heart Association, Inc.)

Distribution of Cardiac Output

The blood flow reserve for a particular organ depends on the distribution of cardiac output as well as the total cardiac output. The apportionment of the cardiac output changes dramatically in exercise, heat stress, and disease, as shown in Table 13-1. At rest almost half the cardiac output of a normal person goes to the kidneys and splanchnic bed for "housekeeping" functions. Skeletal muscle receives only about 20 percent, though it accounts for almost half the body mass. The reverse distribution occurs in light exercise. Heat dissipation in light exercise triples skin flow. Since the skin extracts very little O_2, its contribution to mixed venous blood limits whole body O_2 extraction and $\dot{V}O_2$.

In maximum exercise the muscles received 88 percent of the cardiac output — 22 liters per minute. If there had been no redistribution, muscle flow would have been only 5.3 liters per minute, far less than necessary to accommodate the roughly 50-

Table 13-1
Cardiac Output and Its Distribution in a Normal Person and a Patient with Severe (Grade 3) Mitral Stenosis*

	Normal						Mitral Stenosis			
			Exercise							
	Rest		Light		Maximum		Rest		Exercise (Light)	
	ml/min	% C.O.	ml/min	% C.O.	ml/min	% C.O.	ml/min	% C.O.	ml/min	% C.O.
$\dot{V}O_2$	240		720		2600		150		700	
C.O.	5800		9500		25,000		4000		5800	
Splanchnic	1400	24	1100	12	300	1	800	20	400	7
Renal	1100	19	900	10	250	1	650	16	300	5
Cerebral	750	13	750	8	750	3	650	16	600	10
Coronary	250	4	350	4	1000	4	300	8	500	7
Muscle	1200	21	4500	48	22,000	88	1050	26	3400	57
Skin	500	9	1500	16	600	2	200	5	400	7
Other	500	9	400	1			350	9	200	3

*Differences at rest and with exercise illustrate how disease can compromise the blood flow reserves.
Source: Modified from O. L. Wade and J. M. Bishop, *Cardiac Output and Regional Blood Flow*, Oxford: Blackwell, 1962.

fold increase in muscle $\dot{V}O_2$. Redistributions of cardiac output almost as dramatic as those in exercise accompany emotional stresses, temperature regulation, orthostatic reflexes, and other physiological adjustments.

Clinical Applications

Flow distribution is very difficult to measure, so physicians often fail to think about it. Nevertheless, it plays a major role in pathophysiology. The patient with mitral stenosis considered in Table 13-1 is an informative example. His cardiac output in light exercise was about the same as the normal cardiac output at rest. Muscle flow accounted for almost 60 percent of this. Consequently, renal, splanchnic and cutaneous flows were very low, and comparable to values observed in normal persons during maximal exercise. Similar flow distributions are observed in congestive heart failure. Poor exercise tolerance, inefficient temperature regulation, and renal and gastrointestinal dysfunction, are due not only to low cardiac output but also to failure to distribute that output appropriately.

References

*1. Åstrand, P. O., and Rodahl, K. *Textbook of Work Physiology* (2nd ed.). New York: McGraw-Hill, 1977. Pp. 180–199, 333–355, 379–387, 404–435.

2. Cournand, A., Baldwin, J. S., and Himmelstein, A. *Cardiac Catheterization in Congenital Heart Disease*. New York: Commonwealth, 1949.

3. Ganz, W., Donoso, R., Marcus, H. S., Forrester, J. S., and Swan, H. J. C. A new technique for measurement of cardiac output by thermodilution in man. *Am. J. Cardiol.* 27:392, 1971.

4. Hales, J. R. S., Rowell, L. B., and King, R. B. Regional distribution of blood flow in awake heat-stressed baboons. *Am. J. Physiol.* 237:H705, 1979.

5. Lassen, N. A., Henricksen, O., and Sjersen, P. Indicator Methods for Measurement of Organ and Tissue Blood Flow. In *Handbook of Physiology*, Section 2. Circulation — Vol. III. Peripheral Circulation and Organ Blood Flow, Part 1. Bethesda, Md.: American Physiological Society, 1983.

6. Sasaki, Y., and Wagner, H. N. Measurement of the distribution of cardiac output in unanesthetized rats. *J. Appl. Physiol.* 30:879, 1971.

7. Vatner, S. F., Higgins, C. B., and Franklin, D. Regional circulatory adjustments to moderate and severe chronic anemia in conscious dogs at rest and during exercise. *Circ. Res.* 30:731, 1972.

*8. Wade, O. L., and Bishop, J. M. *Cardiac Output and Regional Blood Flow.* Philadelphia: Davis, 1962. Pp. 3–7, 26–107.

III : Filtration and Determinants of Transport

14 : Starling's Filtration Principle, Updated

About 75 years ago, Starling showed that the concentration of protein is several times greater in the plasma than in the intercellular spaces. The corresponding difference in colloid osmotic pressure would cause water to flow from interstitium to blood, and from cells to interstitium. The force that opposes this tendency to tissue dehydration is the capillary blood pressure. Conversely, the tendency of hydrostatic pressure to "squeeze" fluid out of the capillary is opposed by the colloid osmotic pressure. This chapter and the next are concerned with the mechanisms by which a balance between hydrostatic and osmotic forces is achieved, and with the consequences of imbalance caused by stress or disease.

The capillary pores described in Chapter 10 are really minute vessels for bulk Poiseuille flow of filtrate (Q_F), so

$$Q_F = C_F \cdot \Delta P.$$

C_F, the *capillary filtration coefficient*, is the conductance of all pores in a single capillary, or in a population of capillaries. The pressure term is the difference between transmural hydrostatic and transmural osmotic pressures:

$$Q_F = C_F\,[(P_{cap} - P_{IF}) - (\pi_{cap} - \pi_{IF})],$$

where π is the colloid osmotic pressure, *cap* is capillary, and *IF* is interstitial fluid. Positive pressures produce filtration; negative pressures produce reabsorption. We shall first consider each of the preceding determinants, then their interaction.

The Capillary Filtration Coefficient

Poiseuille's law applied to transcapillary fluid flow can be rewritten as follows:

$$C_F = Q_F/\Delta P = K'A^2/l.$$

r^4 is replaced by the square of the aggregate pore cross-sectional area, A. Viscosity, channel length, and the numerical constants in the Poiseuille relation are assembled into a new constant, K'. Thus C_F can be determined if Q_F and ΔP are known. Such results are expressed per 100 g of tissue to normalize for A and l in the population of capillaries. Q_F can be

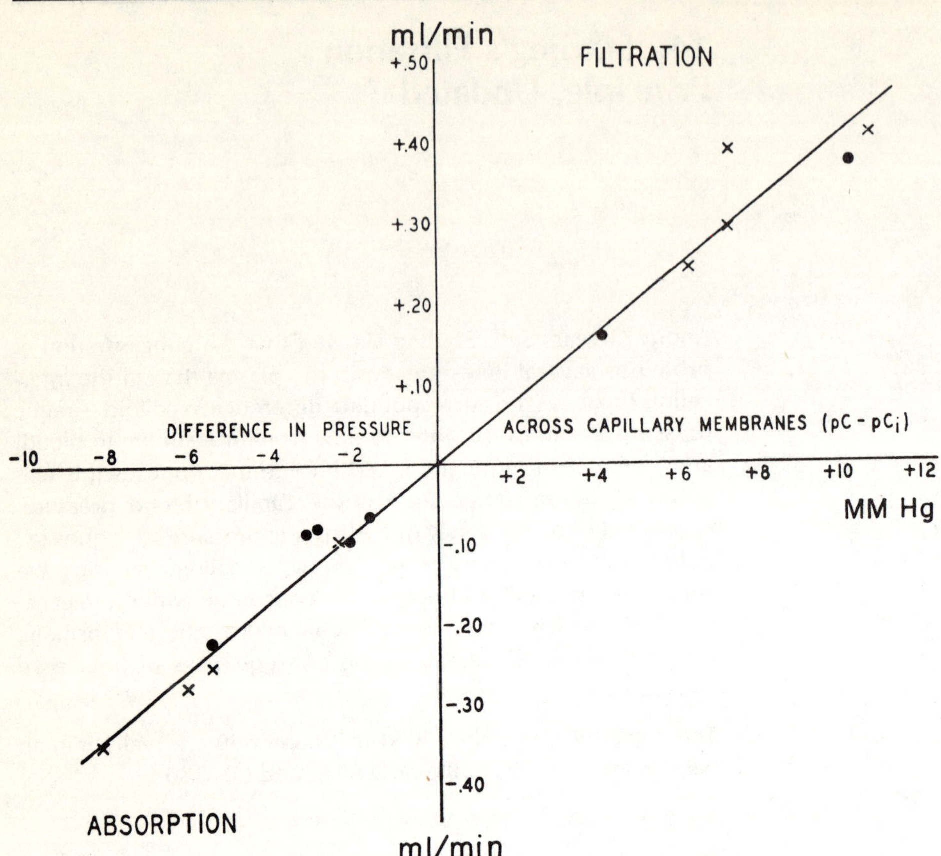

Figure 14-1
Fluid balance in perfused cat limb. Circles represent results with normal perfusate; crosses indicate results when plasma oncotic pressure was increased threefold. (From J. Pappenheimer and A. Soto-Rivera, *Am. J. Physiol.* 152:471, 1948.)

measured as change in organ weight; ΔP can be varied by raising or lowering venous pressure. Results from an isolated, perfused cat limb are shown in Figure 14-1. The slope corresponds to a C_F of 0.014 ml/min · torr per 100 gm. The circles and crosses show results before and after increasing π_{cap} threefold by adding albumin to the perfusate. Since all points fall on the same line, the rate of filtration is independent of the magnitude of pressure and depends on only the *net difference* between hydrostatic and osmotic pressures. Such data prove that the principle put forward by Starling is correct.

C_F has been measured for single capillaries by use of micropipettes. C_F proved to be about 10 times greater at the venous end than at the arterial end. This promotes reabsorption at normal venous pressure. It also explains why high venous pressure has such a large effect on filtration rate and edema formation. Capillaries are hardy: C_F is unaffected by cyanide, anoxia, and change in pH. Since C_F for an individual capillary remains constant under most circumstances, changes in C_F usually denote a change in the number of perfused capillaries per volume of tissue, or the *capillary density*. For example, C_F for a limb increases several-fold during muscle contraction, because of recruitment of capillaries that had not been perfused at rest.

The Oncotic Pressures

The osmotic pressure of protein is less than 0.5 percent of the total osmotic pressure of plasma. Only this small component, called the *oncotic pressure*, influences filtration, because the concentration of small molecules would be the same in blood and interstitial fluid if protein were not present.

Oncotic Pressure of Blood (π_{cap})

The osmotic pressure of an ideal solution is given by van't Hoff's law:

$$\pi = C \cdot R \cdot T,$$

where C is concentration, R the molar gas constant, and T the absolute temperature. The relation between oncotic pressure and the concentration of plasma proteins is shown in Figure 14-2. Deviation from the linearity predicted by van't Hoff's law is due to the Gibbs-Donnan equilibrium. Since plasma proteins are negatively charged at physiological pH, they retain cations, chiefly Na^+, within the blood. These osmotically active cations greatly decrease the concentration of protein required to generate the normal π_{cap} of 25 torr. The phenomenon is caused by binding of water molecules to the charged proteins. As protein concentration increases, the amount of osmotically active solvent decreases.

The nonlinearity in Figure 14-2 acts as a *factor of safety* to stabilize plasma volume.[1] For example, excessive water loss from the body (dehydration) increases the concentration of plasma proteins. The resulting increment in plasma oncotic pressure is greater than would be expected for an ideal solution as shown by the dashed arrow in Figure 14-2. This increases the tendency for fluid to move into the capillary in defense of blood volume. Conversely, hemodilution results in greater reduction of plasma oncotic pressure than would occur otherwise, thereby decreasing the tendency for further absorption from the interstitium.

[1] The same phenomenon stabilizes the volume of the fragile red cells; the hemoglobin concentration in a red cell is about 15 mM!

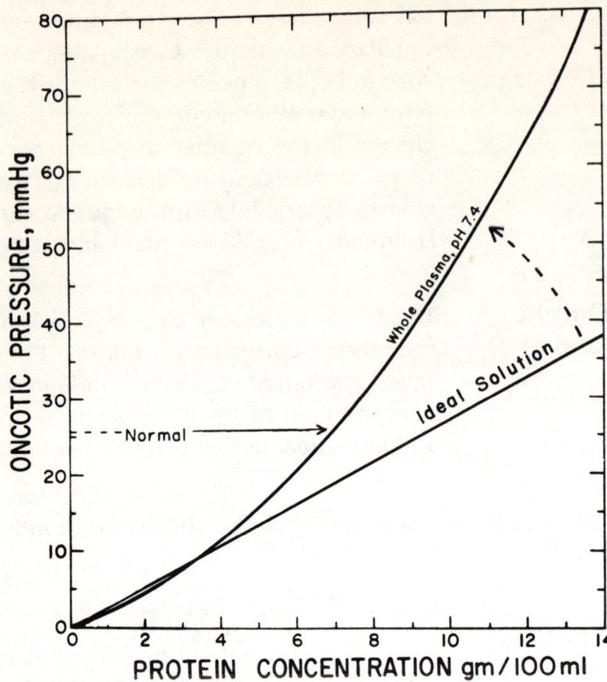

Figure 14-2
Oncotic pressure curves for plasma proteins at 37°C. (From E. M. Landis and J. R. Pappenheimer. In W. F. Hamilton and P. Dow (eds.), *Handbook of Physiology*, Section 2: Circulation. Washington, D.C.: American Physiological Society, 1963. Vol. II, p. 961.)

The anomalous behavior of plasma proteins is particularly striking at high concentrations. In glomerular capillaries, where 20 to 25 percent of the entering plasma is filtered, concentrations reach 9 percent or more. The corresponding oncotic pressure is about 45 torr, almost twice that in systemic capillaries. The steep rise in oncotic pressure along the glomerular capillary limits the fraction of plasma volume that can be filtered, and the high oncotic pressure in peritubular capillaries is a major factor promoting reabsorption of water from the filtrate.

The Oncotic Pressure of Interstitium (π_{IF})

In the course of 24 hours, about half the plasma albumin leaves the circulation and is returned via the lymph. The extravascular circulation of protein is not merely a leak, but a transport mechanism for antibody and hormones that bind to albumin. The average concentration of protein in interstitial fluid is about 1 gm per 100 ml. This small concentration has an effective oncotic pressure of 5 to 10 torr, because the fiber networks in the interstitium reduce the effective concentration of water.

P_{IF} and the Mechanical Properties of the Interstitium

The extracellular extravascular space is best described as a gel. It contains collagen and elastic fibers and polysaccharide fibers. These fibers give it the properties of a solid; that is, when deformed it "remembers" its original shape and returns to it. The gel strongly resists hydrodynamic flow of water but does not significantly impede diffusion of water or small molecules.

The magnitude of P_{IF} is uncertain because of limitations of techniques used to measure it, but there is general agreement that the shape of the pressure–volume relation of the interstitium is as described in Figure 14-3. At the low interstitial fluid volumes characteristic of normal tissue, the tendency to outward filtration is opposed by the low compliance of the interstitium. However, when P_{IF} exceeds 10 to 15 torr, the gel is disrupted, compliance of the interstitium increases, and fluid can accumulate rapidly with little further increase in P_{IF}. Compliance decreases again at large interstitial fluid volumes because of counterpressure by skin or fascia.

P_{cap}, Vasomotion, and Normal Fluid Balance

The determinants thus far considered remain constant on the time scales of most physiological stresses, so fluid balance usually depends on P_{cap}. Until recently, P_{cap} was thought to exceed π_{cap} at the arterial end of a capillary and drop below π_{cap} toward the venous end. This concept predicts a very precarious balance, whereas clinical experience demonstrates that the balance is remarkably stable in health. The situation was clarified by recent measurements of pressure along actively perfused and unperfused capillaries. In the example shown in Figure 14-4A, the

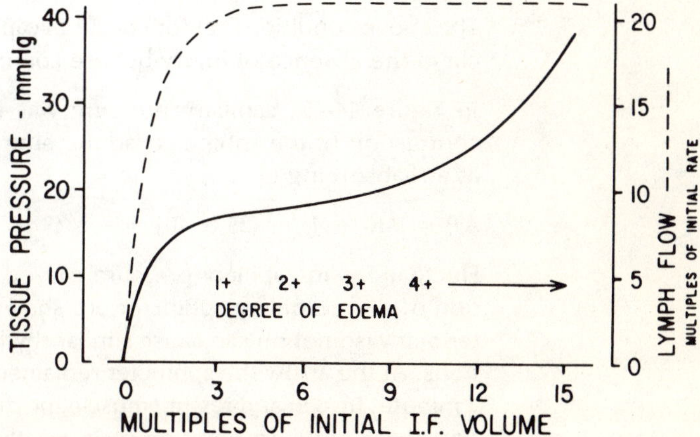

Figure 14-3
Schematic pressure-volume relation for interstitium (*continuous curve, left ordinate*) and lymph flow in a dog's limb as a function of interstitial fluid (I.F.) volume (*dashed curve, right ordinate*).

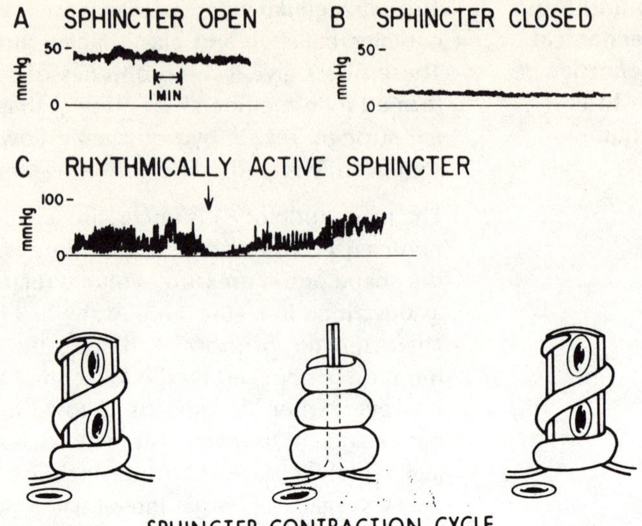

Figure 14-4
Top, pressure at arterial ends of capillaries in wing of unanesthetized bat. (Recordings provided by Dr. Curt Wiederhielm.) Bottom, Contraction cycle of a precapillary sphincter.

measuring pipette was inserted when the precapillary sphincter and upstream arterioles were relaxed. Under these conditions arteriolar resistance was low, and P_{cap} was well above π_{cap} from the arterial to the venous end. Consequently, filtration occurred along the entire capillary. The net balance was as follows:

$$\Delta P = [(\underset{P_{cap}}{45} - \underset{P_{IF}}{1}) - (\underset{\pi_{cap}}{25} - \underset{\pi_{IF}}{8})] = +27.$$

The above conditions seldom occur in capillaries of skin or muscle in the absence of injury but are common in the omentum.

In Figure 14-4B, capillary pressure was low because of tonic contraction of the sphincter, so the entire capillary functioned as a reabsorbing unit:

$$\Delta P = [(10 - 1) - (25 - 8)] = -8.$$

Fluctuations in capillary pressure caused by rhythmic contraction of a precapillary sphincter are shown in Figure 14-4C. Arteriolar vasomotion can cause similar rhythmic pressure fluctuations. At the arrow the sphincter remained contracted for about 1 minute. In skin and resting muscle the duration of the contraction phase of the vasomotion cycle greatly exceeds the duration of the relaxation phase, so π_{cap} exceeds P_{cap} at most locations. Consequently, reabsorption predominates in the population of capillaries, and lymph flow is low. The reverse is true of omentum.

Lung and kidney are special cases in that sphincters or their functional equivalents are absent. Under basal conditions the afferent glomerular arteriole is almost fully relaxed and capillary pressure is about 60 torr. Such high pressures are essential to allow filtration along the entire glomerular capillary, because oncotic pressure rises progressively. At the opposite extreme, the low pressure in the pulmonary artery results in pulmonary capillary pressures less than π_{cap} at all locations when a person is recumbent. Fluid balance in the lung is considered in more detail in the next chapter.

References

1. Brenner, B. M., Baylis, C., and Deen, W. M. Transport of molecules across glomerular capillaries. *Physiol. Rev.* 56:502, 1976.
2. Gore, R. W., and McDonagh, P. F. Fluid exchange across single capillaries. *Annu. Rev. Physiol.* 42:337, 1980.
*3. Landis, E. M., and Pappenheimer, J. R. Exchange of Substances Through the Capillary Walls. In W. F. Hamilton and P. Dow (eds.), *Handbook of Physiology,* Section 2: Circulation. Washington, D.C.: American Physiological Society, 1963. Vol. II, pp. 961–999.
4. Laurent, T. C. Physico-chemical properties of interstitial fluid. *Pflügers Arch.* 336:S21, 1972.
5. Lewis, D. H. (ed.). Symposium on lymph circulation. *Acta Physiol. Scand.* [*Suppl.*] 463:9, 1979.
6. Michel, C. C. Fluid Movements Through Capillary Walls. In E. M. Renkin and C. C. Michel (eds.), *Handbook of Physiology,* Section 2: The Cardiovascular System — Microcirculation, Vol. II. Bethesda, Md.: American Physiological Society, 1984.
7. Wiederhielm, C. A., and Weston, B. V. Microvascular, lymphatic and tissue pressures in the unanesthetized mammal. *Am. J. Physiol.* 225:992, 1973.

15 : Control of Filtration; Edema

Hemorrhage and dehydration occur commonly in nature. It is therefore not surprising that evolution has provided powerful defenses against such occurrences. The most critical body fluid compartment is the circulating blood volume, because it is a major determinant of preload and cardiac function. The interstitial fluid and to some extent the intracellular fluid serve as reserves that can be drawn on to expand the blood volume. *Mobilization of these reserves is the principal function of hydrodynamic flow across somatic capillaries.*

Neural Control of Resistance and Capacitance Vessels

In a series of classical experiments, Mellander quantified the effects of sympathetic nerves on arteriolar resistance and venous capacity. Limbs of an anesthetized cat were enclosed in a rigid box called a plethysmograph. A pressure-volume curve was then constructed for the plethysmograph, from which the extent of tissue swelling or shrinkage could be determined. Arterial pressure was held constant throughout. Results are shown in Figure 15-1.

In panel *A* the sympathetic nerves were stimulated six times per second for 30 seconds to induce arteriolar constriction and venoconstriction. Flow and tissue volume fell. The fall in volume means that during the stimulus more fluid left the plethysmograph than entered. This fluid was whole blood stored in the venous capacity. The survival value of blood mobilized from tissue depots by venoconstriction is obvious.

In panel *B* the stimulus was maintained for 2 minutes. Flow reached a stable minimum in about 30 seconds, but tissue volume continued to shrink slowly throughout the stimulation. The upright arrows and numerals indicate the percentage decrease in protein concentration of blood leaving the plethysmograph. Since the blood was diluted, arteriolar constriction must have lowered mean P_{cap} well below π_{cap} thereby producing reabsorption from the interstitium. If the stimulus was continued longer than 3 minutes, reabsorption slowed and then ceased, presumably because π_{IF} increased or P_{IF} decreased enough to balance the fall in P_{cap}, or both. When the stimulus was turned off, there

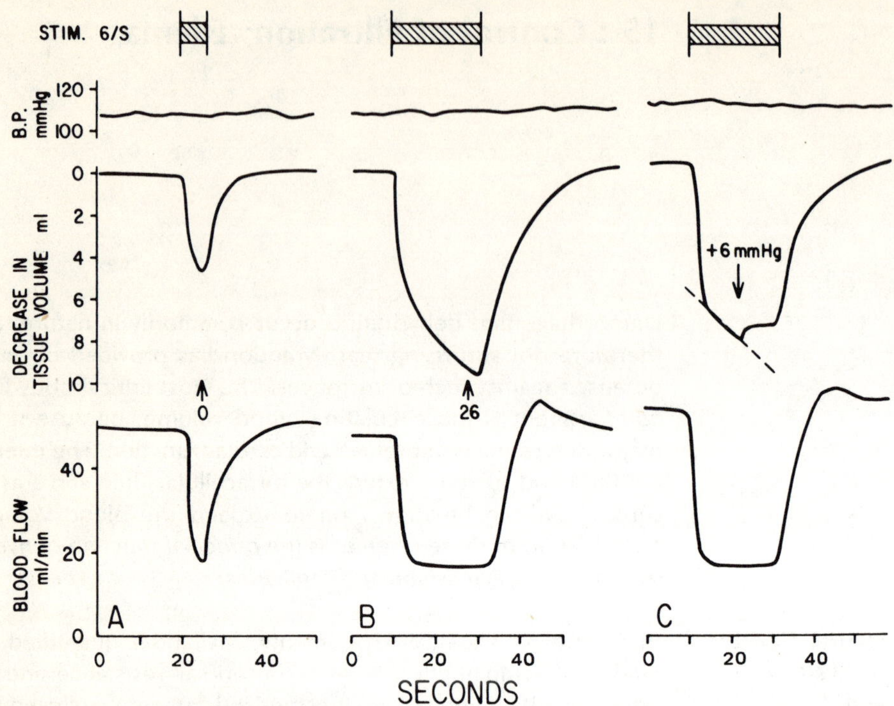

Figure 15-1
Effects of sympathetic nerves on arteriolar resistance, venous capacity, and transcapillary fluid movement. See text for explanation. (Redrawn from data of S. Mellander, *Acta Physiol. Scand.* 50 [Suppl. 176]:1, 1960.)

was an initial rapid increase in tissue volume, as a result of refilling of the venous capacity, followed by a slow increase caused by outward filtration as the arterioles dilated and P_{cap} rose. These interpretations are confirmed in panel *C*. When venous pressure was raised during electrical stimulation by an amount equal to the calculated decrease in P_{cap} (6 torr), absorption of fluid ceased.

Mellander's experiments suggest that the amount of interstitial fluid that can be drawn into the blood during severe hemorrhage is equivalent to half the normal blood volume! There are costs for every benefit: Dilution of blood with interstitial fluid decreases the O_2-carrying capacity of blood. Moreover, much of the fluid that enters the blood comes from the intracellular compartment. Cell dehydration limits the amount of extravascular fluid that can be mobilized without compromise of vital functions. Finally, the vasoconstriction required to shift fluid into the vasculature "throttles" blood flow and cannot be sustained for long periods. Thus redistribution of volume among body fluid compartments is merely a first line of defense against dehydration or hemorrhage — necessary, but not sufficient. Redistributions "buy time" for slower renal controls of Na^+ and water balances. These controls are components of neuroendocrine systems that regulate total fluid volume, as described in Chapters 18 and 25.

Edema

We turn now from reabsorption to excessive filtration. We first consider the safety factors that protect us from edema, then the consequences of edema in the lungs. Our safety factors are large: People with congenital analbuminemia are free of edema even though π_{cap} is less than half normal. Similarly, venous pressure in the foot or in the lung can increase 10 to 15 torr without edema. Safety factors may be categorized as myogenic, interstitial, and lymphatic, as shown in Figure 15-2. The relative importance of these factors depends on the organ, and on the edema-producing stress.

The Myogenic Safety Factor

The most common cause of edema is high venous pressure during orthostatic stress, though in congestive heart failure and certain other disorders venous pressure may be high even when one is recumbent. Venous congestion stimulates reflexes that constrict the upstream arterioles. The rise in resistance lowers P_{cap}. Precapillary sphincters and terminal arterioles are also stimulated, so capillary density and C_F decrease. If supplemented by the muscle venous pump, vasoconstriction is generally effective in preventing orthostatic edema of the legs and feet. Vasoconstriction is insufficient otherwise; pedal edema is common when one is seated and immobile for long periods, as is often

COMPONENTS OF THE "MARGIN OF SAFETY"

1. Myogenic compensations
   a. increase in precapillary resistance
   b. reduction of capillary surface area
2. Interstitial compensations
   a. rise in interstitial fluid pressure
   b. dilution of interstitial proteins
3. Lymphatic compensations
   a. acceleration of fluid removal
   b. washout of interstitial proteins

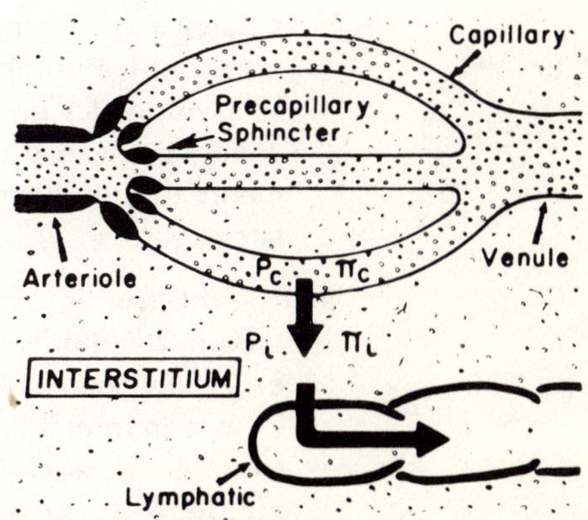

Figure 15-2
Factors of safety against the development of edema. (From H. I. Chen, H. J. Granger, and A. E. Taylor, *Circ. Res.* 39:245, 1976. By permission of the American Heart Association, Inc.)

the case in nursing homes. The reason is that low blood flow initiates local metabolic mechanisms that override the neural vasoconstrictor stimulus. Vasoconstriction is also decreased by inflammation, trauma, anesthesia, deconditioning, and other factors. Under such conditions, interstitial and lymphatic safety factors play the major role.

Interstitial Safety Factors

The normal interstitium is a gel of low compliance. Consequently, very small increments in volume produce pressures large enough to reduce filtration considerably; refer to the continuous curve in Figure 14-3 page 143. Tissue pressure is particularly important because it affects filtration immediately, whereas many minutes are required to achieve maximum rates of lymph flow.

The protein concentration of edema fluid in cardiac failure and hypoproteinemia is less than half that thought to exist in the normal interstitial gel. Simple dilution can therefore decrease π_{IF} by about 5 torr. The foregoing interstitial factors can compensate for a 5- to 10-torr increase in P_{cap} or decrease in π_{cap} at the cost of only slight edema. If this compensation and enhanced lymph flow are insufficient, the gel is disrupted and gross swelling develops. Swelling progresses until the skin or fascia is stressed enough to increase P_{IF} (final slope of pressure-volume curve in Figure 14-3). This last line of defense is unavailable to the lung or to burned skin, because there can be no counterpressure at a free surface. Loss of fluid and protein from burns is a major therapeutic problem.

Lymphatic Compensations

Flow in lymphatic capillaries appears to depend on rhythmic contraction of smooth muscle cells in the major trunks. In the presence of edema, tissue pressure exceeds lymphatic pressure, but lymph flow continues at the maximum rate. The reason lymphatics do not collapse is that they are "anchored" to connective tissue elements of the interstitium by special filaments that hold the lymphatics open as edema fluid accumulates.

The relation between lymph flow and the volume of interstitial fluid in dog limbs is shown in Figure 14-3, dashed curve. Note especially that lymph flow can increase many-fold with little change in interstitial fluid volume. Thus lymphatics tend to *prevent* edema, as well as to diminish the rate and extent of swelling. Indeed, some investigators define edema as an increased rate of transcapillary fluid flow rather than an increase in interstitial fluid volume. Once lymph flow reaches capacity, edema increases rapidly. If peripheral edema is gross enough to be detected by simple observation, lymph flow is already maximal, and almost all safety factors have been expended.

The lymphatics remove protein as well as fluid. This slows edema formation by lowering π_{IF}, and is essential for recovery of normal fluid balance when the edema-producing stress is removed. Elimination of protein is especially important in edema caused by increased capillary permeability, as in trauma, infection, and burns. The protein content of such edema fluid is 3 to 5 percent, and the corresponding π_{IF} is about half π_{cap}. Since inflammation dilates precapillary vessels, P_{cap} is high, and the only restraint on edema formation apart from lymph flow is tissue pressure. The largest increases in tissue volume and the most persistent occur in lymphatic obstruction, because the protein content of such edema fluid is almost the same as that of plasma.

Fluid Balance in the Lungs

The pulmonary interstitium and alveolar spaces must be free of edema for efficient gas exchange. Nevertheless, fluid balance is much more precarious than the low pulmonary artery pressure would suggest. The pressure of the alveolar air is homologous to interstitial fluid pressure in other organs. It cycles about a mean of zero during normal respiration. The oncotic pressure of the pulmonary interstitium is about 8 torr, and in a recumbent person pulmonary capillary pressure is 10 to 15 torr. For these conditions

$$\Delta P = (\underset{P_{cap}}{10 \text{ to } 15} - \underset{P_{IF}}{0}) - (\underset{\pi_{cap}}{25} - \underset{\pi_{IF}}{8}) = -7 \text{ to } -2.$$

Capillaries beneath the visceral pleura are exposed to negative intrapleural pressures of 5 to 8 torr rather than alveolar pressure. Fluid tends to filter out of the subpleural capillaries at all times.

The pulmonary vessels possess little smooth muscle and are not vasoactive under normal circumstances. Since there is no myogenic safety factor, P_{cap} rises several torr during stresses that increase cardiac output. Moreover, when a person is seated or standing, a hydrostatic column increases P_{cap} at the lung bases by 5 to 7 torr. Since the compliance of lung interstitium is large, the principal defense against edema is an exceptionally rich network of lymphatics. These prevent edema until P_{cap} exceeds about 25 torr.

Clinical Application

There are two stages in the development of pulmonary edema. At first, fluid collects in the loose, connective tissue spaces, which act as a sump. The length of the diffusion path for O_2 and CO_2 is increased, but no fluid enters the alveoli, which are lined by an epithelium of very low permeability (equivalent pore radius ≅ 2 nm). Swelling of the interstitium decreases lung compliance, so greater negative pleural pressures are required for inflation. The greater effort required for breathing is perceived as shortness of breath, or *dyspnea*. Fear induced by dyspnea initiates sympathetic drive that increases heart rate, afterload, and myocardial O_2 demand. If the initiating factor is myocardial ischemia or cardiac insufficiency, the added cardiac stress further increases end-diastolic, pulmonary venous, and capillary pressures. If impaired gas exchange decreases arterial O_2 content, cardiac function deteriorates more rapidly. These and other positive feedback mechanisms increase P_{cap} and greatly accelerate transcapillary filtration.

The course of pulmonary edema depends on the rate of onset, because lymph flow takes about an hour to reach a maximum. If edema accumulates slowly, it is generally cleared. If not, or if the filtration rate exceeds lymphatic capacity, fluid breaks out into the alveoli. The patient literally drowns in minutes if treatment is unavailable or ineffective.

References

*1. Chen, H. I., Granger, H. J., and Taylor, A. E. Interaction of capillary, interstitial and lymphatic forces in the canine hind paw. *Circ. Res.* 39:245, 1976.

2. Mellander, S. Comparative studies on the adrenergic neuro-humoral control of resistance and capacitance blood vessels in the cat. *Acta Physiol. Scand.* 50 [Suppl. 176]: 1, 1960.

3. Mortillaro, N. A., and Taylor, A. E. Interaction of capillary and tissue forces in the cat small intestine. *Circ. Res.* 39:348, 1976.

4. Renkin, E. M. Control of Microcirculation and Blood-Tissue Exchange. In E. M. Renkin and C. C. Michel (eds.), *Handbook of Physiology*, Section 2: The Cardiovascular System — Microcirculation, Vol. IV. Bethesda, Md.: American Physiological Society, 1984.

5. Renkin, E., and Fishman, A. *Pulmonary Edema*. Bethesda, Md.: American Physiological Society, 1979.

6. Wiederheilm, C. A. Dynamics of transcapillary fluid exchange. *J. Gen. Physiol.* 52:532, 1968.

16 : Transport of Oxygen and Metabolites

Thus far we have been concerned with pumps, conduits, and flow — *convective transport within* the circulation. For most substances, transport beyond the vascular system depends solely on diffusion. Oxygen is a special case, in that its release from blood is limited by binding to hemoglobin (Hb). Concepts in O_2 transport have changed radically in the past decade. This new knowledge is developed in this chapter and applied in the next.

Diffusion of Small Molecules

Rates of transcapillary diffusion of water-soluble molecules such as glucose, urea, and lactate are incredibly rapid, considering the small fraction of capillary surface area occupied by the aqueous pores through which they move. For example, a 1 percent difference in concentration will suffice to transfer 10 times more glucose across muscle capillaries than is consumed at rest. About 1000 times more glucose diffuses across muscle capillaries each minute than moves through the same pores by hydrodynamic flow. Since transcapillary diffusion is so large, it makes no difference whether net filtration or reabsorption is occurring. Lipid-soluble metabolites traverse the entire endothelial surface, an area at least 1000 times larger than the aggregate area of aqueous pores. Small molecules also readily permeate the interstitium and intracellular space. Thus intermediary metabolism is not limited by capacity for diffusion. This affords maximum latitude to physiological controls of the *rates* at which substances diffuse.

Determinants of Rate of Diffusion

Fick's law[1] states that the rate of diffusion of a substance through area A in direction x is proportional to the concentration gradient:

$$J_s = \frac{ds}{dt} = -D \cdot A \cdot \frac{dc}{dx}.$$

J_s is called the *flux;* note especially that it is a rate, not an amount. In the steady state J_s might correspond to the rate of

[1] Fick's law of diffusion should be clearly distinguished from the Fick principle, which is a statement of mass balance.

consumption of glucose, or rate of production of lactate, and so on. The constant of proportionality between the flux and the concentration gradient is the diffusivity, D, for a particular substance. It varies as the square root of molecular weight, so even large molecules like myoglobin are highly diffusible. As a first approximation, diffusivities are the same in various organs. The term A in Fick's law can be interpreted as the effective capillary surface area. A varies with the functional capillary density and, in the case of O_2, with capillary hematocrit as well. Flux is often normalized for the available area; the quantity J_s/A is called the *flux density*. Notice that an increase in A (and decrease in flux density) decreases the concentration gradient required to achieve a particular flux. The concentration gradient $\left(\frac{dc}{dx}\right)$ is the *driving force* for diffusion and generally is the dominant variable.

Capillary Resistance to O_2 Transport

Fick's law describes the frictional resistance encountered, for example, by glucose in transit of a slit pore. It assumes that the solvent is homogeneous and that the diffusing substance does not react chemically with components of the diffusion path. O_2 reacts with hemoglobin, and its diffusion path is nonhomogeneous because hemoglobin is "packaged" in red cells. These factors *dominate resistance to O_2 mass transfer.* For simplicity, they can be lumped together with frictional resistance as a single, nonlinear resistance for transport (RO_2):

$$RO_2 = \Delta PO_2/\dot{V}O_2$$

Notice the parallel to fluid flow in pipes. For any steady O_2 flux ($\dot{V}O_2$), the ΔPO_2 between two points tells the overall resistance. We shall use this approach to locate the "bottleneck" for O_2 transport.

Capillary O_2 Gradients

Thre are two capillary gradients to think about: a longitudinal O_2 gradient from the arteriolar end to the venular end, and a transcapillary gradient for diffusion from plasma to interstitium. The former sets the intracapillary PO_2 for the latter, as shown in Figure 16-1.

The Longitudinal Gradient

The model in Figure 16-1 consists of a single capillary and the cylinder of tissue it supplies. O_2 bound to Hb is in chemical equilibrium with the small amount of O_2 that can dissolve in plasma. Dissolved O_2 diffuses out of the capillary down the concentration gradient created by O_2 consumption. This lowers PO_2 within the capillary, shifts the equilibrium between free and bound O_2, and allows more O_2 to be released from Hb. Thus as

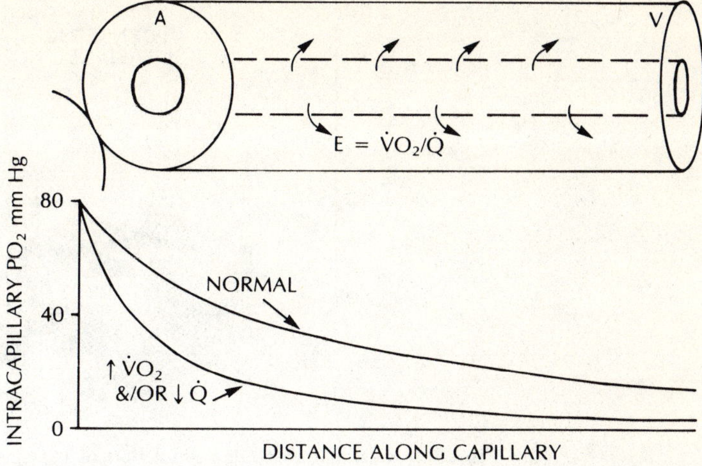

Figure 16-1
Model of longitudinal PO_2 gradients in capillaries. Arrows indicate blood-tissue diffusion of O_2. $\dot{Q}$ represents flow.

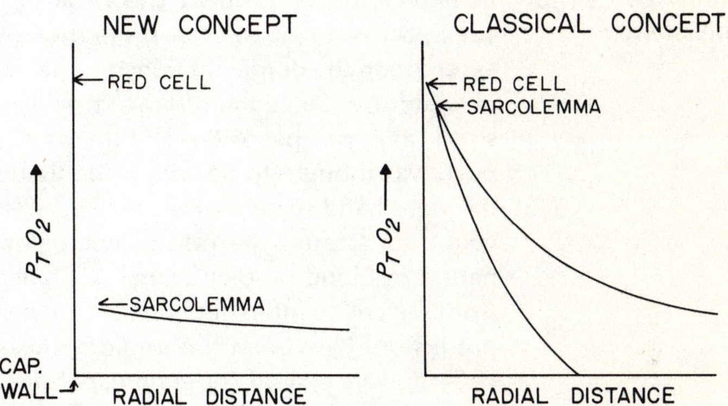

Figure 16-2
Comparison of classical view with current concept of blood-tissue O_2 transport.

a red cell moves along a capillary its O_2 content ($CcapO_2$) falls as the ratio of $\dot{V}O_2$ to flow rate:

$$\Delta CcapO_2 = \dot{V}O_2/\dot{Q}.$$

The fall in $PcapO_2$ that corresponds to the decrease in $CcapO_2$ is greatest near the arterial end, because of the sigmoid shape of the oxyhemoglobin dissociation curve. Typical curves are shown in Figure 17-2, page 164. If $\dot{V}O_2$ increases, or flow decreases, or both, $PcapO_2$ falls more steeply, as indicated in Figure 16-1. *Close coupling of $\dot{V}O_2$ and blood flow* is essential in defending the driving force for outward diffusion, particularly near the venous ends of capillaries.

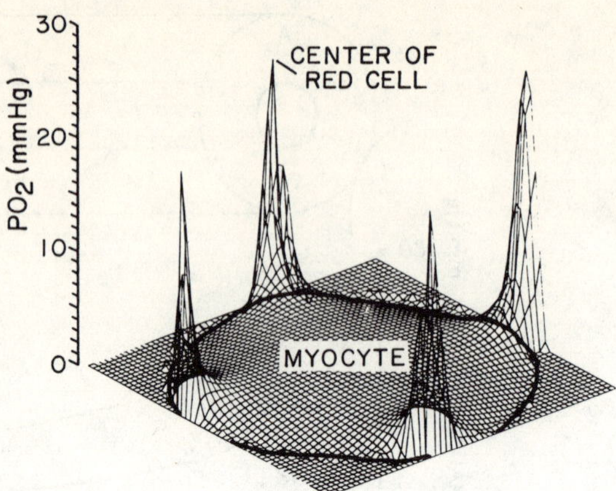

Figure 16-3
Three-dimensional computer simulation of the spatial distribution of PO_2 from four capillaries into an adjacent maximally working red skeletal muscle cell. (From K. Groebe and G. Thews, *Adv. Exp. Med. Biol.* 200:495, 1986.)

From Red Cell to Interstitium

Until recently the capillary was regarded as an extension of tissue space with no special properties of importance. On that assumption the dominant transport parameter is the distance O_2 must diffuse. Since the distance from capillary to interstitium is small, the principal ΔPO_2, and the principal resistance to transport, was thought to lie within the tissue cells, as illustrated in the right hand panel of Figure 16-2. All recent calculations that take into account the role of hemoglobin and the particulate nature of blood predict a large ΔPO_2 across the short distance from red cell to interstitium (*left hand panel,* Figure 16-2). These predictions have been confirmed by measurement. Thus *the red cell–capillary system is the principal site of resistance to blood-tissue O_2 transport.*

A dramatic illustration of this concept is shown in Figure 16-3. The peaks represent calculated PO_2 in four capillaries around a heavily working myoglobin-containing muscle cell 50 μ in diameter. PO_2 falls steeply over the short distance between the interior of a red cell and the sarcolemma. The ΔPO_2 over the long distance from sarcolemma to cell interior is comparatively small. Thus the resistance to O_2 transport (RO_2) from red cell to interstitium is large compared to the RO_2 within a cell.

Flux Density and Transit Time

Why is the drop in PO_2 across the capillary so large? Why is the drop in PO_2 around mitochondria so small? The same O_2 flux crosses the capillary and mitochondrial membranes, but the aggregate surface area of mitochondria in tissues like heart and red skeletal muscle is almost three orders of magnitude larger than the effective capillary surface area. The high O_2 flux per area (flux density) at capillaries is analogous to a large flow being forced through a small orifice — a large pressure drop is required.

The transcapillary O_2 gradient depends not only on diffusion, but also on the chemical reactions that release O_2 from Hb. Because of these reactions, and the low solubility of O_2 in plasma, *red cells do not equilibrate with tissue* in passage through a capillary. The time available for O_2 release is identical to the red cell's capillary transit time. If red cell velocity increases, as in exercise hyperemia, O_2 must be released faster to compensate for the shorter transit time. The increase in O_2 flux requires a larger driving force (ΔPO_2).[2] This is achieved by lowering intracellular PO_2.

Steep transcapillary gradients are not confined to red muscle; they occur whenever high flux density, short capillary transit times, or both demand a large driving force. High flux density can be caused by low functional capillary density or low capillary hematocrit, as well as high $\dot{V}O_2$.

From Cell Membrane to Mitochondria

The principal consequence of a large transcapillary gradient is that the ΔPO_2 from the surface to the interior of a tissue cell is comparatively small. Notice in Figure 16-3 that virtually the entire ΔPO_2 inside the myocyte takes place within a few microns of the capillaries, where O_2 enters at very high flux density. O_2 gradients in individual red muscle fibers have been determined spectroscopically. In accord with Figure 16-3, the *measured* intracellular ΔPO_2 from sarcolemma to cell interior is only 2 to 3 torr in heavy exercise. Thus the resistance of red myoplasm to O_2 transport is about an order of magnitude less than transcapillary resistance.

Shallow intracellular O_2 gradients are particularly remarkable in the large-diameter skeletal-muscle fibers, because intracellular O_2 gradients vary directly with $\dot{V}O_2$ and with the distance O_2 must diffuse. Long diffusion distances within skeletal myocytes are accommodated by a flux of oxymyoglobin molecules in parallel with free O_2. Functions of myoglobin are explained in Chapters 19 and 22. The brain has no need for such an intracellular O_2 carrier, since most brain mitochondria lie just beneath the synaptic membranes that account for the bulk of the O_2 consumed. Diffusion distances are therefore very short. In all organs, capillary recruitment can decrease diffusion distances and minimize intracellular gradients in response to increased O_2 demand. Flux density at the mitochondrion is lower than at any

[2] Recall that flux is a rate.

other point in the O_2 path. Consequently, the ΔPO_2 between cytosol and cytochrome oxidase is negligible — about 0.01 torr at maximal $\dot{V}O_2$.

The Minimum PO_2 to Run the Mitochondria

The biochemical drive on $\dot{V}O_2$ consists of three components: (1) the energy charge, expressed as the ratio of adenosine triphosphate (ATP) to adenosine diphosphate (ADP) and inorganic phosphate (Pi) (ATP/ADP·Pi); (2) the percent reduction of the electron transport chain; and (3) the concentration of free O_2. $\dot{V}O_2$ increases as the energy charge decreases, so ATP consumption and aerobic ATP synthesis are matched automatically. The O_2 affinity of cytochrome oxidase is so high that under most circumstances O_2 is present in great excess. Moreover, as the O_2 concentration falls, cytochrome turnover and $\dot{V}O_2$ are defended by adaptive change in the energy and redox drives. The net effect is shown in Figure 16-4 for a suspension of isolated mitochondria. $\dot{V}O_2$ is constant down to about 0.1 torr, and is half maximal at about 0.05 torr at normal rates of energy turnover. The minimum PO_2 for $\dot{V}O_2$ is the same for tissue in vivo. Thus virtually the entire ΔPO_2 between the air we breathe and cytochrome oxidase can be utilized for O_2 transport.

Hypoxia

Perhaps the most common term in pathophysiology is *hypoxia*. Biochemists define it as O_2-limited electron transport. Physiologists and clinicians use the term in a completely different sense. According to them, hypoxia exists when O_2 availability limits organ function. This condition can be called *tissue hypoxia* and

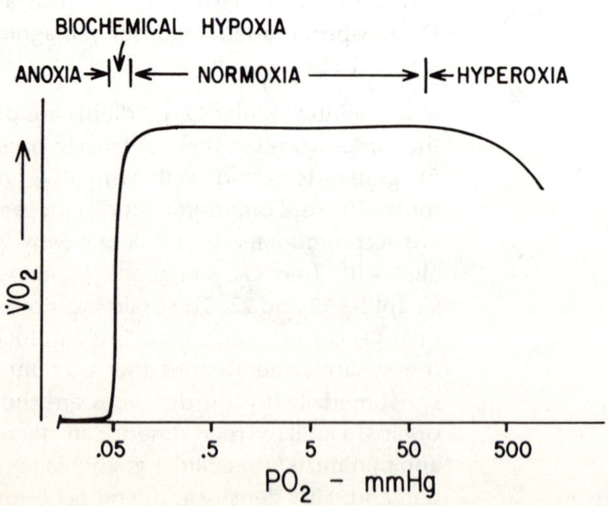

Figure 16-4
Dependence of $\dot{V}O_2$ on PO_2 for a suspension of isolated mitochondria. Note log scale of abscissa.

is caused by heterogeneities in the O_2 delivery system. Heterogeneities result in a probability distribution of intracellular PO_2. To avoid biochemical hypoxia in the cell whose PO_2 is lowest, the population mean must be set well above 0.5 torr. If a large number of O_2-limited cells exist, organ function — mentation, for example — will improve if more O_2 is delivered. Cardiovascular diseases tend to decrease mean O_2 delivery and increase transport heterogeneities. Consequently, the extent to which O_2 delivery can be curtailed without producing tissue hypoxia is diminished. The influence of disease on O_2 transport gradients and safety factors for O_2 transport are considered in the next chapter.

References

1. Clark, A., Jr., Clark, P. A. A., Connett, R. J., Gayeski, T. E. J., and Honig, C. R. How large is the drop in PO_2 between cytosol and mitochondrion? *Am. J. Physiol.* 252:C583, 1987.
2. Clark, A., Jr., Federspiel, W. J., Clark, P. A., and Cokelet, G. R. Oxygen delivery from red cells. *Biophys. J.* 47:171, 1985.
3. Federspiel, W. J. A model study of intracellular oxygen gradients in myoglobin-containing skeletal muscle fiber. *Biophys. J.* 49:857, 1986.
4. Gayeski, T. E. J., Connett, R. J., and Honig, C. R. The minimum intracellular PO_2 for maximum cytochrome turnover in red muscle in situ. *Am. J. Physiol.* 252:H789, 1986.
5. Gayeski, T. E. J., and Honig, C. R. O_2 gradients from sarcolemma to cell interior in red muscle at maximal $\dot{V}O_2$. *Am. J. Physiol.* 251:H789, 1986.

*6. Honig, C. R., Gayeski, T. E. J., Federspiel, W., Clark, A., Jr., and Clark, P. Muscle O_2 gradients from hemoglobin to cytochrome: New concepts, new complexities. *Adv. Exp. Med. Biol.* 169:23, 1984.

17 : Reserves and Safety Factors for O_2 Transport

The object of this chapter is to integrate concepts of O_2 transport by identifying safety factors and reserves. To this end we imagine a sequence of steps from air to mitochondria, each corresponding to a transport process. What each step normally costs us in PO_2 is shown in Figure 17-1.

From Air to Alveoli

The difference between inspired and alveolar PO_2 ($PIO_2 - PAO_2$) is about 55 torr at rest at sea level. This large drop is due to dilution of O_2 with water vapor and CO_2 in the nonexchanging airways of the lung. The rate of alveolar ventilation ($\dot{V}A$) is the product of respiratory frequency, f, and the difference between the total volume of each breath (V_T) and the volume that does not reach the alveoli (dead space volume, V_D):

$$\dot{V}A = f\,(V_T - V_D).$$

$\dot{V}A$ determines PO_2 in the alveoli (PAO_2), and therefore the PO_2 in pulmonary venous and systemic arterial blood (PaO_2). Chemoreceptors detect PaO_2 and $PaCO_2$, which are closely regulated by a negative feedback system with the chest and lungs as effectors. If $\dot{V}O_2$ changes, $\dot{V}A$ changes appropriately, and arterial gas tensions remain nearly constant. The expansion factor for $\dot{V}A$ is about 20-fold, so $\dot{V}A$ almost never limits O_2 transport in health. However, $\dot{V}A$ can be decreased by disease and, to our disgrace, by drug abuse. It is not uncommon to find PaO_2 in the range of 60 torr in otherwise normal people. If PaO_2 falls, safety factors beyond the lung compensate — unless they are compromised or already engaged!

From Alveoli to Arterial Blood

Pulmonary Hemodynamics

Pulmonary arterioles resemble systemic venules: They possess little smooth muscle, and their radii are very large. These characteristics minimize resistance to flow. The pulmonary capillary is not a cylinder but rather two sheets of endothelium that envelope the alveolus. The diffusion distance for O_2 or CO_2 is only 0.1 to 0.5 μm. Sheet flow increases the surface area for exchange, decreases flux density, and minimizes the ΔPO_2 re-

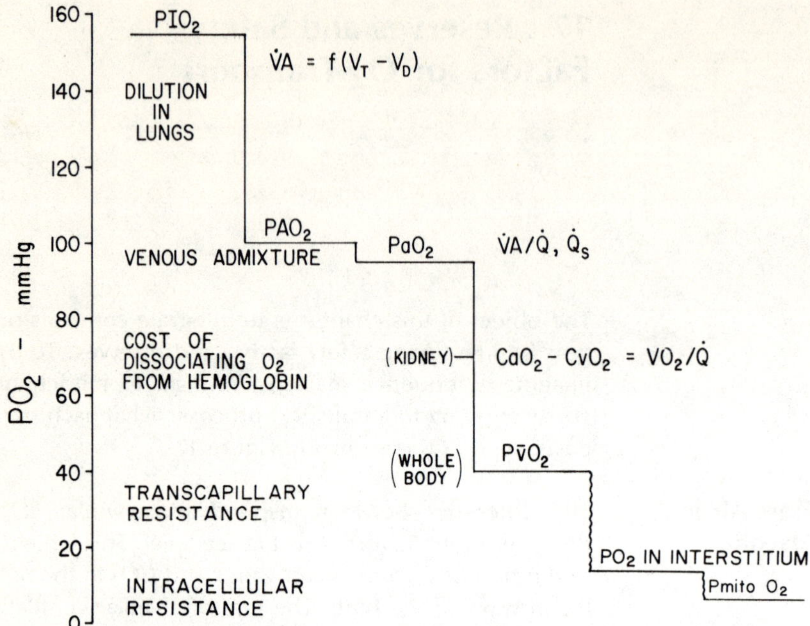

Figure 17-1
Steps in O_2 transport from air to mitochondria, and the mechanism of each step. PO_2 at critical points in the O_2 pathway is shown by horizontal lines, referenced to the ordinate. Values are for normal persons at rest at sea level. The steps from red cell to interstitium and from interstitium to mitochondria (*mito*) are shown as wavy lines to emphasize their variability. The symbols are defined in the text.

quired for diffusion between air and blood. The huge aggregate cross-sectional area of the pulmonary capillary sheets results in low red cell velocities and in transit times more than double the time required to load O_2 onto hemoglobin (Hb) at the prevailing driving force.

The right ventricular output is preferentially distributed to the lower lobes when a person is seated or standing. This flow pattern is largely due to absence of autoregulation or tonic sympathetic neural drive in pulmonary arterioles. Since distention by hydrostatic columns is unopposed, vessel radius and pulmonary blood flow increase with distance below heart level. The underperfused middle and upper lobes of the lung comprise a reserve of additional parallel paths for flow and additional capillary sheets that can be recruited. Recruitment of pulmonary vasculature is a passive process that minimizes the rise in pulmonary arterial pressure when cardiac output increases and maintains mean red cell transit time at about 0.5 s at maximal cardiac output. The pulmonary reserves for transport from air to blood are so large that diffusion per se is seldom the principal cause of hypoxemia.

Matching Ventilation and Perfusion

Ventilation and perfusion are nonuniformly distributed within the lung. Because of regional differences in lung compliance, alveoli near the pleura and at the apex are ventilated more than alveoli near the hilum or the bases. In contrast, flow to the base of the lung is generally greater than to the apex. The match between ventilation and perfusion can be described by the ratio of $\dot{V}A$ to flow ($\dot{Q}$). The $\dot{V}A/\dot{Q}$ ratio varies from about 3 in the upper lobes to 0.6 in the lower lobes; the average for the whole lung is 0.8. $\dot{V}A/\dot{Q}$ inequality can be regarded as a physiologic shunt of venous blood into the systemic circulation. Quantitative descriptions of the $\dot{V}A/\dot{Q}$ ratio are available in any textbook of respiratory physiology. A small anatomical shunt ($\dot{Q}_s$) of bronchial and cardiac venous blood also contributes to the normal alveolar-arterial (A-a) gradient of 5 to 10 torr.

Clinical Application

Mismatch between $\dot{V}A$ and $\dot{Q}$ is chiefly responsible for arterial hypoxemia in primary pulmonary disease and in pulmonary edema caused by cardiac insufficiency. The physiological shunt in these conditions seldom lowers PaO_2 below 50 torr. However, in children with anatomical venoarterial shunts, PaO_2 can be as low as 35 to 40 torr for years. The fact that these children are comfortable at rest demonstrates that even severe hypoxemia need not be accompanied by tissue hypoxia. Mark off the above A-a gradients on Figure 17-1 to appreciate the magnitude of transport reserves beyond the lung. A reserve is like your savings account: If you spend it you do not have it for an emergency. Think of what a PaO_2 of 35 torr costs as you read further.

Arterial to Venous Blood; Role of the Oxyhemoglobin Dissociation Curve

The step from arterial to *mixed* venous blood (PaO_2-$P\bar{v}O_2$) is normally about 55 to 60 torr. To understand the mechanism of this step we must be thoroughly familiar with the O_2 carrier function of hemoglobin (Hb).

Dissolved O_2

The dashed line adjacent to the abscissa in Figure 17-2 illustrates the linear relation between dissolved O_2 and PO_2 for blood at 37°C:

$$O_2 \text{ dissolved} = 0.0029 \text{ vol \%/torr}$$

Dissolved O_2 accounts for only 1.5 percent of total arterial O_2 content at normal [Hb] and PaO_2. It is of the utmost importance, however, for it *determines the affinity of Hb for O_2.*

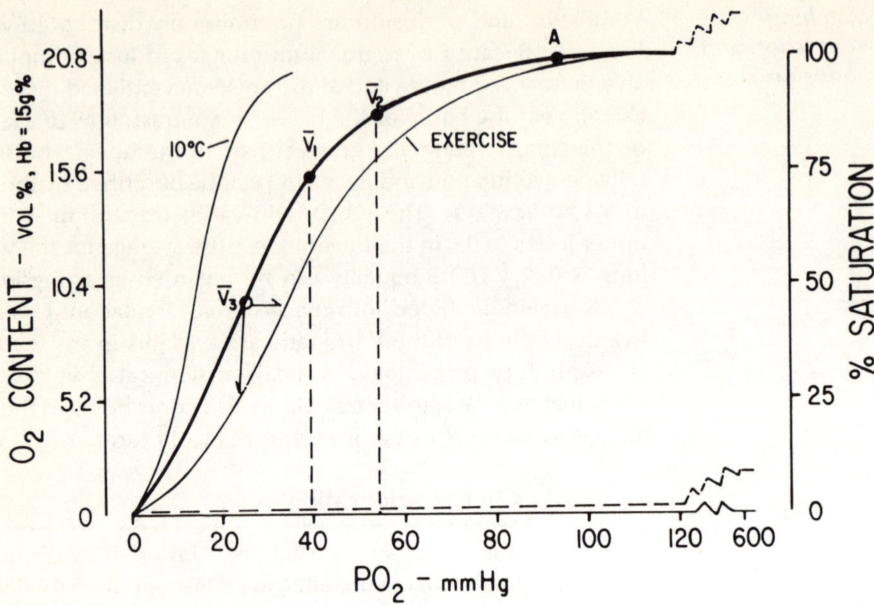

Figure 17-2
Oxyhemoglobin dissociation curves for normal human blood containing 15 g Hb/100 ml. The curve labelled *exercise* was drawn on the assumption that $P\bar{v}CO_2$ = 70 torr, pH_v = 7.15, and temperature = 39°C.

Clinical Application

O_2 Therapy

O_2 at high pressure is often used therapeutically. The theoretical maximum PaO_2 in normal persons breathing pure O_2 is about 670 torr at sea level, but such a value can seldom be approached in disease. Even at 670 torr the content of dissolved O_2 is only 2 vol %, or 10 percent of total CaO_2, assuming [Hb] is normal. Since the extra *amount* of O_2 that can be transported at high PaO_2 is small, PO_2 drops very steeply along arterioles and capillaries until the functional range of Hb is reached. Thus raising PaO_2 has little effect on mean capillary PO_2. Indeed, high PaO_2 may actually lower mean capillary PO_2, because O_2 tends to constrict arterioles and decrease blood flow. Capillary density also decreases in hyperoxemia, particularly in myocardium. Finally, O_2 at high tensions has a direct histotoxic action, especially on the lungs. In view of the foregoing, *the only valid reason for raising* PIO_2 *is to ensure normal saturation of Hb.* This should be achieved by keeping PaO_2 between 80 and 100 torr.

O_2 Combined with Hb

Normal blood contains about 15 g of Hb per 100 ml. However, some of this Hb is oxidized to ferrihemoglobin (methemoglobin) or combined with carbon monoxide. Such forms do not transport O_2. Methemoglobin can be produced by exposure to nitrites and a host of other oxidants. CO is a particularly important hazard; blood of smokers who use three packs of cigarettes a day may contain up to 20 percent carboxyhemoglobin! CO and O_2 compete for the same binding site, but the affinity of Hb for CO is much greater. Spectrophotometers that determine the percentage of carboxyhemoglobin and methemoglobin, total Hb, and percent saturation with O_2 are available in most clinical laboratories. After subtracting nonfunctional Hb, one can calculate O_2 capacity of blood using 1.39 ml O_2 per gram of Hb.

The Hb molecule contains 4 heme groups. The iron atom of each heme can hold one O_2 molecule. O_2 binding promotes more binding, so the first heme to be oxygenated has the lowest affinity for O_2 and the fourth heme has the highest. This positive cooperativity gives rise to the characteristic sigmoid shape of the dissociation curve.

$$Hb_4 + 4O_2 \rightleftarrows Hb_4O_8$$

In the lungs, diffusion of O_2 into the capillary raises $PcapO_2$ and shifts the equilibrium to the right. In the tissue, diffusion of O_2 out of the capillary lowers $PcapO_2$ and shifts the equilibrium to the left.

Role of Blood Flow

Arterial blood is up to 96 percent saturated and contains about 20 vol % at normal [Hb] and PaO_2; refer to Figure 17-2, point *A*. The average O_2 extraction for the whole body is about 5 vol % at rest. To release this amount of O_2, PO_2 must fall to 40 torr; see point $\bar{V}_1$. Extraction is the ratio $\dot{V}O_2/\dot{Q}$, so if cardiac output doubled but $\dot{V}O_2$ remained the same, only half as much O_2 would have to be released from each milliliter. Consequently, $P\bar{v}O_2$ would rise from 40 torr to 55 torr; see point $\bar{V}_2$. The same reasoning can be applied to flow and PvO_2 in the individual organs, except that organ flow can vary proportionately more than cardiac ouput. *The blood flow is the first line of defense* against anoxia because it defends the driving force required to overcome the large transcapillary resistance to O_2 transport, discussed in Chapter 16.

The Extraction Reserve

Notice in Figure 17-2 that most of the O_2 offered to the various organs is not utilized; $C\bar{v}O_2$ is only 25 percent less than CaO_2 at rest despite a large drop in PO_2. The unused O_2 is a *reserve of extraction*. Flow and extraction are multiplicative, not additive, determinants of $\dot{V}O_2$, so a modest increase in extraction has a large effect. The cost is lower end-capillary PO_2; compare $\overline{V}_1$ and $\overline{V}_3$.

The extraction reserve is highly organ-specific. For example, the kidney receives about one-fifth the cardiac output under basal conditions. Because of this enormous flow, it extracts only 1.5 vol %, despite its high $\dot{V}O_2$. The corresponding renal PvO_2 is about 65 torr, as compared with 40 torr for mixed venous blood. When renal blood flow is curtailed, however, as in exercise, renal O_2 extraction can increase many-fold from its low initial value. At the opposite extreme, the unstressed heart extracts 10 to 12 vol %, so coronary PvO_2 is only about 25 torr. Blood flow per gram of myocardium is by no means low; it is merely low *relative to* $\dot{V}O_2$. The heart's small extraction reserve renders it particularly flow-dependent.

Plateau of the Dissociation Curve

The flat portion or plateau of the dissociation curve is a major safety factor against hypoxemia from any cause. Note in Figure 17-2 that blood is at least 90 percent saturated until PaO_2 drops below 60 torr. Consequently, PaO_2 can fall 95 − 60 = 35 torr with little change in O_2 content. This safety factor alone is sufficient to defend CaO_2 against hypoxemia in most clinical situations. Since it is "built into" the Hb molecule it is recruited automatically. The cost is intolerance for additional hypoxemia. For example, if a drug-intoxicated patient with hypoventilation and PaO_2 of 60 torr develops a lung infection, as often happens, $\dot{V}A/\dot{Q}$ decreases, the A-a gradient increases, and arterial saturation falls precipitously. Proper preventive medicine requires that the physician be aware that the *patient's status is precarious if the arterial point is at the inflection of the dissociation curve*.

Steep Slope of the Dissociation Curve

If PaO_2 is normal, the steep slope of the dissociation curve is a safety factor in that it minimizes the large step in PO_2 from arterial to venous blood. Notice in Figure 17-2 that PO_2 must fall 55 torr to release 5 vol % if PaO_2 is 95, but only 8 torr if PaO_2 is 35 torr. The actual fall can be even less than 8 torr if there is sufficient time for adaptive change in the O_2 affinity of Hb.

O_2 Affinity and the Bohr Effect

The PO_2 at which Hb is 50 percent saturated (P_{50}) is a measure of O_2 affinity. The P_{50} of Hb in blood of normal human adults is 26 torr at pH 7.4 and 37°C. Fetal Hb differs from adult Hb in that two of its four polypeptide chains are of the γ rather than β type. This shifts the dissociation curve of fetal hemoglobin to the left; its P_{50} is 20 torr. A low P_{50} is adaptive in that it promotes loading at the placental tension of about 40 torr. On the other hand, a left-shifted dissociation curve lowers the PO_2 in systemic capillaries. The fetus tolerates low capillary and tissue PO_2 because of its high capacity for anaerobic metabolism. It rapidly loses this capacity, however, after birth. Greater dependence on O_2 requires replacement of fetal Hb with adult Hb. Replacement is 90 percent complete in three months.

Hemoglobin is one of the best examples of allosteric control of protein function. CO_2 reacts with Hb to form carbaminohemoglobin, which has less affinity for O_2. CO_2 also generates H^+ from dissociation of H_2CO_3. H^+ binding to oxyhemoglobin decreases O_2 affinity and releases bound O_2. These changes, called the Bohr effect, shift the dissociation curve to the right. Temperature also modifies O_2 binding. Thus we must imagine not one dissociation curve but a family of curves, depending on PCO_2, pH, and temperature.

Affinity changes are particularly adaptive in heavy exercise. At point $\bar{V}_3$ in Figure 17-2, blood at 37°C and normal PCO_2 and pH would be 48 percent saturated. If temperature, pH, and PCO_2 in exercise were 39°C, 7.15, and 70 torr, respectively, the P_{50} would be 37 torr instead of 26 torr. The net effect could be to increase extraction, as shown by the vertical arrow. Notice that release of this extra O_2 costs nothing in capillary PO_2. Alternatively, the curve shift could raise PO_2 in muscle capillaries and increase $P\bar{v}O_2$, as shown by the horizontal arrow. In most cases both extraction and capillary PO_2 would rise.

The Bohr shift is also important in pulmonary capillaries. Loss of CO_2 to alveolar air increases the affinity of Hb for O_2. At the same time the rise in blood PO_2 reduces affinity of Hb for CO_2. Thus the two respiratory gases promote each other's transport.

2,3-Diphosphoglycerate

Polyphosphate anions bind to allosteric groups in the β chains and stabilize the deoxy- configuration of Hb. The most important of these anions is 2,3-diphosphoglycerate (2,3-DPG), an intermediate in glycolysis. Any condition associated with low tissue PO_2 stimulates production of 2,3-DPG and shifts the dissociation curve to the right. Figure 17-3 illustrates a maximal change that raises $P\bar{v}O_2$ 9 torr. To achieve the same increase in $P\bar{v}O_2$ without a curve shift would require a 40 percent increase in cardiac output! The shift is largest between 20 and 40 torr, so organs with large extractions derive maximum benefit, and loading of Hb in the lungs is unaffected. After a week in a blood bank the 2,3-DPG concentration falls sharply, and the dissociation curve shifts to the left. Use of large volumes of such blood can be dangerous because capillary PO_2 must fall to lower than normal values to release the required amount of O_2.

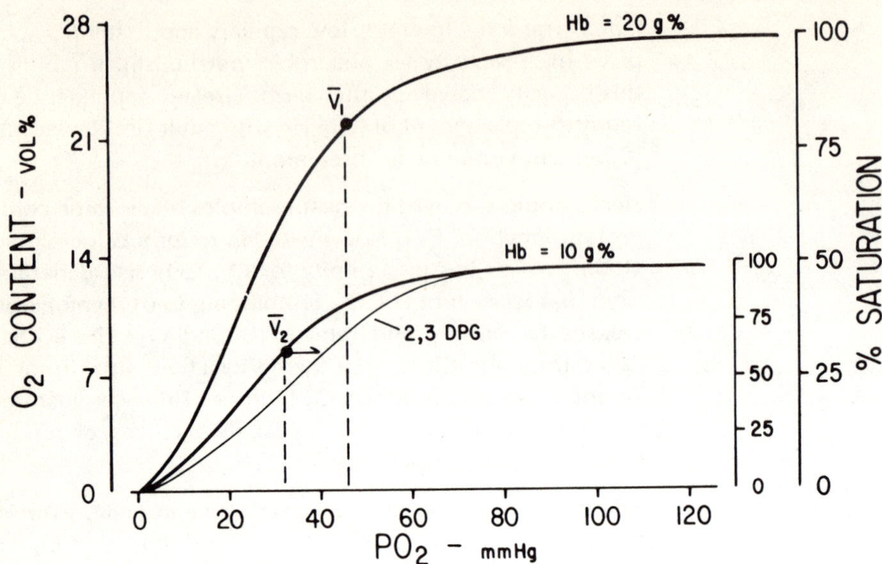

Figure 17-3
Oxyhemoglobin dissociation curves in anemia (*10 g* Hb per 100 ml) and polycythemia (*20 g* Hb per 100 ml). Note differences in scales of ordinates. Symbols and conditions are defined in the text.

Clinical Application

Polycythemia and Anemia

The rate of production of erythrocytes in the bone marrow can be increased about sixfold. This reserve capacity is mobilized in certain types of anemia, and in arterial hypoxemia, by a low-molecular-weight glycoprotein called erythropoietin. Dissociation curves for polycythemia (Hb = 20 g/100 ml) and anemia (10 g/100 ml) are shown in Figure 17-3. O_2 content (*left ordinate*) applies to both curves. The percent saturation is independent of [Hb], so a compressed saturation scale is required in anemia. If we assume a mean extraction of 5 vol %, $P\bar{v}O_2$ at the higher [Hb] (*point* $\bar{V}_1$) would be 46 torr. This is 6 torr higher than if the [Hb] were 15 g per 100 ml because less O_2 must be extracted from each red cell. The percent saturation is therefore higher and corresponds to a higher $P\bar{v}O_2$. Alternatively, a person with a high [Hb] could have a normal $P\bar{v}O_2$ despite lower than normal cardiac output.

The reverse of the above logic can be applied to anemia. In this case each red cell must release a higher percentage of its O_2, so change in percent saturation and $PcapO_2$ is larger for the same O_2 extraction. Compensation for anemia relies largely on increased flow to decrease the O_2 flux per red cell. If the anemia is chronic, 2,3-DPG contributes to adaptation. One should bear in mind the need for extra flow in anemia in evaluating the impact of a relatively small decrease in [Hb] in those whose flow reserves are compromised.

A change in [Hb] is usually accompanied by proportional change in hematocrit. Recall from Chapter 7 that viscosity and resistance are about 50 percent greater than normal at a hematocrit of 60% and rise very steeply above that value. Consequently, cardiac work often increases greatly in polycythemia, even though cardiac output tends to be lower. The fall in viscosity in anemia is relatively small, and its effect on cardiac work is more than offset by the concomitant increase in heart rate and cardiac output.

The Reserve of Intracellular PO_2

If O_2 offered (the product of flow and CaO_2) decreases, or O_2 extraction increases, or both, $PcapO_2$ falls. Cell PO_2 must fall as well, to maintain the transcapillary *difference* in PO_2 required to support the flux. For example, mean intracellular PO_2 in red skeletal muscle is about 30 torr at rest and falls to about 5 torr in moderate exercise. The 25-torr drop in cell PO_2 helps compensate for the drop in $PcapO_2$ that accompanies the increase in O_2 extraction in exercise. *Since the critical* PO_2 *for* $\dot{V}O_2$ *is less than 0.5 torr, low cell* PO_2 *relative to blood is by no means deleterious.* Quite the contrary; it is an essential adaptation to high $\dot{V}O_2$.

The sole function of an intracellular PO_2 greater than about 0.5 torr is to permit diffusion from the cell surface to the cell interior. Recall from Figure 16-3 that the ΔPO_2 from sarcolemma to remote mitochondria is only a few torr in myoglobin-containing cells. Other strategies for minimizing the intracellular ΔPO_2 include small cell size, peripherally distributed mitochondria, and high capillary density.

The Capillary Reserve

Intracellular PO_2 is determined by the transcapillary resistance to O_2 transport, RO_2, as well as by the transcapillary ΔPO_2. RO_2 is shown as a wavy line in Figure 17-1 to indicate its strong dependence on flux density and red cell transit time. RO_2 can be greatly reduced by increasing capillary hematocrit, perfusing more capillaries, or both. Capillary recruitment also shortens the intracellular diffusion path and thereby decreases the ΔPO_2 from cell surface to cell interior.

The capillary reserve is particularly important in heart, brain, and skeletal muscle, which must adapt to large changes in $\dot{V}O_2$. Capillary growth expands the capillary reserve in persons with chronically low PaO_2 and in physiological hypertrophy of heart and skeletal muscles. In pathological cardiac hypertrophy, however, and in many cancers, growth of tissue cells outpaces capillary growth, and the capillary reserve is compromised.

Reserves and safety factors for O_2 transport are summarized below:

1. The expansion factor for $\dot{V}A$ is much greater than for $\dot{V}O_2$.
2. Cardiac output can increase three- to fivefold in health.
3. Cardiac output can be redistributed to sites of high $\dot{V}O_2$.
4. The Hb dissociation curve is flat above 60 torr.
5. The Hb dissociation curve is steep below 50 torr.
6. The O_2 affinity of Hb can decrease in defense of $PcapO_2$.
7. Extraction can be increased by lowering $PcapO_2$.
8. The main resistance to O_2 transport can be reduced by capillary recruitment and increased capillary hematocrit.
9. Intracellular PO_2 can fall almost to zero in defense of the transcapillary PO_2 gradient, because
10. Mitochondria require only 0.01 torr for maximum $\dot{V}O_2$.
11. In heart and skeletal muscle, myoglobin facilitates O_2 diffusion and stabilizes intracellular PO_2.

You probably *understand* the ideas in Part III perfectly. However, you do not *know* them, because you have not yet used them to solve problems. Plan to spend as much time on the problems as on the text.

References

1. Cole, R. Skeletal muscle function in hypoxia: Effect of alteration of intracellular myoglobin. *Respir. Physiol.* 53:1, 1983.
2. Grover, R. F., Wagner, W. W., Jr., McMurty, I. F., and Reeves, J. T. Pulmonary Circulation. In J. T. Shepherd and F. M. Abboud (eds.), *Handbook of Physiology,* Section 2: The Cardiovascular System, Vol. III. Peripheral Circulation and Organ Blood Flow, Part 1. Bethesda, Md.: American Physiological Society, 1983.
3. Hurtado, A. Animals in High Altitudes: Resident Man. In D. B. Dill, E. F. Adolph, and C. G. Wilber (eds.), *Handbook of Physiology.* Washington, D.C.: American Physiological Society, 1964. Pp. 843–858.

*4. Kreuzer, F., and Hoofd, L. Facilitated diffusion of oxygen and carbon dioxide. In: L. E. Fahri and S. M. Tenney, (eds.), Handbook of Physiology, Section 3: The Respiratory System. Volume IV: Gas Exchange. Bethesda, Md. American Physiological Society, 1987.

5. Reneau, D. D., and Silver, I. A. Some effects of high altitude and polycythaemia on oxygen delivery. *Adv. Exp. Med. Biol.* 94:245, 1978.

*6. Thomas, H. M., Lefrak, S. S., Irwin, R. S., Fritts, H. W., Jr., and Caldwell, P. R. B. The oxyhemoglobin dissociation curve in health and disease: Role of 2,3-diphosphoglycerate. *Am. J. Med.* 57:331, 1974.

IV : Regional Circulation and Vasomotor Mechanisms

18 : Mechanisms of Vasomotor Control

This chapter is concerned with the properties of vascular smooth muscle and with neural and non-neural mechanisms of vasomotor control.

Vascular Smooth Muscle

Ultrastructure and the Length-Tension Relation

In smooth muscle, long, thin filaments composed of actin and tropomyosin are collated into bundles by structures homologous with the Z discs. The similarity of the length-tension relation in smooth muscle to that of striated muscle strongly suggests a sliding filament mechanism, but linearly repetitive filament arrays comparable to sarcomeres have not been identified in the former. A further uncertainty is the locus and state of aggregation of myosin. Cells suitably fixed in situ contain single myosin molecules or myosin dimers. On the other hand, thick filaments up to 8 μm long (!) can be found in smooth-muscle cells fixed under different conditions. Either arrangement, long filaments or dimers, is consistent with the unique length-tension relation of smooth muscle.

The length dependence of tension development for bovine mesenteric vein is shown in Figure 18-1. The salient feature for all smooth muscle is the enormous range of lengths over which they function. This range allows for large changes in the volume of hollow organs. The shaded region indicates the comparatively small range of lengths imposed on striated muscle by its precise sarcomere structure.

Mechanochemistry

Regulation of smooth muscle tension depends on Ca^{++} and a 20,000-dalton component of myosin; troponin is not required. The Ca^{++} dependence of smooth muscle tension is shown by the solid curve in Figure 4-2, page 42. The curve is less steep than its counterpart in striated muscle. This wide regulatory range for Ca^{++} confers on smooth muscle a large *reserve of contractility.*

Attached cross-bridges are largely responsible for resistance to shortening in muscles generally. Bridges are broken by myosin

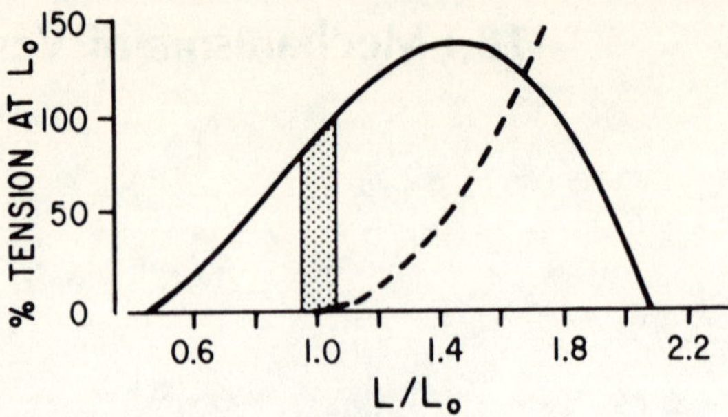

Figure 18-1
Length dependence of tension development in bovine mesenteric vein. Solid curve = length vs. active tension; dashed curve = length vs. passive tension; L_o = resting length. Shaded area indicates operating range for skeletal muscle in vivo. (Modified from R. J. Paul and J. W. Peterson, *Am. J. Physiol.* 228:915, 1975.)

ATPase, so the velocity of shortening depends on the ATPase activity of myosin. Smooth-muscle myosin splits ATP very slowly. This allows maintenance of tension at low rates of energy turnover. Thus a smooth muscle is specialized to contract slowly and maintain tension economically.

Resting Potential, Permeabilities, and Conduction

Resting potentials in vascular smooth muscles range from -30 to -60 mV, whereas E_{K^+} is about -90 mV. The discrepancy is partly due to low P_{K^+}. P_{Na^+} is about the same as in striated muscle and Cl^- appears to be passively distributed. Since the ratio P_{Na^+}/P_{K^+} is high at rest, neurohumoral mediators could control E_m and excitability by modulating g_{K^+}. E_m in smooth muscle is not simply a diffusion potential; it depends, in part, on an electrogenic Na^+-K^+ pump. Poisoning the pump increases excitability and induces contractions. Vascular muscle contains few nexuses, and the space constant is only 100 μm or less in arterioles. The fact that the cells are poorly coupled permits independent contraction and relaxation in adjacent vessels.

Action Potential and Excitation-Contraction Coupling

Some vessels exhibit spontaneous electrical activity; two examples are shown in Figure 18-2. The recording in *A* shows action potentials about 200 ms in duration arising from a typical pacemaker potential. The recording might well have been obtained from the sinoatrial node. The underlying mechanisms are also similar: Smooth muscle action potentials are unaffected by tetrodotoxin, are blocked by Ca^{++} channel antagonists, and are more sensitive to replacement of $Ca^{++}{}_o$ than $Na^+{}_o$. The mechanism of the pacemaker potential is not known.

In contrast to heart muscle, smooth-muscle tension long outlasts the action potential, so *summation of tension (tetanus) is*

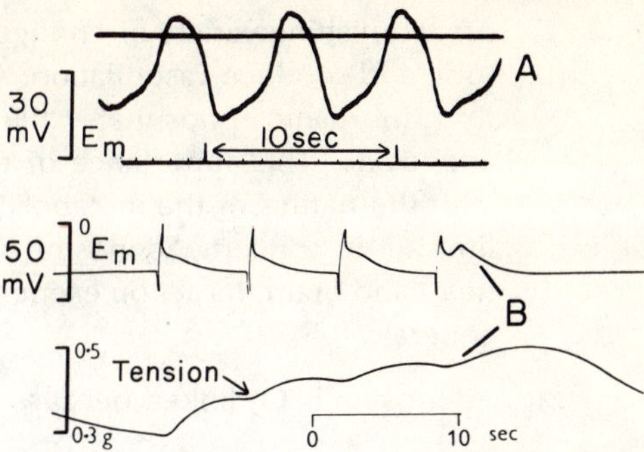

Figure 18-2
A. Spontaneous action potentials in cutaneous venule of frog. Similar recordings were obtained from small arteries. (From S. Funaki, *Nature* 191:1102, 1961.) B. Electrical activity in turtle vein (*top trace*) causes summation of tension (*bottom trace*). (Modified from I. C. Roddie, *J. Physiol.* [Lond.] 163:138, 1962.)

possible; see Figure 18-2*B*. Peak tension in smooth muscles of this type therefore depends on the frequency of action potentials and the duration of the action potential train. Repetition of trains is generally due to slow oscillations in E_m caused by the Na^+-K^+ pump. It is important to realize that small depolarizations can induce tension even without action potentials. Smooth-muscle contraction caused by either spontaneous action potentials, oscillations in E_m, or both partly accounts for tension in the vessel wall and resistance to flow. This intrinsic, non-neural component of active tension and resistance to blood flow is called *basal tone*.

Non-neural Controls of Vasomotor Tone

The Bayliss Response and Autoregulation

Smooth muscle resists stretch by contracting (increasing basal tone). Decreased stretch decreases basal tone and induces relaxation. This behavior is termed the myogenic, or Bayliss response. The usual cause of a change in length of vascular smooth muscle is a change in pressure. For example, a rise in arterial pressure stretches arterioles. Without active compensation, flow would increase greatly since resistance varies as radius to the fourth power. Instead, flow tends to remain constant as arterial pressure is varied over a wide range. An example is shown in Figure 20-3, page 207. This behavior is termed *autoregulation*. Autoregulation is important because the background stability that it creates permits nerves and metabolites to adjust flow and flow distribution in support of organ function.

Metabolic Controls

An astonishing variety of endogenous metabolites inhibit basal tone and produce vasodilation. A partial list includes CO_2, H^+, K^+, inorganic phosphate (Pi), adenine nucleotides, and adenosine. The importance of each varies among organs and with the nature of the metabolic stress. Often several metabolites act in concert. Adenosine seems particularly important in heart and brain. Its action exemplifies local metabolic control in general.

Adenosine is O_2 linked because it is derived from ATP:

$$\text{ATP} \xrightarrow{\text{ATPase}} \text{Pi} + \text{ADP} \rightarrow \text{to mitochondria, or}$$

$$\text{2ADP} \xrightleftharpoons{\text{myokinase}} \text{ATP} + \text{AMP}.$$

At low O_2 demand, the rate of ATP utilization is matched by the rate of oxidative phosphorylation in the mitochondria, and little AMP is produced. As O_2 demand increases, the myokinase equilibrium shifts to the right. AMP does not diffuse out of cells because of its charge, so its intracellular concentration rises. The enzyme 5′-nucleotidase is widely distributed in cell membranes:

$$\text{AMP} \xrightarrow{\text{5'-nucleotidase}} \text{Pi} + \text{adenosine}.$$

Adenosine is uncharged so it can cross cell membranes and diffuse to vascular smooth muscle. Adenosine and possibly other dilator metabolites may also be generated within the smooth-muscle cell itself. The action of adenosine is terminated by reuptake or by deamination to inosine, which is not vasoactive.

Mechanisms of Neural Control

The effect of stimulating the adrenergic nerve to an isolated pulmonary artery is shown in Figure 18-3*A*. Note that tension increases markedly without any change in E_m whatsoever. This *nonelectrical* activation can be duplicated with norepinephrine and various drugs; indeed, norepinephrine can induce contraction in some fully depolarized smooth muscles. Neurally induced nonelectrical smooth-muscle contraction is accompanied by a trivial change in Ca^{++} influx and is caused by release of Ca^{++} from an internal store. The amount of release depends on the amount stored, as determined by active transport across the sarcolemma. The transport mechanism discussed in Chapter 4 is directly applicable.

Not all vessels respond in this way. In some, norepinephrine and adrenergic nerves cause classical electrical activation; see Figure 18-3*B*, which is a recording from a cell in the guinea pig

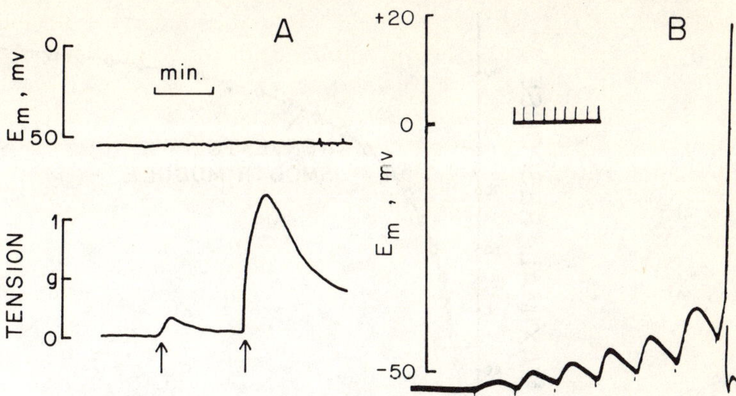

Figure 18-3
A. No electrical activity whatever is observed in pulmonary artery in vitro when the sympathetic nerve is stimulated at arrows (*top trace*). Despite electrical quiescence, stimulation evokes substantial tension (*bottom trace*). (Modified from C. Su, J. A. Bevan, and R. C. Ursillo, *Circ. Res.* 15:20, 1964. By permission of the American Heart Association, Inc.) B. Membrane potential of a smooth-muscle cell during repetitive stimulation of the hypogastric nerve; time marker = 100 ms. (From G. Burnstock and M. E. Holman, *J. Physiol.* [Lond.] 155:115, 1961.)

vas deferens. These cells behave like vascular muscle but yield better recordings. Each stimulus gives rise to a slow, nonregenerative nerve-muscle junction potential. Successive stimuli are larger (facilitation) and arise from a less negative potential until a smooth-muscle action potential is elicited. Most sympathetic nerves release norepinephrine from their endings and induce smooth-muscle contraction and vasoconstriction. *Such noradrenergic fibers are chiefly responsible for reflex regulation of arterial pressure.* A smaller population of special sympathetic nerves relax vascular muscle in skin and skeletal muscle. Relaxed vessels dilate because of passive distension by arterial pressure. Vasodilator nerves are thought to release acetylcholine, dopamine, or peptide transmitters that hyperpolarize the smooth-muscle membrane. Sympathetic vasodilator fibers fire only in support of specific functions. They are not involved in the reflex regulation of blood pressure.

Most sympathetic vasoconstrictor nerves exhibit action potentials even under basal conditions. Such nerves are said to be tonically active, and their discharge frequency is termed *sympathetic tone.* The relationship between sympathetic tone and smooth-muscle contraction is shown in Figure 18-4, curve *A.* (Curve *B* will be considered later.) Tension rises sharply at low frequencies, and half-maximum tension occurs at about 1 nerve action potential per second. Vasomotor nerves discharge at

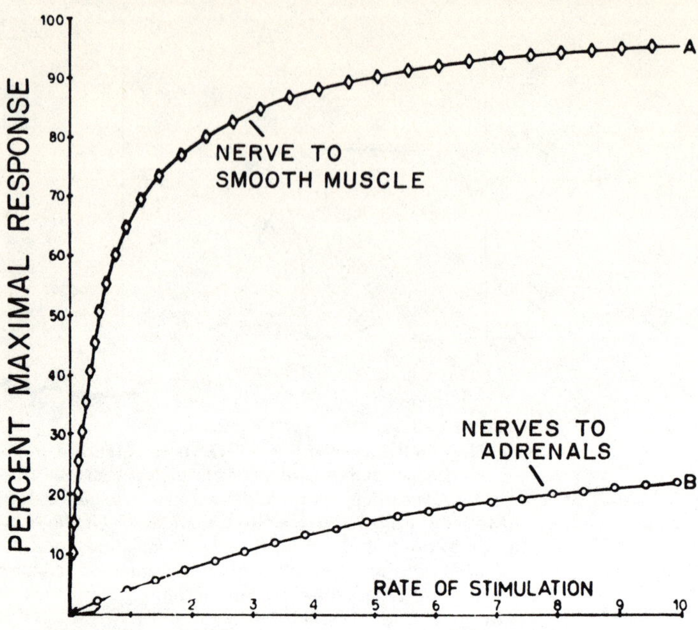

Figure 18-4
Frequency-response relation for nictitating membrane when stimulated via its nerves (*curve A*) and when stimulated indirectly by catecholamines released from the adrenal medulla (*curve B*). (Modified from O. Celander, *Acta Physiol. Scand.* 32 [Suppl. 116]:1, 1954.)

about 0.5 to 3.0 per second under most circumstances, so either constriction or dilation can be produced by varying sympathetic tone. It is important to recognize that *the principal mechanism for vasodilation during postural and baroreceptor reflexes is simply less sympathetic vasoconstriction.*

Interplay of Sympathetic Tone and Basal Tone

Sympathetic tone is superimposed on the basal tone of smooth muscle. The separate effects of the two determinants of resistance to blood flow are shown schematically in Figure 18-5. Sympathetic and basal tone largely determine the distribution of cardiac output. The heart and brain are metabolically active organs in which flow per gram must be large at all times. In these organs sympathetic tone is low, and flow is regulated mainly by non-neural controls of basal tone. In contrast, basal tone is low in organs concerned with environmental exchanges (gastrointestinal tract, lung, kidney), or absent altogether (thermoregulatory vessels in the skin of the face and digits). This provides maximum latitude to the central nervous system to regulate flow in the interests of the whole organism. For example, in persons supine and at rest, sympathetic tone to the renal vessels is very low, and basal tone is absent. Consequently, resistance is almost at a minimum. This explains why the kidney, which ac-

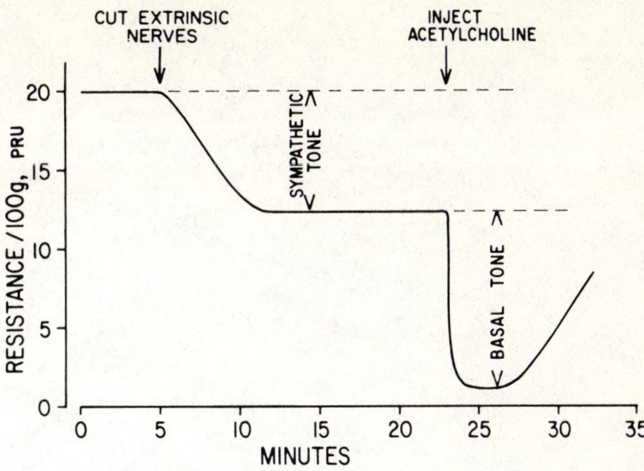

Figure 18-5
Components of resistance to blood flow.

counts for only 0.5 percent of body weight, receives about 20 percent of the cardiac output. During heavy exercise in human beings, sympathetic tone in the kidney increases markedly and renal blood flow is limited to a smaller fraction of cardiac output.

Metabolic and central neural controls operate as a system of checks and balances. Neural controls defend arterial pressure and optimize blood flow distribution in support of behavior. In so doing they may override local controls. On the other hand, metabolic controls can override neurally induced vasoconstriction to prevent ischemic injury.

Neural Pathways

Sympathetic preganglionic fibers originate in the intermediolateral column of the spinal cord and emerge in the ventral roots. Most synapse in the paravertebral sympathetic chains. However, about a third of all sympathetic fibers to limb vessels, and a smaller fraction to vessels of the trunk, do not enter the sympathetic chains. They travel instead with the spinal nerves and synapse in minute ganglia along the way. Sympathetic synapses are cholinergic, even though the final postganglionic neuron usually releases norepinephrine from its endings. Sympathetic synapses are subject to long-term modulation by slow postsynaptic potentials that may last several minutes! Such sustained responses are unusual in neurophysiology and help to explain the long duration of certain autonomic responses.

Sympathetic postganglionic fibers form a plexus in the vascular adventitia. In Figure 18-6*A*, an arteriolar branch in dog gracilis muscle is outlined by noradrenergic fibers. Near the smooth-

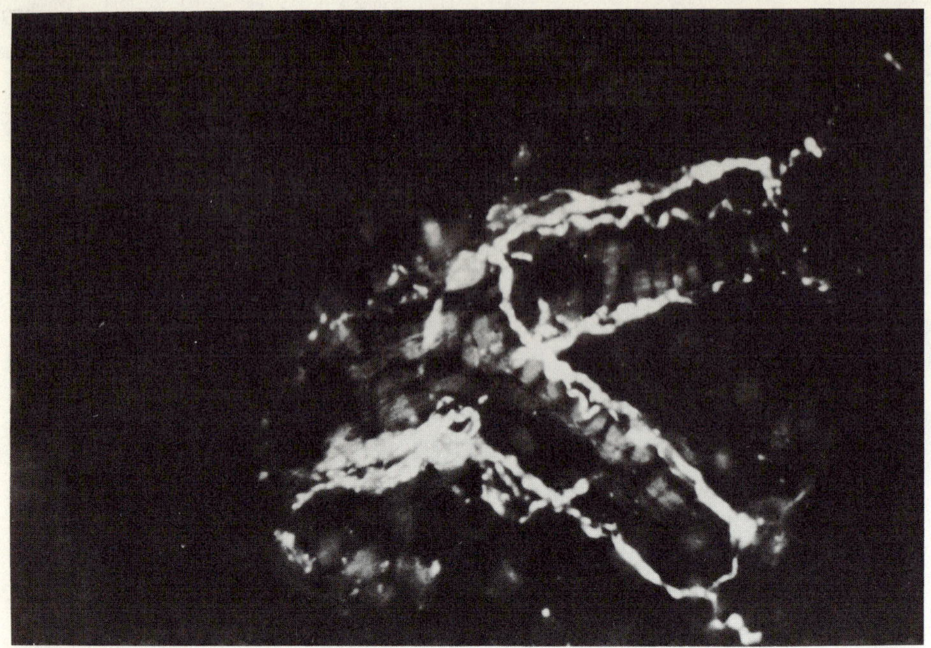

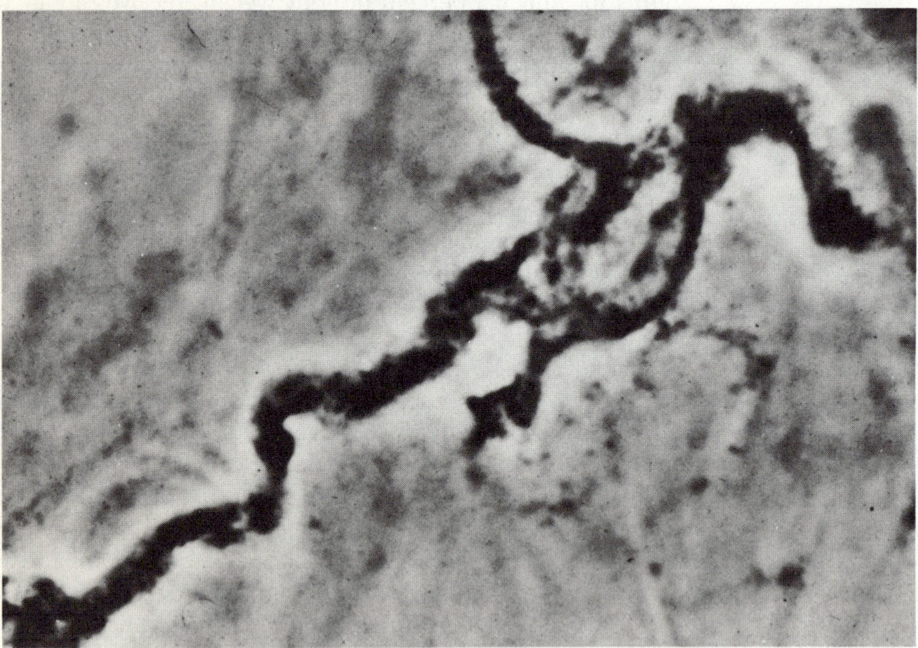

Figure 18-6
A. A rich adrenergic plexus outlines the bifurcation of an arteriole in dog gracilis muscle. The fibers are visualized by means of norepinephrine fluorescence, which appears white in the photograph. B. A neuronal cell body in an arteriole is outlined by a histochemical stain specific for acetylcholinesterase (Courtesy Dr. E. A. Schenk, University of Rochester School of Medicine, Rochester, N.Y.)

muscle cells the unmyelinated fibers exhibit varicosities 0.5 to 1.0 μm in diameter. Varicosities contain high concentrations of norepinephrine, packaged in small vesicles for release by nerve action potentials. Varicosities are particularly abundant in arterioles 25 to 100 μm in diameter. Recall that these arterioles are particularly important for control of blood flow.

Intrinsic Vasomotor Nerves

Parasympathetic vasomotor fibers originate in the brainstem, or the lateral gray matter of the sacral segments of the spinal cord, and synapse close to or within the organs innervated. The main fact to remember about these nerves is that they play no role in the reflex regulation of arterial pressure. They provide for arteriolar dilation in erectile tissue and in salivary and enteric glands.

If the nerves to an organ are cut, the peripheral ends degenerate and disappear within a few days. Vasomotor responses in such organs were therefore assumed to be non-neural. That assumption is no longer justified, since neuronal cell bodies have been found by histochemical techniques in the adventitia of small arteries and arterioles in all organs and animal species examined. An example is shown in Figure 18-6*B*, from an extrinsically denervated dog gracilis muscle. The synaptic connections and electrical properties of intrinsic vasomotor nerves are not known. Indirect evidence suggests, however, that they are involved in local vasodilator mechanisms.

Denervation Hypersensitivity

Receptors for norepinephrine are confined to patches of cell membrane adjacent to adrenergic nerve terminals. If the adrenergic nerve is destroyed, the entire cell surface becomes responsive to norepinephrine. The same mechanism occurs at cholinergic synapses. Proliferation of receptors accounts for the marked increase in sensitivity to acetylcholine or norepinephrine that accompanies denervation. Denervation supersensitivity limits the effectiveness of sympathectomy in treatment of hypertension and vasospastic disorders, for the vessels become highly responsive to circulating catecholamines.

Blood-borne Vasoactive Agents

Catecholamines

Action potential frequency recorded in the sympathetic nerve to the adrenal gland itself is less than 3 per second under normal circumstances and reaches 10 per second only in extremis—asphyxia, for example. Figure 18-4, curve *B*, shows how much smooth-muscle tension can be developed if the nerves to both adrenals are stimulated electrically. Even at 10 per second, tension is less than 20 percent of that observed when the membrane responds to norepinephrine released from its own sympathetic motor nerve (*curve A*). Similarly, levels of circulating catecholamines observed in conscious dogs during heavy exercise or hemorrhage do not notably increase cardiac contractility. Thus Walter B. Cannon's notion of the adrenal medulla as "the loud pedal of the sympathetic nervous system" is simply not correct. Sympathetic responses are far more specific, as emphasized in Chapters 23 and 26.

The true function of the adrenal medulla is in regulation of intermediary metabolism, and in this way it plays a supportive, though nonessential, role in circulation. Catecholamines increase the rate of O_2 consumption, accelerate glycolysis, raise glucose and lactate concentrations in blood, increase lipolysis, promote clotting, and modify the absorption of Na^+, Ca^{++}, and glucose from the intestine. Thresholds for these and other metabolic effects are 5 to 100 times less than the minimum blood concentrations required to modify circulation.

Angiotensins and Aldosterone

The kidney is a major endocrine organ. The anatomy of its secretory apparatus is shown in Figure 18-7. The juxtaglomerular cells (really modified smooth muscle) synthesize, store, and release into the blood an acid protease called *renin*. Renin's only biological effect is to cleave the decapeptide angiotensin I (AI) from an α-globulin substrate found in plasma. An enzyme in vascular endothelium rapidly converts AI to the octapeptide angiotensin II (AII). The lungs are particularly rich in converting enzyme; from 60 to 100 percent of AI is converted in a single passage. AII is among the most powerful vasoconstrictor substances known for the renal, cutaneous, and splanchnic beds. Its influence in skeletal muscle varies among species, and it has little effect on pulmonary, coronary, cerebral, and postcapillary vessels. AII is a weak cardiac stimulant; doses that raise arterial pressure usually decrease cardiac output because of reflex bradycardia. AII is degraded by various peptidases into angiotensin III (AIII) and inactive compounds.

It is unfortunate that the angiotensins were named before all their physiological effects were discovered. We now know that their principal function in vivo is in the maintenance of water and electrolyte balance and the regulation of blood volume. Angiotensins selectively stimulate synthesis and release of aldosterone by the adrenal cortex. Aldosterone plays an essential role in water and electrolyte balance by promoting the retention of sodium and excretion of potassium, chiefly by the kidney. Angiotensins cross the blood-brain barrier via special capillaries beneath the lining of the third and fourth ventricles. There they

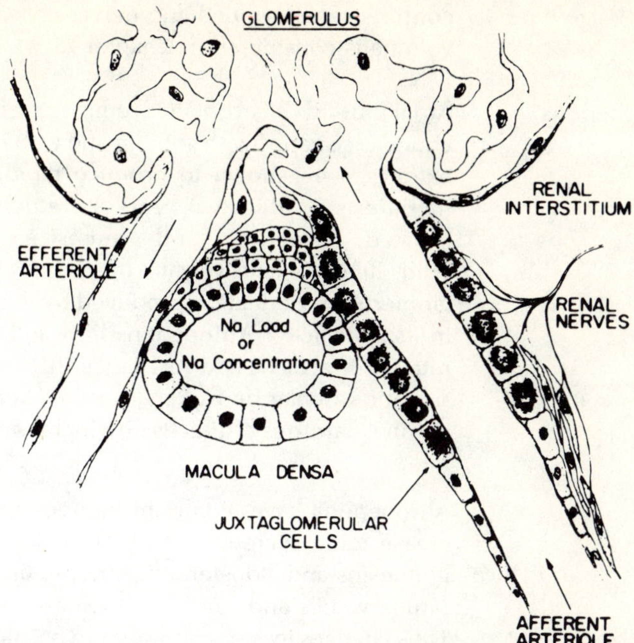

Figure 18-7
Juxtaglomerular apparatus. Granules in juxtaglomerular cells contain renin. Renal nerves end on both the juxtaglomerular cells and the adjacent smooth muscle of the afferent arteriole. (From J. O. Davis, *Circ. Res.* 28:301, 1971. By permission of the American Heart Association, Inc.)

stimulate neuroendocrine structures that promote drinking and the release of antidiuretic hormone by the pituitary. In the absence of Na^+ depletion, the metabolic effects of angiotensins are manifest at concentrations well below those required for vasoconstriction. Thus the angiotensins, like the catecholamines, play no direct role in regulation of arterial pressure under normal circumstances. Nevertheless, they affect arterial pressure indirectly through defense of fluid balance and blood volume. The biological half-lives of AII and AIII are about 60 and 30 s, respectively. In contrast, the half-life of renin is 15 to 30 minutes. Consequently, the principal control of the entire peptide cascade is the rate of renin release.

There are three independent stimuli to renin release: (1) Renin secretion is inversely proportional to the rate of sodium chloride delivery to the distal renal tubule. (2) Renin secretion is enhanced by decreased arterial pressure in the kidney. (3) An increase in firing rate in the renal sympathetic nerves promotes renin release through direct secretomotor innervation of the juxtaglomerular cells. Consequently, fear, anxiety, exercise, orthostatic stress, and decreased circulating blood volume are all powerful stimuli to release of renin. The regulatory system that controls renal sympathetic nerve activity in defense of blood volume is considered in Chapter 25.

Atriopeptins

Atrial muscle cells contain prominent secretory granules whose abundance varies with sodium and water balance. In 1981, atrial extracts were shown to produce rapid, massive diuresis and natriuresis. Within two years the *atriopeptin* hormones were isolated, sequenced, and synthesized. Labelled atriopeptins bind almost exclusively to the renal arteries, arterioles, and glomeruli. Vasodilation produced by these hormones is unique in its specificity: Atriopeptins have little or no effect on heart rate, contractility, and resistance in coronary, splanchnic, and somatic vascular beds. Renal vasodilation could produce diuresis and natriuresis directly, by increasing glomerular filtration rate.

Atriopeptins have important indirect actions as well. They decrease renin secretion and thereby lower plasma levels of angiotensins and aldosterone. Atriopeptins also bind to posterior pituitary cells and can inhibit release of antidiuretic hormone. Thus changes in water and sodium balance are brought about by *reciprocal neuroendocrine controls.*

Clinical Application

Vasomotor Effects of Angiotensins in Na^+ Depletion

Salt depletion greatly elevates the plasma concentration of angiotensins. Na^+ depletion may occur in vomiting, diarrhea, and profuse sweating and in patients treated with diuretics or low-Na^+ diets. The effect of endogenous angiotensins on the ability of a normal person to tolerate orthostatic stress is shown in Figure 18-8. In a person with a normal Na^+ intake (*salt repleted,* left panel), tilting from the supine to the upright position increased heart rate. Pulse pressure fell, but mean pressure remained the same. Since angiotensins are difficult to measure in blood, the response of the renin-angiotensin system was assayed as change in the activity of plasma renin. Plasma renin activity (*PRA* in Figure 18-8) and plasma aldosterone (*PA*) were significantly increased. After 30 minutes the subject was returned to the supine position. PRA returned to normal in 30 minutes. A half hour thereafter, upright tilt was repeated in the presence of a highly specific converting enzyme inhibitor (*C.E.I.* in Figure 18-8). Since angiotensin I could no longer be converted to angiotensin II, PRA increased markedly, but PA remained low. Hemodynamic responses were unchanged, showing that angiotensins are not required for pressure regulation under normal circumstances.

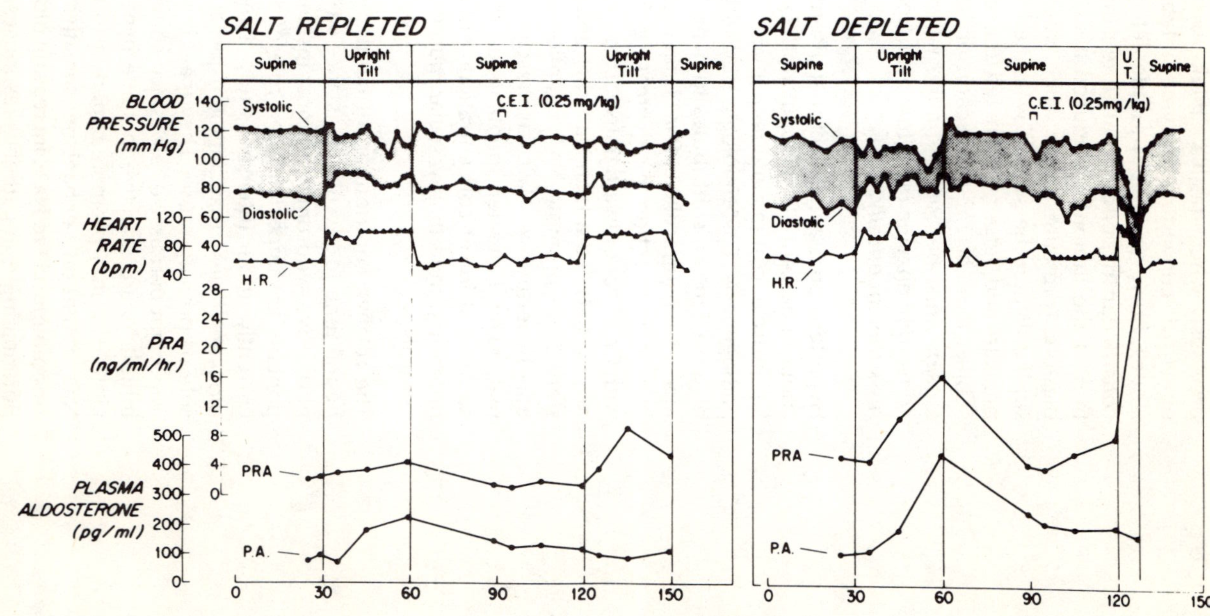

Figure 18-8
Tolerance to orthostatic stress is the same in the presence and absence of angiotensin when sodium stores are normal (*left panel*). After sodium depletion (*right panel*), the same stress causes hypotension and fainting. Abbreviations are defined in the text. (From J. Sancho, R. Re, J. Burton, A. C. Barger, and E. Haber, *Circulation* 53:400, 1976. By permission of the American Heart Association, Inc.)

The same subject was retested after 3 days on a diet containing 10 mEq Na^+ and 100 mEq K^+ (*salt depleted,* right panel, Figure 18-8). This time tilt produced much larger changes in PRA and PA, but the hemodynamic response was similar to that observed previously when the Na^+ intake was normal. The effect of converting enzyme inhibition demonstrates, however, that in salt-depleted states, vasoconstriction depends on angiotensins. Administration of the inhibitor produced a significant fall in diastolic pressure even when the subject was supine. When the subject was tilted upright, mean pressure and pulse pressure fell dramatically and the subject fainted. *The interaction of Na^+ and angiotensins must be borne in mind when one is using converting enzyme inhibitors or angiotensin antagonists therapeutically.*

Mechanisms Underlying Hypertension

Hypertension is a multifactorial disorder that affects about 15 percent of the population. Excessive vascular muscle contraction is a major factor in the pathogenesis. Epidemiologic studies indicate that a high Na^+ intake contributes to hypertension in humans. High intracellular $[Na^+]$ can promote smooth-muscle contraction by decreasing E_m, competing with Ca^{++} for outward transport, or modifying $P_{Ca^{++}}$ or P_{K^+}. Rats fed a high-Na^+ diet and given adrenal steroids to promote Na^+ retention become markedly hypertensive. Vascular muscles from such animals exhibit greater spontaneous rhythmicity and contract at lower concentrations of Ca^{++}, K^+, and norepinephrine than vascular muscles from normal controls.

The relative contribution of basal and sympathetic neural tone to vascular resistance varies among hypertensive syndromes. In most instances both components are important. The role of angiotensins is currently under intensive study. Effects of specific blockers reveal that angiotensins are seldom the sole or primary cause. They may, however, play an important permissive role, since converting enzyme inhibitors are effective in some hypertensives. Angiotensins may promote hypertension by increasing Na^+ retention, enhancing sensitivity of vascular smooth muscle to Na^+, increasing blood volume, or potentiating sympathetic responses. Atriopeptins lower arterial pressure in some animal models of hypertension. Their role as direct vasodilators and as antagonists to angiotensins in human hypertension remains to be determined.

References

1. Atlas, S. A., Volpe, M., Sosa, R. E., Laragh, J. H., Camargo, M. J. F., and Maack, T. Effects of atrial natriuretic factor on blood pressure and the renin-angiotensin-aldosterone system. *Fed. Proc.* 45:2115, 1986.

2. Burnstock, G., and Bell, C. Peripheral Autonomic Transmission. In J. I. Hubbard (ed.), *The Peripheral Nervous System*. New York: Plenum, 1974.

3. Crass, M. F., and Barnes, D. C. *Vascular Smooth Muscle: Metabolic, Ionic and Contractile Mechanisms*. New York: Academic, 1982.

*4. Davis, J. O., and Freeman, R. H. Mechanisms regulating renin release. *Physiol. Rev.* 56:1, 1976.

5. Peach, M. J. Renin-angiotensin system: Biochemistry and mechanisms of action. *Physiol. Rev.* 57:313, 1977.

6. Ray, B. S., and Console, A. D. Residual sympathetic pathways after paravertebral sympathectomy. *J. Neurosurg.* 5:23, 1948.

7. Siegman, M. J., Butler, T. M., Mooers, S. V., and Davis, R. E. Chemical energetics of force development, force maintenance and relaxation in mammalian smooth muscle. *J. Gen. Physiol.* 76:609, 1980.

*8. Sparks, H. V., Jr. Effect of Local Metabolic Factors on Vascular Smooth Muscle. In *Handbook of Physiology,* Section 2: The Cardiovascular System—Vascular Smooth Muscle, Vol. II. Bethesda, Md.: American Physiological Society, 1980.

9. Van Breemen, C., Aaronson, P., and Loutzenhiser, R. Sodium-calcium interactions in mammalian smooth muscle. *Pharmacol. Rev.* 30:167, 1979.

10. Young, M. A., Hintze, T. H., and Vatner, S. F. Correlation between cardiac performance and plasma catecholamine levels in conscious dogs. *Am. J. Physiol.* 248:H82, 1985.

19 : The Coronary Circulation

Atherosclerosis is epidemic wherever a large segment of the population is exposed to stress, tobacco, and a luxus diet. In the United States, coronary artery disease is responsible for about one-third of deaths from all causes among people between 40 and 60 years of age. The reason atherosclerosis is so life-threatening lies in the physiology of the coronary and cerebral circulations, summarized in Tables 19-1 and 20-1.

The Coronary Vessels

The Macromesh

The heart is supplied by the right and left coronary arteries, which arise just distal to the aortic valve. The relative importance of the two main arteries is genetically determined. In fortunate people, neither is dominant, and their branches anastomose freely. The large arteries penetrate the wall from epicardium to endocardium, perpendicular to the long axes of the circumferentially oriented muscle fibers. At each level, branches give rise to arcades of highly branched arterioles. High flow is essential for cardiac function, yet a large vasodilator reserve is required for adaptation to stress. The exceptionally short lengths of coronary arterioles minimize resistance and permit substantial vasoconstrictor tone under basal conditions.

The Micromesh

Each terminal arteriole gives rise to a sheaf of interconnected capillaries. There are about three times as many coronary capillaries per volume of tissue as in red skeletal muscle; about half are actively perfused at rest. The abundance of coronary capillaries minimizes both O_2 flux density and red cell velocity. A large component of flow is perpendicular to the long axis of the capillaries, via branches and anastomoses. Consequently, the red cell flow path from arteriole to venule greatly exceeds the length of a single capillary. Relatively low velocities and long path lengths prolong red cell transit times. The foregoing capillary adaptions lower the ΔPO_2 required for blood-tissue O_2 transport and permit high O_2 extraction even at maximal rates of

Table 19-1
Summary of Physiology of Normal Coronary Circulation

Characteristics and Requirements
$\dot{V}O_2$/g is always high
Anaerobic capacity is small relative to ATP demand
Therefore, flow/g must always be large
Large capillary area is required
Cardiac $\dot{V}O_2$ may increase fivefold, so
Flow and capillary density must be closely coupled to $\dot{V}O_2$
Problems
Blood flow/g is low relative to $\dot{V}O_2$/g, so
Extraction is large at rest, and extraction reserve is small
Vascular compression increases resistance in systole, so
Coronary flow occurs mainly in diastole
Time for diastolic flow decreases if heart rate increases
Systolic resistance increases from epicardium to endocardium, causing
Transmural gradients in vasodilator reserve and capillary reserve
Adaptations
Flow and $\dot{V}O_2$ tend to change proportionately, so
Extraction does not increase during moderate work
Small myocytes permit high capillary density
Flow and capillary density are higher in subendocardium
Metabolic controls are more powerful than neural controls
Myoglobin promotes O_2 extraction, facilitates diffusion, and buffers PO_2
Coronary collaterals compensate for local obstruction

coronary blood flow. Thus the coronary O_2 exchanger is admirably designed for high $\dot{V}O_2$.[1]

Clinical Application

Should a large vessel become occluded, some cells may not survive. Around them is a zone of injured but viable tissue. Recent experiments indicate that this so-called border zone is less than 1 mm wide, so the line of demarcation between normal and dead tissue is very sharp. This is hardly surprising; since mitochondria function normally to a PO_2 of about 0.1 torr, the transition between normoxia and anoxia must take place over a short distance. Around the border zone is a much larger region (on the order of centimeters) precariously supplied by collaterals. These collaterals connect the vascular bed distal to the site of obstruction to unoccluded portions of the

[1] If you did not follow the reasoning in the preceding paragraph reread Chapter 16, pages 154 to 157 before continuing.

macromesh. Collaterals initially have little or no vasodilator reserve, and their resistance even at maximum dilation is much higher than that of normal pathways. Consequently, if normal vessels dilate, as in exercise, flow will be diverted away from collaterals. The same would occur in hypotension. The phenomenon has been called "coronary steal." Tissue at risk of becoming anoxic if flow decreases, or $\dot{V}O_2$ increases, constitutes a large *hemodynamic* border zone. It is to be distinguished clearly from the small biochemical border zone. Growth of new collaterals begins in days and is complete in about six months. New collaterals may become so abundant that flow in the region they supply is normal, even during moderate exercise.

A system of small vessels connects the ventricular lumen with the main capillary bed. Though luminal vessels account for only 2 percent of ventricular flow, they supply the chordae tendineae and the main branches of the Purkinje net. In people with coronary occlusion, luminal vessels maintain viability of a 0.5- to 1.0-mm rim of tissue beneath the endocardium. This luminal supply minimizes the incidence of valve dysfunction, conduction disorders, and arrhythmias.

Myocardial Metabolism

The heart accounts for roughly 12 percent of whole body energy turnover under basal conditions, even though it is only 0.5 percent of body weight. About 80 percent of cardiac energy turnover is attributable to contraction per se. Since virtually all this energy is derived from aerobic metabolism, cardiac $\dot{V}O_2$ is enormous — about 8 ml/100 g · min in the unstressed heart. For comparison, the $\dot{V}O_2$ of resting skeletal muscle is about 0.2 ml/100 g · min. The expansion factor for myocardial $\dot{V}O_2$ is 3 to 4 in young adults and 5 to 6 in well-trained athletes. The $\dot{V}O_2$ of maximally working hearts is 40 to 50 ml/100 g · min, 250-fold greater than that of resting skeletal muscle, and far greater than that of any other maximally working organ or tissue. This incredible performance requires high flow to maximize O_2 offered and an efficient capillary O_2 exchanger to maximize O_2 extraction. A maximally working dog heart can extract 90% of the O_2 in coronary arterial blood and lower coronary venous PO_2 to 10 torr without anoxic loci in the myocytes!

The heart is not particular about its fuel: It oxidizes glucose, lactate, keto-acids, fatty acids, and certain amino acids in proportion to their concentrations in arterial blood. Under normal

Table 19-2
Summary of Determinants of Myocardial O_2 Supply and Demand

I. Determinants of O_2 demand
   A. Wall tension
      1. Diastolic volume (preload)
      2. Ventricular systolic pressure (afterload)
   B. Heart rate
   C. External work
   D. Sympathetic drive
   E. $\dot{V}O_2$, nonbeating heart
II. Determinants of O_2 supply
   A. Pressure gradients
      1. Aortic systolic pressure minus systolic tissue pressure
      2. Aortic diastolic pressure minus diastolic tissue pressure
      3. Transmural distribution of tissue pressure
   B. Diastolic time
   C. O_2 offered (flow times CaO_2)
      1. Total coronary resistance
      2. Vasodilator reserve
      3. Heart rate
      4. Collaterals
      5. [Hb]
      6. PaO_2
   D. O_2 extracted
      1. $PcapO_2$ minus $PcellO_2$
      2. Transcapillary resistance to O_2 transport
      3. Capillary reserve
   E. Intracellular O_2 distribution
      1. Capillary density
      2. Functions of myoglobin

circumstances the heart derives about two-thirds of its energy from fatty acids. Glycogen and anaerobic enzymes are distributed throughout the myocardium but are of particular importance for Purkinje fibers. In sharp contrast to skeletal muscle, the heart can incur only a small O_2 debt and can function anaerobically for only a few beats. Nevertheless, when O_2 limits ATP production, the heart breaks down glycogen and produces substantial amounts of lactate. Since the critical cardiac metabolite is O_2, coronary physiology is largely concerned with the dynamic balance between O_2 supply and demand. This "bank account" thinking is summarized in Table 19-2.

Myocardial O_2 Demand

The determinants of O_2 demand are considered individually in Chapter 1, pages 13 to 14. The following relates that information to the coronary circulation.

Wall Tension

Active wall tension is by far the largest item in the heart's energy budget. It depends on preload, afterload, and heart rate. A convenient, though empirical, index of total tension is the area under the systolic portion of the left ventricular pressure curve.

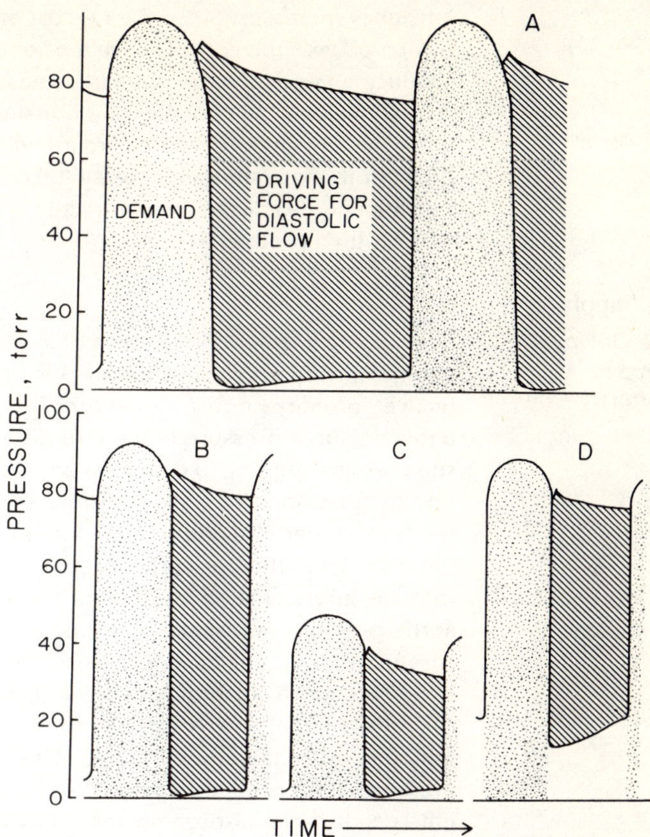

Figure 19-1
Stippled areas indicate the systolic tension-time integral, which is strongly correlated with O_2 demand. Shaded areas approximate the mean driving force for coronary blood flow. A. normal heart. B–D. Tachycardia shortens diastolic time and decreases the driving force. C. Hypotension lowers both demand and driving force. D. Driving force is reduced by high ventricular end-diastolic pressure. E. Effect shown is manifest mainly in subendocardium.

This area multiplied by heart rate is termed the *tension-time product*. This product and O_2 demand increase in tachycardia and aortic valve disease.

Metabolic Repair, External Work, and Ca^{++} Transport

The $\dot{V}O_2$ of the nonbeating heart represents the cost of maintenance and repair. It is surprisingly large — about 10 times the $\dot{V}O_2$ of resting skeletal muscle. Moreover, this obligatory O_2 demand can double in cardiac hypertrophy. External work amounts to only about 15 percent of total energy demand. During normal exercise, cardiac output and external work increase with little change in preload or afterload, so mechanical efficiency increases. Since the O_2 *cost of external work is small compared with the cost of active tension,* exercise that does not produce a large increase in heart rate is not a severe stress for cardiac patients. In contrast, emotional upsets can be very taxing if accompanied by tachycardia and increased sympathetic drive. Both these stresses increase the cost of Ca^{++} transport to activate and deactivate the contractile system, and increase the tension-time product as well.

O_2 Supply

The Driving Force for Coronary Flow

The beating heart inhibits its own blood supply, because muscle contraction squeezes and compresses coronary vessels. The effective coronary perfusion pressure is therefore the difference between aortic pressure tending to distend the vessels and tissue pressure tending to compress and narrow them. Because of this compression, the bulk of systolic coronary flow merely distends the superficial arteries and does not penetrate deeply into the wall. The effective coronary perfusion pressure can therefore be approximated by the difference between the mean aortic pressure in diastole and the mean intraventricular pressure in diastole. The latter serves as an estimate of tissue pressure. This approximation is shown as the shaded areas in Figure 19-1. Recall that tachycardia shortens diastolic time proportionately more than systolic time. This decreases the diastolic pressure–time product (Figure 19-1 B). The diastolic pressure-time product can also be decreased by a fall in aortic diastolic pressure (Figure 19-1 C) or by a rise in ventricular diastolic pressure (Figure 19-1 D). If the driving force for coronary flow falls, flow must be defended by appropriate change in coronary vascular resistance.

Coronary Resistance and Vasodilator Reserve

There are normally two components of coronary resistance: an extravascular component resulting from systolic compression and an intravascular component produced by vasomotor tone. The former accounts for one-fourth to one-third of the total. The throttling effect of systole is shown in Figure 19-2. A flow probe was placed on the left anterior descending coronary artery of a dog. Flow decreased sharply during isovolumic contraction, remained low throughout systole, and rose to a maximum in early diastole.

Diastolic flow is controlled by vascular smooth muscle. If tissue pressure, hypotension, or tachycardia reduces the diastolic pressure–time product, active vasodilation lowers the intravascular component of resistance to compensate. Tachycardia is a good example: *Total coronary flow increases linearly with heart rate* in normal persons, despite decreased diastolic time, be-

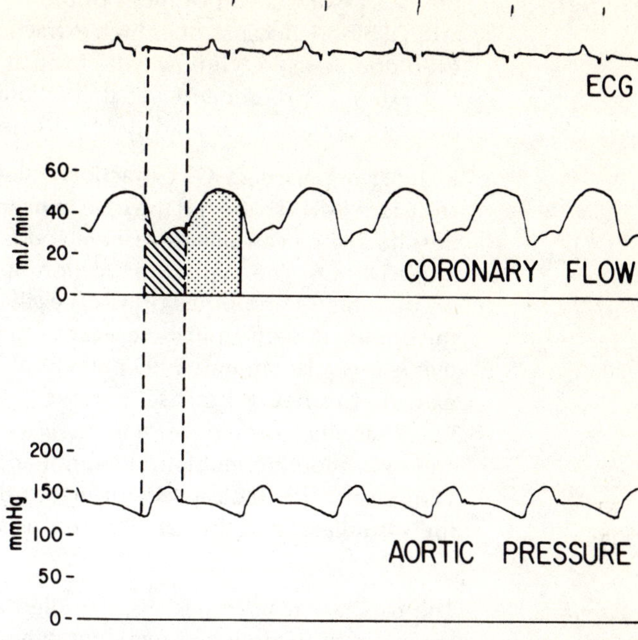

Figure 19-2
Electrocardiogram, aortic pressure, and blood flow in left anterior descending coronary artery of anesthetized dog. Systolic flow is shown as shaded area; diastolic flow, as stippled area.

cause of vasodilation brought about by metabolic controls. The example illustrates the importance of an adequate vasodilator reserve. All too often, however, the vasodilator reserve is heavily engaged at normal heart rate because of atherosclerosis. A sclerotic segment of a large coronary artery is a *fixed resistance in series* with arteriolar resistance. The ΔP across the narrowed arterial segment lowers coronary arteriolar pressure just as effectively as if aortic pressure had fallen because of hemorrhage. The decrease in driving force for flow is compensated for by lowering resistance of downstream arterioles. When the lumen of a conduit artery is about one-fourth normal, the vasodilator reserve is exhausted, resistance is fixed, and the stenosis is said to be critical.

Blood Flow and O_2 Extraction

Under basal conditions, coronary flow is about 80 ml/100 g · min in resting, conscious dogs and in humans. Its expansion factor is roughly the same as for $\dot{V}O_2$. In health, the two variables change in direct proportion. If $\dot{V}O_2$ doubles, flow doubles, and so on. This holds O_2 extraction (the ratio $\dot{V}O_2/\dot{Q}$) constant. The longitudinal intracapillary gradient in O_2 content therefore remains constant except during very heavy work. Tight coupling between flow and $\dot{V}O_2$ is of the utmost importance, for even at rest the heart extracts half or more of the O_2 delivered to it by the arterial blood. Because of its high extraction, the heart could not even double its $\dot{V}O_2$ if flow were fixed at the resting value. *It is this extreme flow dependence* that accounts for the devastating effect of occlusive coronary artery disease.

In most organs high O_2 extraction reflects inability to deliver sufficient flow. This is not the case in heart; its extraction is high despite a large vasodilator reserve and is the same over a wide range of $\dot{V}O_2$. The high O_2 extraction of myocardium depends on the unique properties of its O_2 exchanger, which minimize the dominant transcapillary resistance to O_2 transport. So effective is this adaptation that 90 percent of the O_2 offered can be extracted in heavy exercise without tissue hypoxia! Thus the heart has a large *reserve of transcapillary O_2 conductance*. Flow and extraction are multiplicative, not additive, determinants of $\dot{V}O_2$, so the aerobic capacity of myocardium depends on both the vasodilator and the capillary reserves.

The Capillary Reserve

The capillary reserve has been studied in rat hearts in situ by means of stop-motion cinematography. Intercapillary distance (ICD) is measured directly from the photomicrographs, and the corresponding capillary densities are calculated; see Figure 19-3. Each data point represents mean ICD for one rat. In normoxemia, capillary density is about 2300 per square millimeter, roughly double that in dogs. The rat heart requires more capillaries because its O_2 exchanger must support a much larger O_2

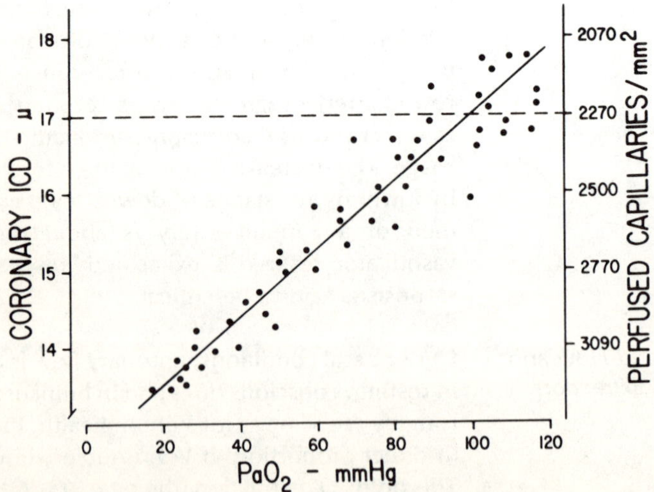

Figure 19-3
Effect of arterial PO_2 on measured mean intercapillary distance (*ICD*) and calculated capillary density in rat hearts beating in situ. Scale of right ordinate is not linear.

flux. Hypoxemia causes precapillary vessels to relax and recruits segments of the capillary network from the reserve. Notice that ICD decreases linearly between a PaO_2 of 120 and 20 torr. This linear relation extends well above the tension required to saturate hemoglobin, indicating that capillary control responds to PO_2 rather than to O_2 content. Under normal circumstances, PaO_2 is held constant by chemoreceptor reflexes, and ICD reflects local tissue PO_2.

Disease can compromise transport by encroaching on the capillary reserve. Sclerosis of small vessels or rigid, impacted erythrocytes can permanently delete capillaries from the array. In pathological hypertrophy, capillary growth does not keep pace with the growth of muscle fibers. Recruitment can compensate for these changes, but at the cost of depleting the reserve. In an animal model of hypertrophy, cardiac failure occurred when the capillary reserve was fully utilized at rest but the heart continued to grow.

Intracellular PO_2 *and the Role of Myoglobin*

Recall that the driving force for blood-tissue O_2 transport is the difference between $PcapO_2$ and intracellular PO_2. The heart's high O_2 extraction results in low $PcapO_2$. To maintain the required driving force, intracellular PO_2 must be uniformly low. Myoglobin accomplishes this, while ensuring a constant O_2 supply at mitochondria. Myoglobin saturation and the PO_2 in equilibrium with myoglobin are shown in Figure 19-4. Mean intracellular PO_2 was approximately 5 torr, whereas coronary venous

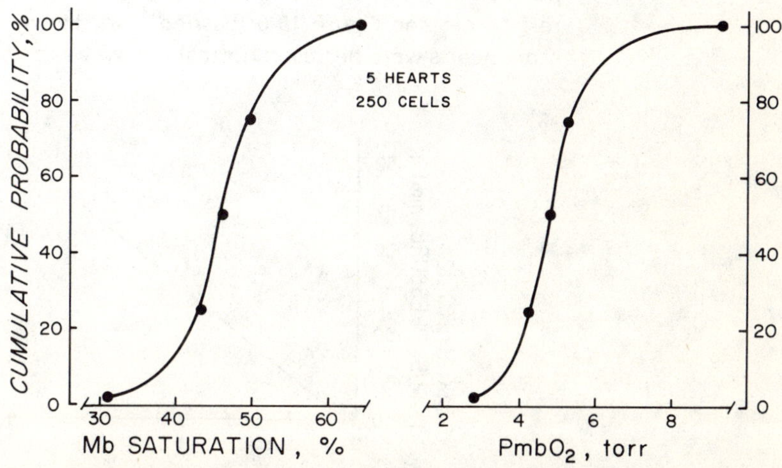

Figure 19-4
Myoglobin (*Mb*) saturation and PO_2 in 250 individual subepicardial canine myocytes. Ordinate indicates percentage of cell population in which saturation or PO_2 is equal to or less than corresponding values on the abscissa. (Measurements were made in collaboration with Dr. T. E. J. Gayeski.)

PO_2 was 25 to 30 torr. Almost identical PO_2 distributions are observed in 5 species, and presumably in humans as well. Moreover, PO_2 distributions are almost the same at near-maximum heart rates and over a wide range of preload and afterload. Thus the vasodilator and capillary reserves are remarkably successful in maintaining the balance between O_2 supply and demand in the stressed but otherwise normal heart.

Notice that PO_2 was extremely uniform; half the cells were between 4 and 5 torr, and none were below 2 torr. The minimum PO_2 for cytochrome turnover is approximately tenfold less than 2 torr, so cell PO_2 is low relative to blood but high relative to biochemical requirements. Uniformity of cell PO_2 depends on close capillary spacing and on the functions of myoglobin as PO_2 buffer and facilitator of intracellular O_2 diffusion. These functions of myoglobin are developed in Chapter 22, pages 228 to 229.

Gradients from Epicardium to Endocardium

Systolic tissue pressure increases almost linearly with depth beneath the epicardium. It approaches but does not exceed ventricular pressure at the endocardial surface; see Figure 19-5. Since vessels are collapsible, systolic flow is restricted throughout the myocardium and approaches zero in the innermost layers of the wall. To learn the effect of the epicardial-endocardial tissue pressure gradient on the distribution of *systolic* blood flow, a pneumatic occluder was placed around the circumflex coronary artery. Total flow could be limited to systole by timing occlusion and release appropriately. As expected, flow closely paralleled the epicardial-endocardial gradient in extravascular resistance; see Figure 19-6 (*dashed line*). However, when the same hearts were perfused normally, flow was actually higher in

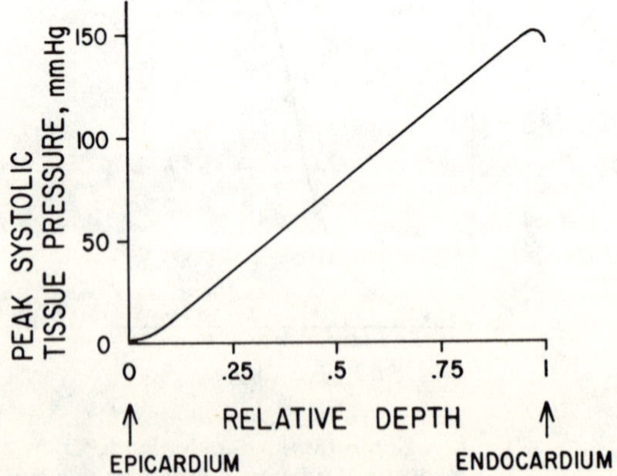

Figure 19-5
Transmural gradient in myocardial tissue pressure in the dog.

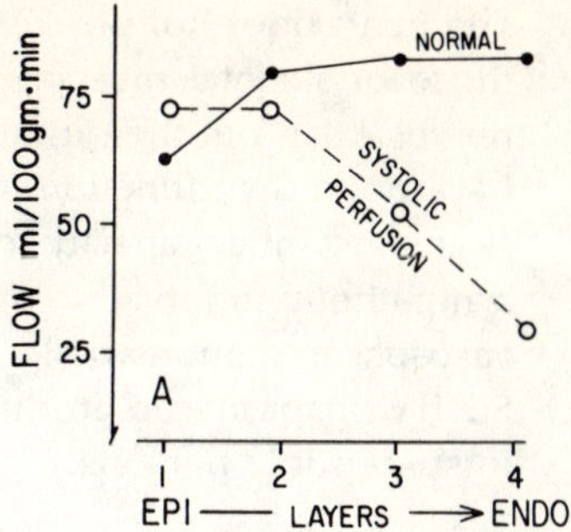

Figure 19-6
Transmural distribution of blood flow is nearly uniform under normal circumstances (*solid line*) but decreases with depth when flow is limited to systole (*dashed line*). (Data of D. S. Hess and R. J. Bache, *Circ. Res.* 38:5, 1976. By permission of the American Heart Association, Inc.)

the subendocardium (Figure 19-6, *solid line*). Higher flow to deep myocardium is required because $\dot{V}O_2$ is about 25 percent higher in deep myocardium.

Compensation for the epicardial-endocardial gradients in extravascular resistance and $\dot{V}O_2$ is complete in normal animals. Transmural differences in intracellular PO_2 are small, and concentrations of creatine phosphate, ATP, and lactate are uniform across the wall, even at near-maximal heart rates. This successful adaptation depends mainly on an epicardial-endocardial gradient in vasomotor tone brought about by metabolic controls. Capillary density and myoglobin concentration are also greater in the subendocardium. The cost is smaller vasodilator and capillary reserves in deep myocardium. It is no coincidence that the subendocardium is particularly prone to ischemic injury, and that the extent of necrosis (death of tissue) after coronary occlusion increases with depth beneath the epicardium.

Control of Coronary Circulation

Metabolic Mechanisms

The smooth muscle of coronary vessels is controlled mainly by dilator metabolites. In the heart, these substances are responsible for the tight coupling between $\dot{V}O_2$ and flow, for autoregulation, for equalizing transmural flow, and for setting an appropriate capillary density. Mechanisms of circulation-metabolism coupling are not fully understood. A large body of evidence indicates that *adenosine* is an important vasodilator metabolite in myocardium. Adenosine is O_2-linked because it is derived from ATP, as explained in Chapter 18. However, other metabolites, including O_2 itself, appear to play a role.

Neural Controls

The heart does not possess sympathetic vasodilator nerves like those of skeletal muscle. Cardiac parasympathetic vasodilator nerves exist, but their influence on resistance is small, and they have no known function. Coronary arteries and arterioles possess substantial capacity for sympathetic vasoconstriction. This sympathetic innervation appears responsible for stress-related vasospasm demonstrable by angiography in awake humans. Such vasospasm can produce ischemia and cardiac pain (angina) in susceptible persons.

Sympathetic stimulation elicits large changes in heart rate, tension development, and $\dot{V}O_2$. The effects of antiadrenergic drugs and of chronic cardiac denervation suggest that sympathetic nerves augment coronary flow mainly by increasing metabolic demand.

Coronary Circulation in Exercise

Evolution has had ample time to develop the reserves that protect our most vital — and unpaired — organ. The capacity of these reserves is illustrated in Figure 19-7. Coronary hemodynamics were monitored in racing sled dogs during competition. Data from implanted transducers were telemetered to receivers on the sled. The huge increase in pulse pressure (*top trace*) reflects high stroke volume and power output, but mean aortic pressure did not increase. Heart rate doubled in 5 and remained about 300 per minute throughout the run. Though the diastolic

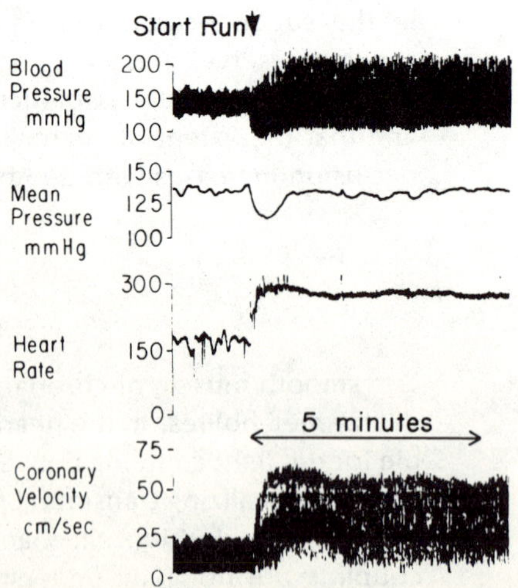

Figure 19-7
Changes in coronary hemodynamics at onset of a race. Running began at arrow, but animal was excited beforehand. (From R. L. Van Citters and D. L. Franklin, *Circ. Res.* 24:33, 1969. By permission of the American Heart Association, Inc.)

pressure–time product decreased, measured flow velocity in the circumflex coronary artery rose fivefold in 15 seconds! Moreover, the animals possessed unused vasodilator reserve and could continue to run at that near-maximal heart rate for several hours. Small wonder that the stress of valvular heart disease or hypertension is well tolerated for many years, even in deconditioned humans.

Clinical Application

In a sense this entire chapter could be considered clinical application, since the effects of disease are so clearly related to normal physiology. The pathophysiology of coronary circulation has been clarified by studies of animal models of disease.[2] Results demonstrate that imbalance between O_2 supply and demand can develop without obstruction of coronary vessels. This can happen in hypoxemia, hypotension, hypertrophy, anemia, and hypermetabolism. In all these conditions, injury is often limited to the subendocardium, where the flow and capillary reserves are smallest. Occlusion of a large artery generally produces a transmural infarction. The extent and distribution of irreversible injury depend on the flow and capillary reserves in tissue supplied by collaterals. Though physicians cannot undo an occlusion, they can protect vulnerable tissue in the hemodynamic border zone by decreasing O_2 demand and by dealing with functional conditions that limit O_2 supply.

References

1. Brown, A. M. Motor innervation of the coronary arteries of the cat. *J. Physiol.* (Lond.) 198:311, 1968.

2. Buckberg, G. D., Fixler, D. E., Archie, J. P., and Hoffman, J. I. E. Experimental subendocardial ischemia in dogs with normal coronary arteries. *Circ. Res.* 30:67, 1972.

3. Downey, J. M., Downey, H. F., and Kirk, E. S. Effects of myocardial strains on coronary blood flow. *Circ. Res.* 34:286, 1974.

4. Drake-Holland, A. J., Laird, J. D., Noble, M. M., Spaan, J. A. E., and Vergroesen, I. Oxygen and coronary vascular resistance during autoregulation and metabolic vasodilation in the dog. *J. Physiol.* (Lond.) 348:285, 1984.

*5. Feigl, E. O. Coronary physiology. *Physiol. Rev.* 63:1, 1983.

6. Gibbs, C. L., and Chapman, J. B. Cardiac mechanics and energetics: Chemomechanical transduction in cardiac muscle. *Am. J. Physiol.* 249:H199, 1985.

7. Griggs, D. M., Jr. Blood flow and metabolism in different layers of the ventricular wall. *Physiologist* 22:36, 1979.

[2]These experiments well demonstrate the importance of research now threatened by misguided legislation.

8. Heineman, F. W., and Grayson, J. Transmural distribution of intramyocardial pressure measured by micropipette technique. *Am. J. Physiol.* 249:H1216, 1985.

9. Honig, C. R., and Gayeski, T. E. J. Comparison of intracellular PO_2 and conditions for blood-tissue O_2 transport in heart and working red skeletal muscle. *Adv. Exp. Med. Biol.* 215:309, 1987.

10. Kirk, E. S., Urschel, C. W., and Sonnenblick, E. H. Problems in Cardiac Performance: Regulation of Coronary Blood Flow and the Physiology of Heart Failure. In A. C. Guyton and C. E. Jones (eds.), *Cardiac Physiology.* Baltimore: University Park Press, 1974. Pp. 300–314.

11. Klocke, F. J., and Ellis, A. K. Control of coronary blood flow. *Annu. Rev. Med.* 31:489, 1980.

12. Lambert, P. R., Hess, D. S., and Bache, R. J. Effect of exercise on perfusion of collateral-dependent myocardium in dogs with chronic coronary artery occlusion. *J. Clin. Invest.* 59:1, 1977.

13. Olsson, R. A. Local factors regulating cardiac and skeletal muscle blood flow. *Annu. Rev. Physiol.* 43:385, 1981.

14. Schaper, W. *The Collateral Circulation of the Heart.* Amsterdam: North Holland, 1971.

15. Stone, H. L. Control of the coronary circulation during exercise. *Annu. Rev. Physiol.* 45:213, 1983.

16. Thomas, J. X., Jr., Jones, C. E., and Randall, W. C. Neural Modulation of Coronary Blood Flow. In W. C. Randall (ed.), *Nervous Control of Cardiovascular Function.* London: Oxford University Press, 1984.

20 : The Cerebral Circulation

The essential features of circulation in the brain are summarized in Table 20-1. As in the heart, the frame of reference is the instantaneous balance between high O_2 demand and determinants of O_2 supply. The brain differs from myocardium, however, in its extreme anatomical, metabolic, and functional heterogeneity; it is, in fact, a population of "miniorgans." The principal adaptation to this heterogeneity is an exceptional capacity to redistribute flow between active and inactive loci.

$\dot{V}O_2$ and Total Brain Blood Flow

Venous concentrations of N_2O or xenon in blood from the internal jugular vein can be used to measure total cerebral blood flow by use of the Fick principle, as described in Chapter 13. The brain accounts for about 15 percent of the cardiac output and 20 percent of total body $\dot{V}O_2$, even though it is only 2 percent of body weight. Total cerebral blood flow is 90 to 100 ml/100 g · min before puberty, drops to about 55 ml/100g · min in young adults, and remains constant thereafter in healthy, vigorous persons. Cerebral flow and $\dot{V}O_2$ are substantially reduced by anesthesia and cerebrovascular disease.

Heterogeneity of Flow and Metabolism

Redistribution of Blood Flow

The regional distribution of cerebral flow changes dramatically with neuronal activity. In no other organ is flow redistribution so essential for normal function. The relation between brain function and circulation is best studied in conscious humans, who can vary local neural activity on demand. To measure regional flow, a gamma emitter such as ^{85}Kr or ^{133}Xe is injected into a carotid artery, and disappearance rates are measured with a battery of well-collimated detectors positioned over the skull. Mathematical analysis allows one to distinguish between flow to nerve fibers (white matter) and cell bodies (gray matter) within a particular region. Results so obtained are shown in Figure 20-1.

In the awake, resting state, flow is distributed mainly to the frontal lobe, which is largely concerned with thinking and in-

Table 20-1
Summary of Circulation in the Brain

Characteristics and Requirements
1. $\dot{V}O_2$/g is always high in certain loci
2. Local $\dot{V}O_2$ can increase several-fold
3. There is no O_2 store; glycolysis cannot meet energy demand, so
4. Flow/g and capillary density must be high in active tissue
5. There is no intracellular O_2 carrier, so diffusion distances must be short
6. Total flow, flow distribution, and diffusion distance must be closely coupled to $\dot{V}O_2$
7. Rigid cranium necessitates constant intracranial volume
8. Extracellular fluid volume must be small and constant
Problems
1. Cerebrospinal fluid (CSF) pressure rises if intracranial volume increases
2. High CSF pressure compresses vessels and increases resistance
3. In erect humans cerebral perfusion pressure is about 20 percent less than aortic pressure
Adaptations
1. Low vasomotor tone
2. Large capacity for redistribution of flow within the brain
3. Intrinsic neural controls initiate prompt vasodilation at active loci
4. Well-developed autoregulation of blood flow
5. Powerful metabolic controls
6. Blood-brain barrier
7. Increase in CSF pressure increases arterial perfusion pressure

trospection — perhaps the subject was wondering why he volunteered for the measurements. This pattern changed immediately in response to stimulation or activity. Voluntary contraction of the muscles of the hand and forearm increased flow to those portions of the motor cortex and sensory cortex concerned with that hand and arm. Flow in corresponding regions of the opposite brain hemisphere, which controls the contralateral arm, did not change. Reasoning increased flow to the precentral and postcentral regions. Reading aloud activated blood flow in occipital cortex (vision), temporal cortex (audition), and in sensory, motor, and frontal cortex concerned with control of speech. Hyperemia and brain function are so closely related that computer maps of local flow can be used to determine which cortical loci are activated by pain, thinking, emotion, or behavior!

Regional Metabolism

Computer-assisted tomography based on positron-emitting isotopes such as $^{15}O_2$ (positron emission tomography, or PET) permits safe, quantitative determinations of local $\dot{V}O_2$ and glucose

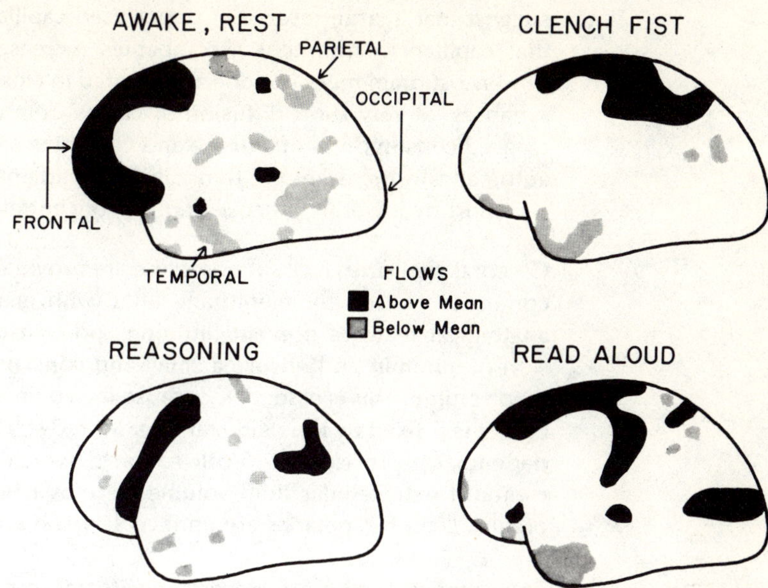

Figure 20-1
Outlines of dominant cerebral hemisphere in humans. Dark shading represents flows more than 20 percent greater than the mean. (Modified from D. H. Ingvar, *Brain Res.* 107:181, 1976.)

uptake; flow can be measured as well. $\dot{V}O_2$ of cerebral gray matter depends on both location and neural activity. It varies from 3 to 15 ml/100 g · min. Thus $\dot{V}O_2$ at certain active loci is almost double the $\dot{V}O_2$ of the unstressed heart. $\dot{V}O_2$ of white matter is about 1.5 ml/100 g · min, and is spatially and temporally uniform. The difference between white and gray matter reflects the low energy cost for conduction of action potentials and the high cost of synaptic activity. As in the heart, flow varies linearly with $\dot{V}O_2$, so intracapillary PO_2 is well maintained. Glucose utilization is also linearly related to flow. Precise coupling between flow and the consumption of glucose is essential because the brain relies on glucose oxidation almost exclusively. Since the metabolism of critical neurons is so high, cessation of flow for only 5 to 10 seconds will cause loss of consciousness, and 5 minutes of ischemia will produce irreversible damage. The $\dot{V}O_2$ of the vital medullary centers is substantially less than that of the cortex and basal ganglia. Consequently, people who survive prolonged hypoxemia or ischemia are often left with parkinsonism or intellectual impairment.

Capillaries and the Blood-Brain Barrier

Gray matter is provided with as many capillaries as myocardium — up to 3500 per square millimeter. White matter contains about one-fourth as many. Qualitative observations in animals suggest that a large reserve of unperfused capillaries exist and that capillary recruitment accompanies increases in regional flow. Most brain mitochondria are situated in close proximity to synapses, at very short diffusion distances from capillaries. Increased consumption of glucose and O_2 during synaptic activity automatically increases the transcapillary gradients required for transport by lowering glucose and O_2 concentrations in cells.

Cerebral capillaries lack slit pores and are provided with a thick, continuous basement membrane lined with glial cells. These anatomical features prevent filtration and transcapillary diffusion of albumin and ensure a small and constant extracellular fluid volume. This is essential, because the volume of the cranial contents is fixed by the rigid cranium. Moreover, brain function depends on precise cell-to-cell contacts, which could be disrupted if extracellular fluid volume were as labile as in other organs. Lymph capillaries are unnecessary and are not present.

The absence of slit pores severely limits transcapillary diffusion of small water-soluble molecules. Transport of essential nutrients such as glucose and organic wastes requires carrier-mediated systems in the endothelium. Nonmetabolizable solutes such as sucrose, certain ions, and many drugs lack carriers and are virtually excluded from the cerebral extracellular space. The foregoing permeability characteristics have led to the concept of a *blood-brain barrier*, which affords a unique environment for neuronal function.

Control of Cerebral Circulation

Autoregulation and Metabolites

The cerebral vessels autoregulate blood flow very effectively, as shown in Figure 20-2. Cerebral flow tends to remain nearly constant as arterial pressure varies between 80 and 180 torr, provided PO_2 and PCO_2 are normal.

The main metabolic controls of cerebrovascular resistance are PO_2, PCO_2, H^+, adenosine, and K^+. The latter is important only during very intense neuronal activity — seizures, for example. CO_2 is generally the dominant control; its powerful influence on cerebral circulation is shown in Figure 20-3. The range of total flow is smaller in brain than in most other organs reflecting strong reliance on regional redistribution. Consequently, a maximal CO_2 stimulus increases total flow by only a factor of 2. Note that hypocapnia is accompanied by vasoconstriction; when $PaCO_2$ is 20 torr, flow is roughly halved. This accounts for the

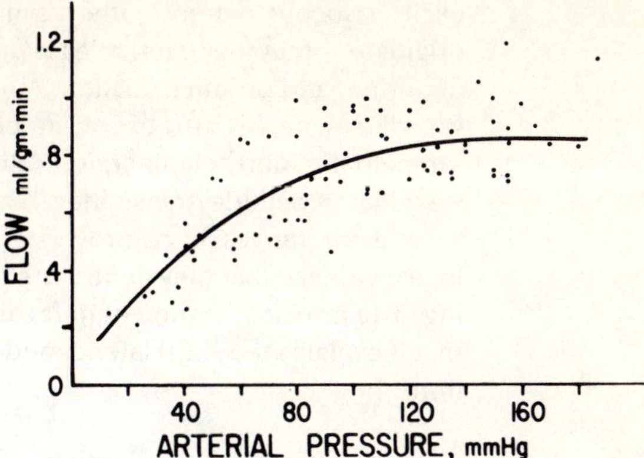

Figure 20-2
Brain displays good autoregulation of blood flow when $PaCO_2$ is normal. (Modified from A. M. Harper, *Acta Neurol. Scand.* [*Suppl.*] 14:94, 1965.)

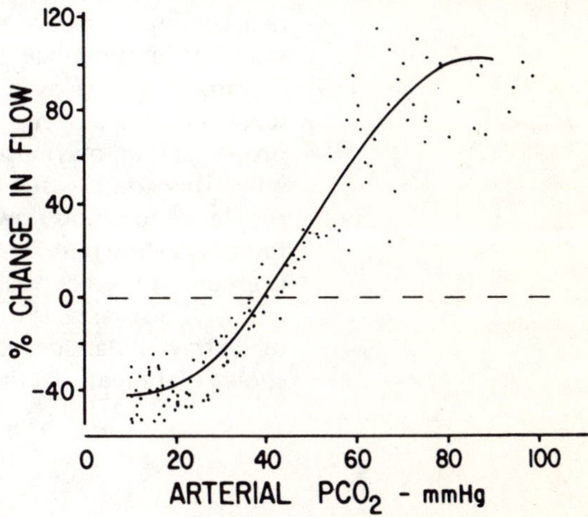

Figure 20-3
Effect of $PaCO_2$ on cerebral blood flow in normotensive dogs. Note small vasodilator reserve and vasoconstriction during hypocapnia. (Modified from A. M. Harper, *Acta Neurol. Scand.* [*Suppl.*] 14:94, 1965.)

dizziness and even loss of consciousness that can be brought about by voluntary hyperventilation.

In conscious animals the magnitude and time course of resistance during hypoxemia parallel the fall in extracellular pH and the concentration of lactate in cortical tissue. The vasodilator effect of both hypoxemia and CO_2 appears to be brought about by extracellular H^+, generated by lactic or carbonic acids.

Neural Controls

The cerebral vessels are supplied with adrenergic nerve fibers. Some of these originate in the superior cervical ganglion and elicit vasoconstriction. Other sympathetic vasomotor fibers originate within the brain, release dopamine rather than norepinephrine, and produce dilation. A population of nonadrenergic vasodilator nerves also exists; at least some of these are parasympathetic and cholinergic. Others appear to release a vasodilator peptide transmitter. The function of the cerebral vasodilator nerves is controversial, and direct electrophysiologic evidence that they contribute to vasomotor control is lacking. The principal argument in favor of the neural hypothesis is that it explains the short latency and rapid initial rate of vasodilation.

Clinical Application

The Problem of the Rigid Cranium

The cranium is rigid and the brain is incompressible, so the total volume of the cranial contents must be kept virtually constant to avoid change in intracranial pressure. Increases in arterial volume during vasodilation are small and are compensated for by reciprocal decreases in venous volume. In disease, however, space-occupying lesions or excess cerebrospinal fluid may raise intracranial pressure markedly. This compresses blood vessels and increases resistance to blood flow. The effect of various brain tumors is shown in Figure 20-4. Cerebrospinal fluid pressure in normal people is 10 to 15 cm H_2O. At 45 cm H_2O, resistance is roughly twice normal because of extravascular compression. The dashed line shows that mean arterial pressure increases linearly

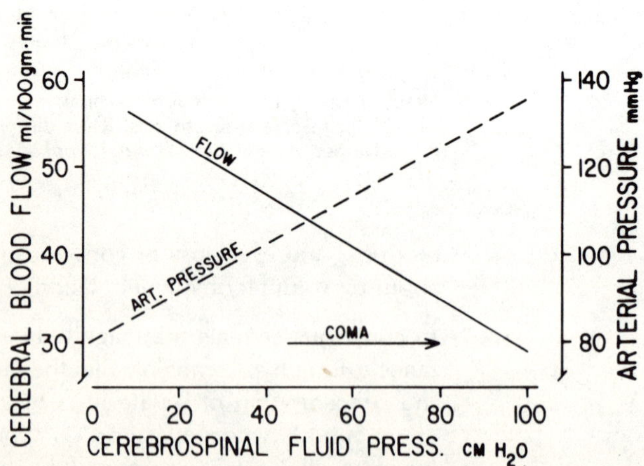

Figure 20-4
Effect of cerebrospinal fluid pressure on systemic arterial pressure and cerebral blood flow in patients with intracranial tumors. (Replotted from data of S. S. Kety, H. A. Shenkin, and C. F. Schmidt, *J. Clin. Invest.* 27:493, 1948.)

with cerebrospinal fluid pressure. This partly compensates for the higher resistance and minimizes the decrease in flow. Nevertheless, at 45 cm H_2O, flow is roughly two-thirds normal. Patients with higher pressures and lower flows are generally comatose. Flow is compromised to a greater extent if intracranial pressure rises rapidly, as in subdural hemorrhage.

Systemic hypertension and bradycardia caused by high intracranial pressure is called the Cushing reflex. The large cerebral vessels possess stretch receptors, whose discharge frequency reflects the difference between arterial pressure tending to distend the vessel and cerebrospinal fluid pressure tending to compress it. If cerebrospinal fluid pressure rises, the effect on the receptors is the same as if blood pressure had fallen. The resulting change in discharge frequency increases sympathetic vasoconstrictor discharge. Pressure-sensitive sites within the substance of the lower brainstem also contribute to the Cushing reflex.

Deleterious Flow Redistributions

Tissue around an occluded artery is supplied by collaterals. Should arterial pressure fall, autoregulatory vasodilation in the healthy tissue will divert flow from the collaterals, whose resistance is fixed at a minimum value. Vasodilation caused by a rise in $PaCO_2$ (hypoventilation) or injection of a vasodilator drug would have a similar effect. The phenomenon is termed *intracerebral steal.* A similar phenomenon occurs in the heart. The aware physican realizes that injured tissue has limited factors of safety and takes steps to prevent deleterious flow redistribution.

References

*1. Heistad, D. D., and Kontos, H. A. Cerebral Circulation. In J. T. Shepherd and F. M. Abboud (eds.), *Handbook of Physiology,* Section 2: The Cardiovascular System, Vol. III, Part 1. Bethesda, Md.: American Physiological Society, 1983.

2. Kety, S. S., Shenkin, H. A., and Schmidt, C. F. The effects of increased intracranial pressure on cerebral circulatory functions in man. *J. Clin. Invest.* 27:493, 1948.

*3. Lassen, N. A., Ingvar, D. H., and Skinhoj, J. Brain function and blood flow. *Sci. Am.* 239(4):62, 1978.

4. Raichle, M. E. Measurement of local cerebral blood flow and metabolism in man with positron emission tomography. *Fed. Proc.* 40:2331, 1981.

5. Siesjo, B. K., Berntman, L., and Nilsson, B. Regulation of microcirculation in the brain. *Microvasc. Res.* 19:158, 1980.

6. Sokoloff, L. Relation between physiological function and energy metabolism in the central nervous system. *J. Neurochem.* 29:13, 1977.

21 : The Splanchnic Circulation

The vessels of the liver, spleen, and gastrointestinal tract constitute the splanchnic circulation. Flow to each component can be adjusted individually.

Total Splanchnic Flow and Blood Volume in Adaptation to Stress

Total splanchnic flow averages 25 percent of the cardiac output at rest, or about 1.5 liters per minute in a 70-kg person. Its expansion factor is about 3, but maximum vasodilation occurs only in certain gastrointestinal infections. The average O_2 extraction is 3 to 4 vol %, roughly the same as resting skeletal muscle. Because of its high flow relative to $\dot{V}O_2$, the splanchnic circulation can be curtailed for short periods without causing ischemic damage. Splanchnic vasoconstriction plays an important role in defending arterial pressure during postural adjustments, exercise, and heat stress in humans. This vasoconstriction is not overridden by the ingestion or digestion of food. Redistribution of flow from the splanchnic to the somatic bed is not a major contributor to exercise hyperemia in normal individuals, but in patients with low cardiac output flow diverted from the splanchnic bed may account for half the increment available to working muscle.

The splanchnic bed contains 20 to 25 percent of total blood volume, or about 1200 ml. Almost half this volume is in the liver, and most of the rest in the gastrointestinal veins. The postcapillary splanchnic vessels are at least as well innervated as the arterioles. During exercise or orthostatic stress, reflexly mediated splanchnic venoconstriction shifts volume into the thorax in support of ventricular filling and stroke volume. Blood mobilized from the splanchnic reservoirs can compensate for about half the volume lost in a moderate hemorrhage in humans.

The Gastrointestinal Circulation

Blood Flow

The stomach and intestine consist of a smooth-muscle compartment and a secretory-absorptive mucosal compartment, separated by a nerve plexus. The flow in muscularis and mucosa is on the order of 10 and 40 ml/100 g · min, respectively, in the postabsorptive state. During digestion and absorption, flow to the muscularis tends to decrease, whereas flow to the mucosa may increase up to fourfold. This enormous flow prevents excessive hemoconcentration and high blood viscosity during secretion, and minimizes changes in portal venous osmolality during absorption.

Vasomotor Control

The mechanisms of secretion–blood flow coupling are not the same in various parts of the gastrointestinal tract and are still incompletely understood. Flow to salivary glands, pancreas, and much of the intestine is controlled by peptide neurotransmitters, notably vasoactive intestinal peptide, and by gastrointestinal hormones such as gastrin and cholecystokinin. Metabolites and products of digestion also play a role.

Vasodilation during digestion depends on both physical and psychological stimuli. Results of experiments on dogs are summarized in Figure 21-1. Miniature pressure and flow transducers and equipment for telemetry were installed, and after recovery from the operation, the effect of feeding was studied in a carefully controlled environment. Anticipation and ingestion of food increased cardiac output more than 50 percent and raised blood pressure about 30 percent. Thus eating is a major cardiac stress if the cardiac output reserve is limited; recall the concepts in Figure 13-6, page 131.

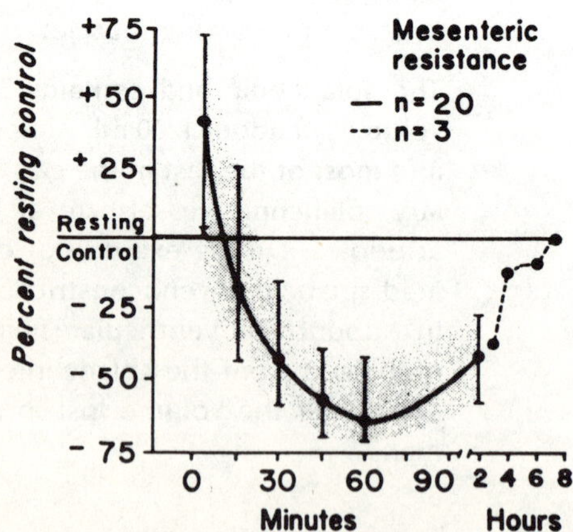

Figure 21-1
Average mesenteric resistance during eating and digestion in dogs. Food was presented at time 0 and ingested in 5–10 min. Vertical lines denote ranges. (From S. F. Vatner, D. Franklin, and R. L. Van Citters, *Am. J. Physiol.* 219:170, 1970.)

Systemic changes subsided and mesenteric resistance began to fall about 10 minutes after eating. Intestinal blood flow was maximal within an hour, and subsided in 3 to 4 hours. A somewhat smaller and less well sustained vasodilation was observed in fasted, muzzled dogs that could see and smell the food but could not eat it.

The Countercurrent Mechanism in Intestinal Villi

The intestinal epithelium is thrown up into fingerlike projections, or *villi*. These increase the surface area for absorption several-hundred-fold. Each villus is supplied by a terminal arteriole that runs from the base to the tip, where it breaks up into a dense net of capillaries. These are specially adapted for water and solute transport by their high hydraulic conductivity (C_F). They are closely applied to the intestinal epithelium and drain from the tip of the villus toward the base. Thus the direction of flow in the capillaries is opposite to that in the arteriole, as shown in the left panel of Figure 21-2. The ascending and descending limbs of the *countercurrent loop* are separated by only 15 μm. Small molecules can diffuse this distance in a very small fraction of the transit time of plasma through the villus.

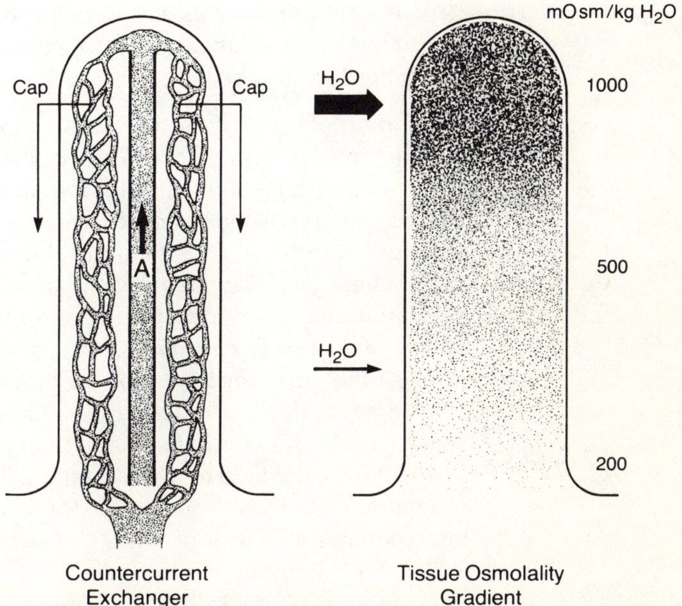

Figure 21-2
Left, Arrows indicate opposite direction of flow in the central arteriole and the surrounding capillaries. Right, Shading represents a gradient in tissue osmolality from the tip to the base of the villus. Water absorption from the intestinal lumen parallels the tissue osmolality gradient.

Because of the anatomy just described, water-soluble substances in the intestinal lumen readily diffuse into the capillaries. A variable amount diffuses down concentration gradients between the capillaries and arteriole and enters the arteriolar lumen. The flow then conveys them to the tip of the villus, where they reenter the capillary net. This decreases the concentration gradient for diffusion from the intestinal lumen. The net effect is a functional barrier that slows absorption of highly diffusible substances (urea, for example). Blood osmolality must be maintained within narrow limits. The countercurrent mechanism serves as a factor of safety that prevents sudden, large increases in the osmolality of portal blood.

Lipid-soluble gases such as O_2 and CO_2 diffuse across the entire surface of the villus capillaries into the intestinal lumen. Since the lumen is a virtual sink, substantial amounts could be lost from the blood. The villous countercurrent minimizes such loss by promoting diffusion from the arteriole to the capillaries. The efficiency of the countercurrent exchanger increases with the time available for diffusion. Thus countercurrent shunting is greatest when blood flow is low. In extreme vasoconstriction, arteriovenous shunting of O_2 from the arteriole to the capillaries near the base of the villus may be sufficient to limit the $\dot{V}O_2$ of structures at the tip. This accounts for the susceptibility of the tips of the villi to injury during prolonged ischemia, as in shock and other low flow states.

Absorption of water from the intestine depends mainly on the oncotic and hydrostatic pressures in the interstitium (π_{IF} and P_{IF}). Hydrodynamic flow of water requires an osmotic gradient. The gradient is created by active transport of Na^+ from the intestinal lumen into the interstitium of the villi. The magnitude of the gradient (and the rate of water absorption) is increased by the countercurrent exchanger, because much of the Na^+ that enters capillaries is returned to the tip of the villus via the arteriole. The Na^+ concentration in blood therefore increases from base to tip. High plasma Na^+ impedes removal of Na^+ actively transported into the interstitium and creates an osmotic gradient from the base to the tip of the villus; see the right panel of Figure 21-2. The osmolality of the distal third of the villus interstitium is at least four times that of plasma. Consequently, water absorption can occur even if plasma osmolality is less than the osmolality of the intestinal contents.

Microvascular Pressures and Fluid Balance

Micropuncture measurements indicate that mean transmural hydrostatic pressure in capillaries of the mesentery is about 30 torr. Since transmural oncotic pressure is about 22 torr, the mesentery is an organ for filtration. In contrast, pressure in the capillaries of the villi is normally less than 15 torr, so the mucosal capillaries serve as an absorptive network. Oncotic and hydrostatic pressures are about equal in the muscularis layer. The Starling forces are nearly balanced for the intestine as a whole. Abundant lymphatics play an important role in prevention and removal of edema.

The Hepatic Circulation

The liver microcirculation is formed by sheets of hepatocytes covered on both sides by endothelium. The sheets are arranged radially around a central vein to form a spongelike labyrinth of blood sinusoids; see Figure 21-3. Blood percolates through the labyrinth from the portal inflow at the periphery to the central vein, much like fluid through a chromatographic column. The importance of this anatomy is that the "capillary" surface area is nearly maximal, and the *diffusion distance from blood to mitochondria is at the theoretical minimum*. Increases in metabolic activity must therefore be accommodated by changes in the composition or rate of blood flow or both. The principal

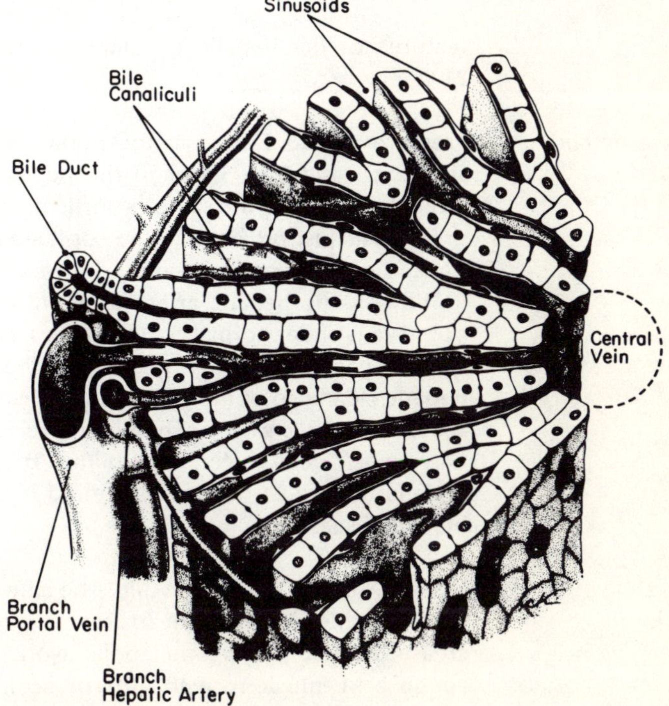

Figure 21-3
Stereographic reconstruction showing confluence of hepatic arteriole and portal venule at the periphery of a lobule, and the interconnected sinusoids. Arrows indicate direction of flow. Note the large surface area of the blood-tissue interface and short diffusion distances. (From W. Bloom and D. W. Fawcett, *A Textbook of Histology*. Philadelphia: Saunders, 1968.)

Table 21-1
Summary of Circulation in the Liver

Hepatic Characteristics and Requirements
$\dot{V}O_2$/g high and increases with metabolic work Increased $\dot{V}O_2$ may not be accompanied by more flow Weak neural and intrinsic controls Hydrostatic pressure in sinusoids is less than plasma oncotic pressure
Problems
About three-fourths of total flow is venous Flow is determined mainly by events in gastrointestinal circulation Flow decreases in erect position
Adaptations
Huge flow when recumbent (25% of C.O.) Hepatic artery supplements O_2 supply Extraction reserve can be almost fully utilized because Large capillary surface area and short diffusion distance Sinusoids are highly permeable, so Transmural difference in oncotic pressure is small

features of the hepatic circulation are summarized in Table 21-1.

Pressure and Flows

Pressure is 8 to 12 torr in the portal vein, 3 to 8 torr in the sinusoids, and 3 to 5 torr in the hepatic vein. Since hepatic arterial pressure is the same as aortic pressure, a steep resistive drop exists just proximal to the confluence of the hepatic arterial and portal venous streams. This intrahepatic resistance limits flow in the hepatic artery to about one-fourth that in the portal vein under normal circumstances. Hepatic blood flow can be measured in humans by applying the Fick principle to the hepatic clearance of the dye Bromsulphalein. Flow ranges from 100 to 130 ml/100 g · min when one is recumbent but falls markedly when one is seated or standing. The effect of position on hepatic flow must be borne in mind in treating patients with hepatic disease.

O_2 Delivery and $\dot{V}O_2$

Liver $\dot{V}O_2$ is 4 to 7 ml/100 g · min. The latter figure is only slightly less than that of beating heart. Moreover, hepatic $\dot{V}O_2$ may increase 2.5-fold during metabolic work (e.g., processing an amino acid infusion), with little or no increase in total flow. Since the average O_2 extraction of the gastrointestinal tract is only 3 to 4 vol %, the O_2 content of portal venous blood is 14 to 16 vol % when the hemoglobin concentration is normal. O_2 offered is supplemented to a varying extent by oxygenated blood from the hepatic artery. Consequently hepatic venous O_2

content is 9 to 11 vol %, and its PO_2 is 25 to 30 torr in recumbent humans. The enormous surface area of the sinusoids results in very low O_2 flux density. Consequently, O_2 in the sinusoids can fall as low as 1 vol % (about 4 torr) without compromising aerobic respiration. Thus the *usable* extraction reserve is at least as large as in organs supplied entirely by arterial blood.

Local and Neural Controls

The hepatic arterial bed shows good autoregulation of blood flow but responds weakly to metabolites. The only important hepatic vasomotor mechanism is the "choke" that controls the mixture of arterial and portal blood. If portal flow decreases, as in exercise, hepatic arterial flow increases and holds O_2 offered almost constant. In contrast, a rise in hepatic venous pressure of only a few torr causes marked, well-sustained hepatic arterial constriction.

Filtration and Hepatic Fluid Balance

Fluid balance across the endothelium of the sinusoids requires that the transmural difference in oncotic pressure be small to match the low transmural hydrostatic pressure. This is accomplished by high permeability; indeed, the hepatic endothelium is discontinuous. As one might expect, the protein concentration of fluid filtered and collected in hepatic lymph is almost the same as that of plasma. Up to half the lymph in the thoracic duct is derived from the liver. Lymph flow and the low compliance of the hepatic capsule constitute the liver's main factors of safety against edema.

Clinical Application

Hepatic cirrhosis and right ventricular failure can markedly increase hydrostatic pressure in the sinusoids. This raises venous pressure throughout the splanchnic bed. In addition, the oncotic pressure of the blood is often low because of impaired protein synthesis in the liver. When the rate of fluid filtration in the splanchnic bed exceeds the reabsorptive capacity of the lymphatics, fluid collects in the abdomen. This fluid is called *ascites*. As much as 15 liters of fluid may accumulate! The abdominal pressure (equivalent to P_{IF}) required to stop ascites formation can be as high as 40 torr. The protein concentration of ascitic fluid ranges from 10 to 60 percent of the plasma concentration. If most of the fluid comes from the liver, its protein concentration will be high, and the rate of ascites formation will not be much affected by the protein concentration and oncotic pressure of the plasma. If the fluid comes mainly from the less permeable gastrointestinal capillaries, however, its protein concentration will be lower, and the rate of ascites formation will be accelerated by hypoproteinemia. Secretion of aldosterone and vasopressin further complicates fluid balance in these patients, by promoting renal retention of salt and water.

References

1. Gore, R. W., and Bohlen, H. G. Microvascular pressures in rat intestinal muscle and mucosal villi. *Am. J. Physiol.* 233:H685, 1977.

2. Granger, D. N., Barrowman, J. A., and Kvietys, P. R. *Clinical Gastrointestinal Physiology*. Philadelphia: Saunders, 1985.

*3. Greenway, C. V. Role of splanchnic venous system in overall cardiovascular homeostasis. *Fed. Proc.* 42:1678, 1983.

4. Groom, A. C., Levesque, M. J., and Brucksweitger, D. Flow stasis, blood gases and glucose levels in the red pulp of the spleen. *Adv. Exp. Med. Biol.* 94:567, 1978.

*5. Lundgren, O. Microcirculation of the Gastrointestinal Tract and Pancreas. In E. M. Renkin and C. C. Michel (eds.), *Handbook of Physiology,* Section 2: The Cardiovascular System — Microcirculation, Vol. IV, Part 2. Bethesda, Md.: American Physiological Society, 1984.

6. Rappaport, A. M. The microcirculatory hepatic unit. *Microvasc. Res.* 6:212, 1973.

7. Shepherd, A. P., and Granger, D. N. *Physiology of the Intestinal Circulation*. New York: Raven, 1984.

8. Vatner, S. F., Franklin, D., and Van Citters, R. L. Mesenteric vasoactivity associated with eating and digestion in the conscious dog. *Am. J. Physiol.* 219:170, 1970.

22 : The Somatic Circulation

Skin and muscle account for about half the body weight. The salient characteristic of circulation in this mass of tissue is the enormous *range* of blood flow required to support temperature regulation and exercise.

Circulation in the Skin

The function of the cutaneous circulation is to maintain heat balance. Heat is an order of magnitude more diffusible than water or O_2. Its transport is therefore limited by the rate at which flow delivers heat to the body surface. True capillaries are not essential; heat diffuses readily to, from, and between arteries and veins.

Vascular Arrangements

The vascular anatomy takes full advantage of the diffusivity of heat. Cutaneous arteries are branches of vessels that supply the underlying muscles. During exercise, arterial blood picks up heat in transit through the muscle and delivers it directly to the skin. The primary mechanism for heat transfer lies in the outermost millimeter of skin; temperature falls precipitously across this short distance. A plexus of arterioles gives rise to wide-bore capillary loops in which blood cools in passage to the epidermis. These loops offer much less resistance to flow than ordinary capillaries. The loops drain into a venous plexus just superficial to the arterioles. Heat diffuses from arterioles to the cooler venules, which have a larger surface area for exchange with the environment. As one might expect, the properties of the heat exchanger vary with vasomotor tone. Fully vasodilated skin loses eight times as much heat per liter of blood as fully vasoconstricted skin. The latter is, in fact, an excellent insulator.

During exercise or heat stress, blood returns via superficial veins. Considerable heat loss occurs in transit, especially in the limbs. Temperature in hand veins, for example, may be several degrees higher than in the brachial vein. In the cold, however, cutaneous venous blood returns almost exclusively via deep veins that run in close proximity to the arteries. Countercurrent heat exchange from arteries to deep veins substantially reduces the amount of heat that reaches cold-exposed skin.

The hands, feet, earlobes, and face are especially important for temperature regulation because of their large surface area. The skin in these regions contains true arteriovenous (AV) shunts 20 to 40 μm in diameter. The shunts carry 200 to 600 times as much flow as conventional capillaries of equal length, and their relatively thick walls do not impede heat transfer. Shunts are particularly numerous in the fingers and toes.

Blood Flow and Heat Transport

The skin of a 70-kg person weighs about 2 kg. In a thermoneutral environment it receives about 25 ml/100 g · min, or 10 percent of the cardiac output. Flow is most temperature-dependent in the digits, where arteriovenous shunts are most abundant. In a person going from a cold to a hot environment, flow in the fingers may vary from 0.2 to 40.0 ml/min per 100 g of skin — a 200-fold change! Total skin flow in adult humans ranges from 20 ml per minute to 8 liters per minute, and heat transfer for the whole body ranges from 0.02 to 30 kcal per minute.

Consequences of Cutaneous Vasodilation

The systemic effects of severe radiant heat stress are shown in Figure 22-1. Data are averages for young men seated at rest in whom skin temperature (*dashed curve, top panel*) was raised to 40.5°C. Cardiac output and regional blood flows paralleled the temperature of the blood (*solid curve, top panel*), and hence the body "core," but were poorly correlated with skin temperature. Increased cardiac output, and flow diverted from various vascular beds together contributed 7.8 liters per minute to skin flow. Increased cardiac output was by far the more important factor; only 15 percent of the increment in skin flow was due to flow redistribution. If cardiac output is limited by disease, however, redistribution becomes proportionately more important for temperature regulation.

The principal function of vasoconstriction in the viscera during heat stress is to maintain arterial pressure despite massive cutaneous vasodilation. Nevertheless, arterial pressure fell. The skin is an effector in the feedback loops that regulate arterial pressure, so cutaneous vasoconstrictor nerves were stimulated. Thus skin flow was the net result of vasodilation induced by thermoregulatory reflexes and vasoconstriction caused by other reflex drives. Because of competing neural influences, the full potential for cutaneous vasodilation cannot be realized, particularly when cardiac output is limited by disease.

Cutaneous veins as well as arteries dilate during heat stress. Pooling in the extensive cutaneous venous plexuses accounts for the initial fall in central blood volume in Figure 22-1. Reflex venoconstriction in defense of cardiac output curtailed cutane-

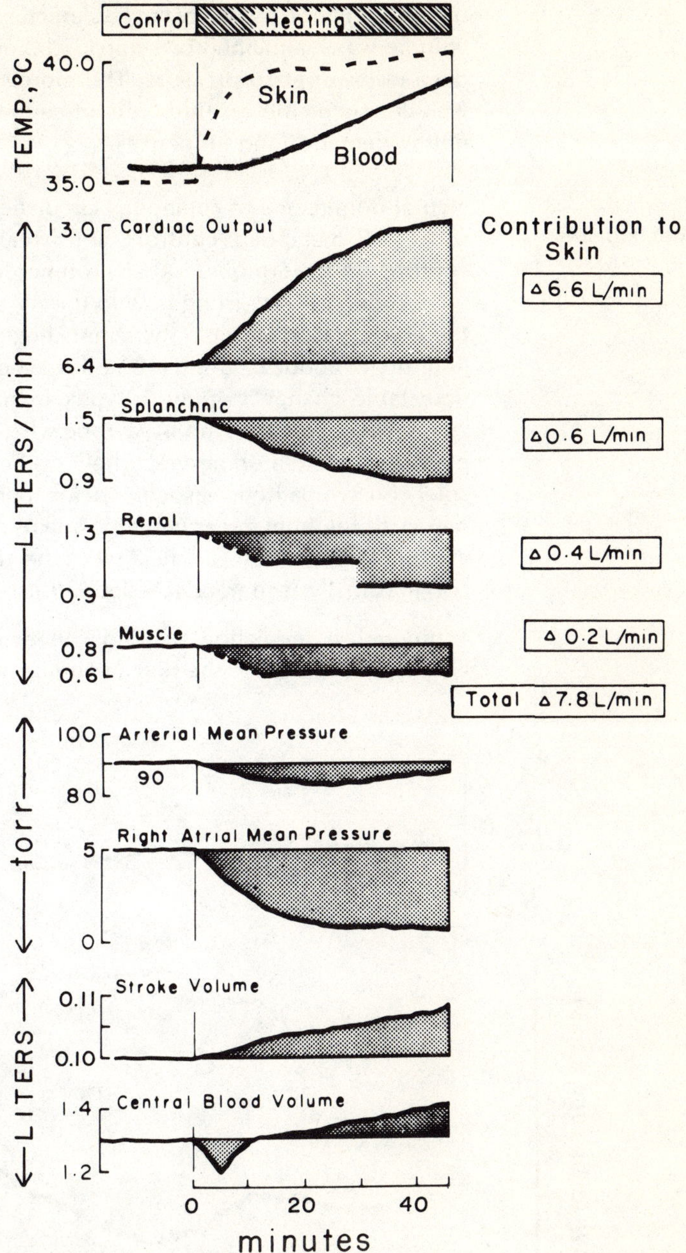

Figure 22-1
Average changes in young men exposed to radiant heat while seated at rest. (Modified from L. B. Rowell, Human Adjustment to and Adaptation to Heat Stress — Where and How? In L. J. Folinsbee, J. A. Wagner, J. F. Borgia, B. L. Drinkwater, J. A. Gliner, and J. R. Bedi [eds.], *Environmental Stress*. New York: Academic, 1978.)

ous venodilation at the cost of less efficient heat transfer. Stroke volume was maintained by sympathetic drive despite tachycardia and lower atrial pressure. Thermoregulation, like exercise, well illustrates the essential role of central integration of competing demands and influences.

Control Mechanisms

Neural dominance of cutaneous circulation is facilitated by absence of metabolic controls and weak autoregulatory responses. In a thermoneutral environment, body temperature is "fine-tuned" by adjusting flow to the AV shunts, particularly in the digits. Vasodilation in the shunts begins at an ambient temperature of about 22°C and is one-third complete before the first detectable change in flow to trunk or forearm skin at about 28°C. The shunts have no basal tone whatever and are not supplied by vasodilator nerves. Their caliber therefore depends solely on sympathetic vasoconstrictor tone. For example, if the nerves to the human ear (which contains numerous AV shunts) are blocked with a local anesthetic, the shunts dilate passively and maximally; see trace labelled *left ear* in Figure 22-2.

Temperature regulation depends on two types of receptors. One type is located in the skin and initiates responses that antic-

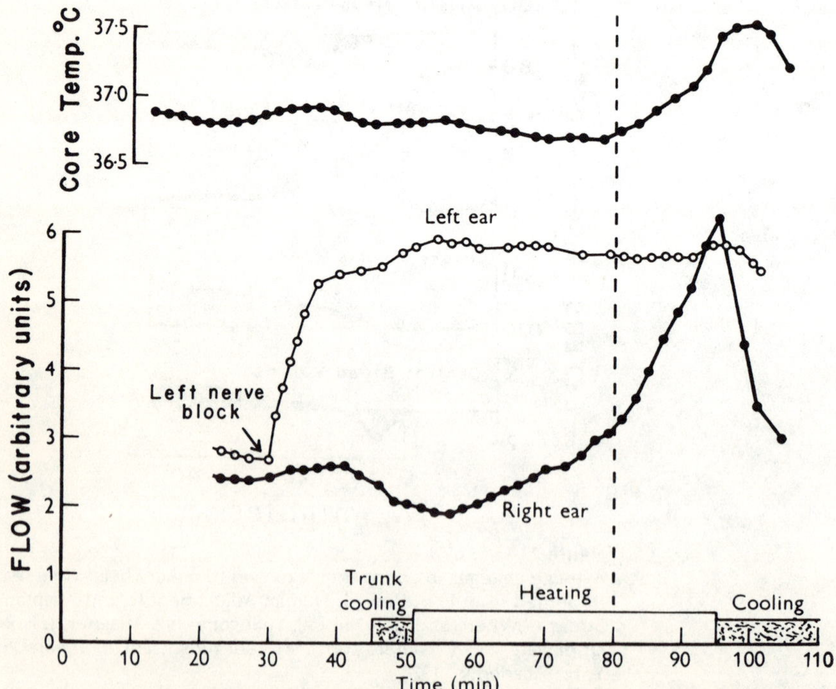

Figure 22-2
Effect of heating and cooling the trunk on auricular blood flow in 10 young men. (Modified from R. H. Fox, R. Goldsmith, and D. J. Kidd, *J. Physiol.* [Lond.] 161:298, 1961. By permission of Cambridge University Press.)

ipate and tend to prevent change in core temperature. The principal effectors are the AV shunts. In the experiment shown in Figure 22-2, briefly cooling the skin of the trunk evoked reflex vasoconstriction in the right ear. This reduces heat loss. Subsequently heating the trunk evoked reflex vasodilation. Dilation of shunts as in the ear dissipated heat and delayed a rise in core temperature (*topmost trace*) until the time indicated by the dashed line.

When prolonged heating raised core temperature (to the right of the dashed line), vasodilation was much larger and more rapid than when only skin receptors were stimulated. A 1°C rise in core temperature from an initial temperature of 37°C produces about 10 times as large an increase in flow to skin of the trunk as a 1°C rise in skin temperature.

The receptors for core temperature are located in the hypothalamus, which controls resistance and sweat secretion throughout the skin via sympathetic nerves. Secretion is mediated by acetylcholine; cutaneous vasodilation depends on a neuropeptide transmitter, possibly vasoactive intestinal peptide (VIP). Interestingly, both acetylcholine and neuropeptide appear to be released from the same special sympathetic nerve endings.

Cold Stress

If a hand is immersed in water at 10°C or less, flow to the exposed fingers may actually cease. The rise in resistance is due to a doubling of viscosity as well as to vasoconstriction. If immersion continues, vasodilation restores flow to about one-third that observed at room temperature. Cold vasodilation coincides with a sensation of pain. The mechanism is probably identical to that responsible for inflammatory responses of the skin to trauma. Axon collaterals from cutaneous pain fibers are thought to release substance P, a peptide transmitter that increases flow and capillary permeability in the injured tissue. The phenomenon is termed the *axon reflex*. It is not a true reflex, however, because it does not involve a synapse. Exposure of the whole body to a cold environment induces cutaneous vasoconstriction, first in the hands and feet, then in the head, and finally in the trunk. Vasoconstriction is well advanced before muscle heat production is increased by shivering.

Circulation in Skeletal Muscle

The salient features of muscle circulation are summarized in Table 22-1.

Blood Flow and Muscle Metabolism at Rest

The $\dot{V}O_2$ of resting human muscle is about 0.2 ml/100 g · min, roughly 1/100 that of certain areas of the brain. Nevertheless, muscle accounts for about 20 percent of the O_2 consumed by the whole body because the muscle mass is enormous — about

Table 22-1
Summary of Circulation in Skeletal Muscle

Characteristics
1. Enormous tissue mass
2. $\dot{V}O_2$ is low at rest
3. $\dot{V}O_2$ can increase more than 50-fold
4. Energy demand changes instantaneously
5. Large glycolytic capacity
6. Physicochemical differences between red and white fibers
Problems
1. Flow and capillary density must be limited in resting fibers
2. Flow and capillary density must increase promptly in active fibers
3. Muscle participates in regulation of temperature and arterial pressure
4. Long intracellular diffusion path
Adaptations
1. Well-developed basal tone and autoregulation
2. Large flow and capillary reserves
3. Large extraction reserve
4. Prompt vasodilation and capillary recruitment during contraction
5. Myoglobin serves as O_2 store, O_2 buffer, and O_2 redistributor

30 kg in a 70-kg person. Flow at rest ranges from 2 to 10 ml/100 g · min, with great variability within and among muscles. O_2 extraction is 2 to 4 vol %, smaller than that of any organ other than skin. Thus muscle flow is high *relative to* $\dot{V}O_2$, even though flow per gram of muscle is very low at rest. Since flow can be curtailed without compromising resting metabolism, the muscle vascular bed is ideally suited to serve as effector in feedback loops that regulate arterial pressure.

Heterogeneity of muscle flow and metabolism is largely due to regional differences in fiber type; see Table 22-2. Most muscles are a mixture of red and white fibers, but only the red fibers are used in performing everyday tasks. They do their work entirely aerobically unless flow is limited by disease. The bulk of a mixed muscle is composed of white fibers, which are used solely for brief, heavy work requiring large tensions. Such tensions produce high tissue pressures, which compress blood vessels and limit flow. Notice in Table 22-2 that the white fibers are well adapted for brief periods of anaerobic work.

Role of Glycolysis

Glycolysis can be "switched on" in milliseconds, whereas about 15 s is required to reach half the steady-state $\dot{V}O_2$ when work begins. Consequently, glycolysis and breakdown of creatine phosphate are the principal sources of ATP in the transition to

Table 22-2
Characteristics of Red and White Fibers*

Feature	Red	White
Mitochondria	Abundant	Sparse
Glycolytic enzymes	Moderate	Abundant
Myoglobin (dog, human)	~0.5 mM	~0
Capillary density	High	Low
Maximum flow	~100 ml/100 gm · min	~50
Contraction velocity	Usually slow	Fast
Tension/motor unit	Low	High
Control	Fine	Coarse
Frequency of use	Regularly	Infrequently
Fraction of mass of mixed muscle	~25%	~75%
Endurance	High	Low

*Experts recognize at least three fiber types; this table conveys only the essentials.

steady work, and in intense, brief efforts using white fibers. In contrast, glycolysis accounts for less than 1 percent of ATP production in *red* muscle fibers during steady work. Nevertheless, the rate of glycolysis in steadily working red fibers increases with $\dot{V}O_2$. Lactate accumulates within red fibers, and additional lactate is released into the venous blood. The relation between lactate efflux from red fibers and the lowest intracellular PO_2 in a large cell population is shown in Figure 22-3. Note that *lactate efflux does not reflect intracellular* PO_2 in red muscle fibers during steady work, and can occur without any hypoxic cells whatever. Glycolysis in pure red muscles, and in mixed muscles performing ordinary tasks, is fully aerobic. Its function is to support *oxidative* ATP production in mitochondria by matching concentrations of mitochondrial substrates to O_2 demand. The amount of O_2 consumed during recovery to replenish glycogen and high-energy phosphate stores is termed the O_2 debt.

Clinical Application

Anoxia is a powerful stimulus to glycolysis, so blood lactate has long been used as an O_2 indicator. For example, arterial lactate is often measured during graded exercise. In both patients and normal subjects, the arterial lactate concentration rises progressively above a threshold work rate. This threshold was formerly interpreted to indicate recruitment of anaerobic glycolysis when the circulation could no longer deliver sufficient O_2 to meet ATP demand. We now know that this concept of an "anaerobic threshold" is erroneous. Changes in arterial lactate in exercise are determined largely by work-related

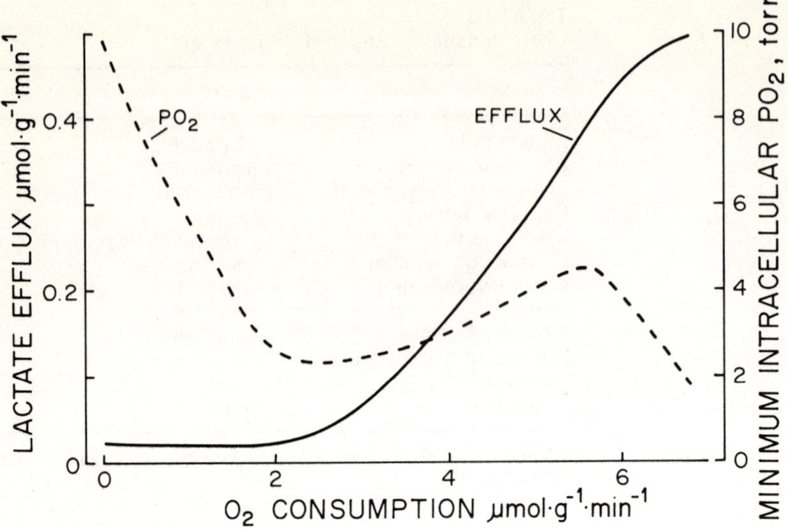

Figure 22-3
Lactate efflux and intracellular PO_2 in dog gracilis muscles performing isometric twitch contraction in situ.

changes in liver metabolism. Moreover, aerobic glycolysis is so large that an anaerobic increment in glycolysis is difficult to recognize even when venous as well as arterial lactate concentrations are available. These facts greatly limit the use of lactate as an O_2 probe in clinical practice.

Flow, Extraction, and $\dot{V}O_2$ in Exercise

Flow increases almost linearly with $\dot{V}O_2$ through about 80 percent of $\dot{V}O_{2max}$. Maximum flow in a mixed muscle during exercise is about 100 ml/100 g · min, roughly the same as for unstressed myocardium. If the capillary reserve is fully mobilized, the O_2 extraction can reach 80%. Maximal muscle $\dot{V}O_2$ is 15 to 20 ml/100 g · min, depending on the type of exercise and physical training.

Exercise Vasodilation

The central problem for muscle circulation is how to limit flow at rest, yet provide sufficient flow for aerobic work. Resistance per 100 g of resting muscle is about 100, 20, and 10 times that in kidney, heart, and splanchnic bed, respectively. At least half this huge resistance is due to basal tone, so active vasodilation as well as decreased sympathetic vasoconstrictor tone is essential in exercise.

Both nerves and metabolites contribute to exercise vasodilation. In certain emotionally charged situations, special extrinsic sympathetic nerves initiate vasodilation in anticipation of exercise.

These nerves are thought to release acetylcholine or a vasodilator peptide from their endings. In most circumstances, however, exercise vasodilation is initiated and maintained by mechanisms "built into" the skeletal muscle. These intrinsic mechanisms are activated by muscle contraction, so they depend on the central nervous system indirectly. Resistance begins to fall in 1 s, and half-maximal flow is achieved in 5 to 10 s. Even a single twitch will often cause a detectable drop in resistance. These and other characteristics suggest that exercise vasodilation is initiated by the intrinsic nerves whose cell bodies lie within the walls of the arterioles; one such nerve is shown in Figure 18-6B.

Intrinsic vasomotor nerves can be blocked with local anesthetics at doses that do not affect contraction of skeletal muscle. After such blockade, exercise vasodilation is delayed and develops more slowly than normal, under the influence of vasodilator metabolites. The identity of these metabolites varies with muscle fiber type and with the duration and intensity of exercise. Candidates include O_2, K^+, adenosine, inorganic phosphate, H^+, CO_2, and substances released from vascular endothelium. In most instances several vasodilator metabolites act in concert.

Role of Capillary Recruitment

O_2 extraction in exercise is chiefly limited by the transcapillary PO_2 gradient. A large gradient is required to overcome transcapillary resistance to O_2 transport, as explained in Chapter 16. This PO_2 gradient varies directly with O_2 flux density and inversely with capillary transit time. Capillary recruitment decreases O_2 flux density by providing additional capillary surface area, and prolongs red cell transit times by increasing the aggregate cross-sectional area of the capillary bed. O_2 flux density is further diminished by the rise in capillary hematocrit that accompanies exercise hyperemia. In the presence of more capillaries and red cells less O_2 need be extracted from each. The fall in flux density decreases the transcapillary PO_2 gradient required to deliver the flux.

Characteristics of capillary recruitment in exercise are shown in Figure 22-4. Measurements were made on dog gracilis muscles at rest and during phasic exercise at 75 percent of $\dot{V}O_{2max}$. The muscles were quick-frozen, and the number of red-cell-containing capillaries per microscope field was determined. Notice the great heterogeneity of local capillary density at rest. The prominent lower tail of the distribution at rest means that at many locations there were few red cells, or none whatever. Functional capillary density increased and became much more homogeneous within 5 s after the onset of exercise. Recruit-

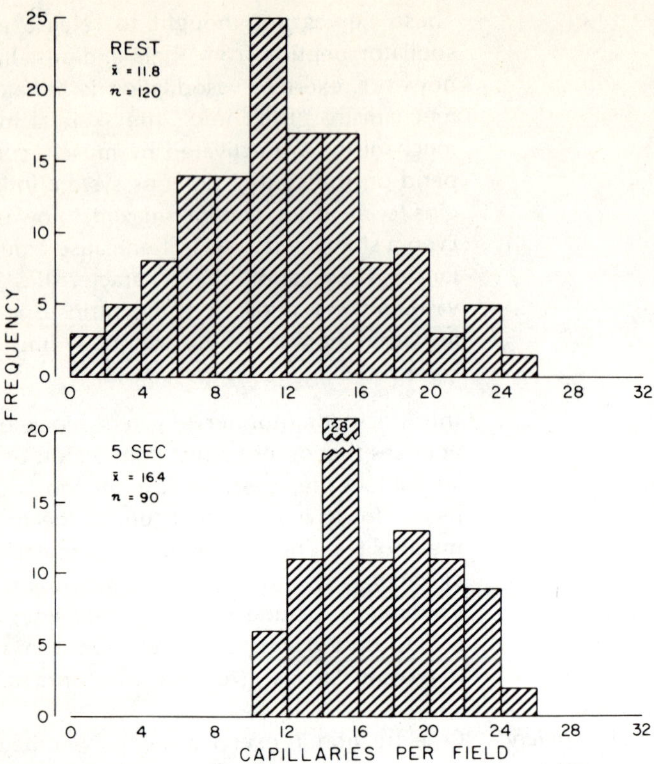

Figure 22-4
Probability distributions for capillary density in 90 randomly selected fields in a pure red muscle. Ordinate indicates frequency of observations for class intervals shown on abscissa.

ment matches the properties of the oxygen exchanger to flow and $\dot{V}O_2$.

Role of Myoglobin

The O_2 affinity of myoglobin (Mb) is five times that of Hb, but about 50 times less than that of cytochrome oxidase. Mb is therefore admirably suited to accepting O_2 from Hb, storing it, and releasing it to the electron transport chain. Mb's oxydissociation curve is shown in Figure 22-5; it applies to all muscles and species. Mb lacks allosteric controls, and each Mb molecule binds only one O_2. When PO_2 exceeds 20 torr, small changes in Mb saturation, and hence total O_2 content, are accompanied by large changes in PO_2. Conversely, below half saturation (5 torr), *Mb acts as a PO_2 buffer*; large changes in saturation and O_2 content are accompanied by small changes in PO_2. Both slopes of the Mb dissociation curve are adaptive.

Mb is an O_2 carrier as well as a PO_2 buffer. A flux of oxymyoglobulin molecules in parallel with free O_2 (so-called Mb-

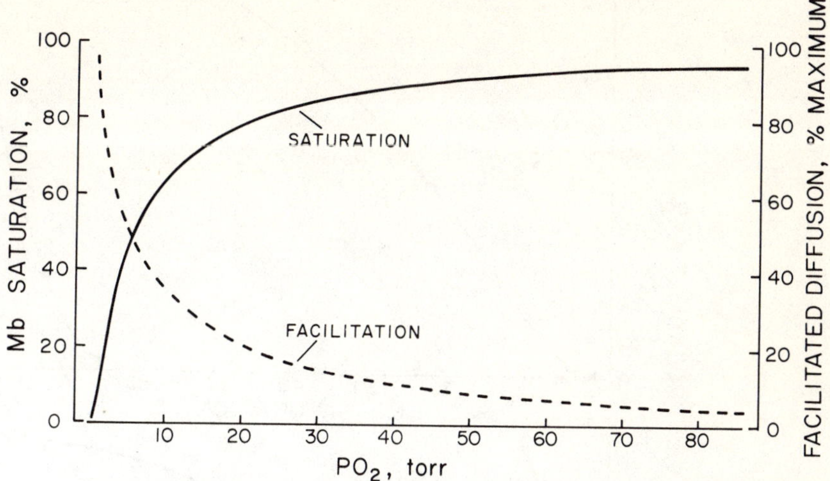

Figure 22-5
Myoglobin (*Mb*) oxydissociation curve (*solid line*) and effect of PO_2 on Mb-facilitated diffusion (*dashed line*).

facilitated diffusion) augments O_2 flux over the long distance from sarcolemma to the cell interior. The Mb-facilitated flux becomes dominant at saturations characteristic of working muscle. Thus the increase in facilitation shown in Figure 22-5 is a major reserve of O_2 transport.

Mb saturation in vivo represents the balance of all determinants of O_2 supply and demand. Figure 22-6 compares Mb saturation and corresponding PO_2 measured in individual myocytes at rest and during maximal work. Results are shown as probability distributions to illustrate local heterogeneity. Mb was more than 60 percent saturated at all locations at rest (Figure 22-6, *top*). At these high saturations PO_2 is poorly buffered; PO_2 ranged from 10 to 53 torr.

The fall in saturation during exercise is accompanied by a large fall in PO_2. This fall helps defend the transcapillary PO_2 gradient against the fall in intracapillary PO_2. In the example shown in Figure 22-6, median cell PO_2 fell to only 1.5 torr. Moreover, the range was very small, largely because of the steep buffer slope of the Mb dissociation curve. Consequently, PO_2 remained high enough to ensure maximal cytochrome turnover at all locations. The buffer and transport functions of Mb are essential; if Mb is destroyed, $\dot{V}O_2$ falls and the muscle promptly fatigues.

In summary, the enormous range of $\dot{V}O_2$ characteristic of red muscle depends on the interaction of flow, Hb, capillary recruit-

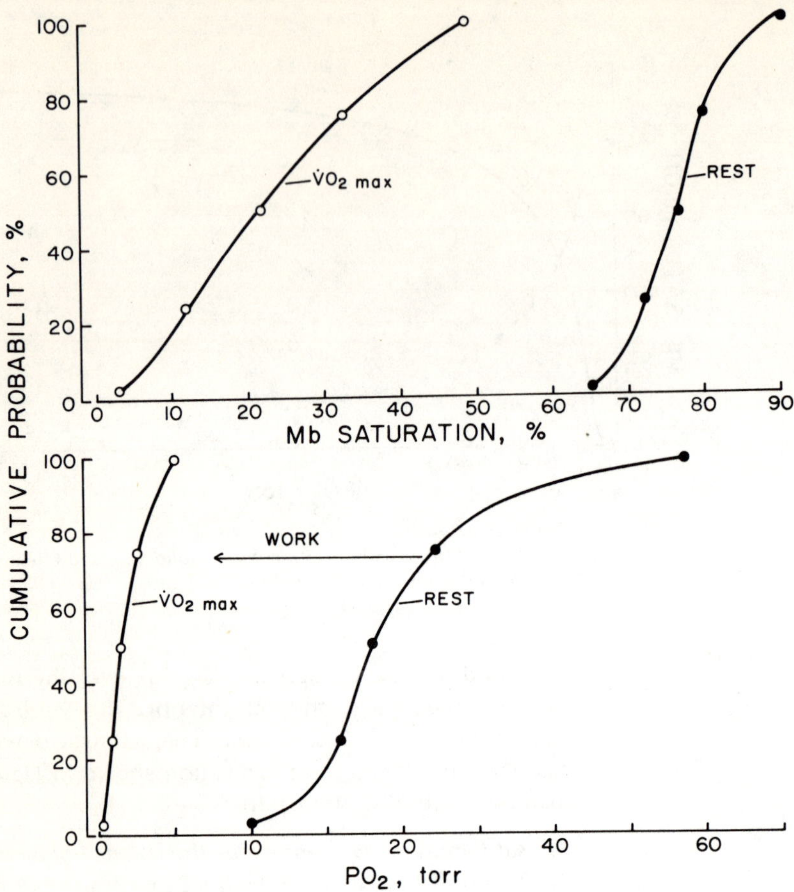

Figure 22-6
Probability distributions of myoglobin (*Mb*) saturation and intracellular PO_2 in a red muscle at rest (*filled circles*) and at maximal $\dot{V}O_2$ during twitch contraction (*open circles*). Ordinate indicates the percentage of the cell population whose PO_2 is equal to or less than the corresponding value on the abscissa. (Measurements were made in collaboration with Dr. T. E. J. Gayeski.)

ment, and Mb as an integrated transport system. Each system component can be compromised, directly or indirectly, by disease.

References

1. Astrand, P. O., and Rodahl, K. *Textbook of Work Physiology*. New York: McGraw-Hill, 1977. Pp. 291–318.
2. Brooks, G. A. Lactate production under fully aerobic conditions: The lactate shuttle during rest and exercise. *Fed. Proc.* 45:2924, 1986.
3. Gayeski, T. E. J., Connett, R. J., and Honig, C. R. Oxygen transport in rest-work transition illustrates new functions for myoglobin. *Am. J. Physiol.* 248:H914, 1985.
4. Gayeski, T. E. J., and Honig, C. R. O_2 gradients from sarcolemma to cell interior in red muscle at maximal $\dot{V}O_2$. *Am. J. Physiol.* 251:H789, 1986.

*5. Granger, H. J., Meininger, G. A., Borders, J. L., Morff, R. J., and Goodman, A. H. Microcirculation in Skeletal Muscle. In: M. A. Mortillaro, (ed.), *Physiology and Pharmacology of the Microcirculation,* Vol. 2. New York: Academic, 1984.

6. Hensel, H. *Thermoreception and Temperature Regulation.* New York: Academic, 1981.

7. Honig, C. R., Odoroff, C. L., and Frierson, J. L. Capillary recruitment in exercise: Rate, extent, uniformity and relation to blood flow. *Am. J. Physiol.* 238:H31, 1980.

8. Johnson, J. M., Brengelmann, G. L., Hales, J. R. S., and Vanhoutte, P. M. Regulation of the cutaneous circulation. *Fed. Proc.* 45:2841, 1986.

9. Rowell, L. B. *Human Circulation Regulation During Physical Stress.* New York; London: Oxford University Press, 1986.

References to Other Regional Circulations

Circulation in lung, kidney, fetus, and placenta is generally considered in those parts of a physiology course that deal with respiration, kidney function, and reproduction. Readers who are not participating in a standard course may find the following references helpful.

Renal Circulation

1. Brenner, B. M., Baylis, C., and Deen, W. M. Transport of molecules across glomerular capillaries. *Physiol. Rev.* 56:502, 1976.
2. Knox, F. G., and Spielman, W. S. Renal Circulation. In J. T. Shepherd and F. M. Abboud (eds.), *Handbook of Physiology*, Section 2: The Cardiovascular System, Vol. III: Peripheral Circulation and Organ Blood Flow, Part 1. Bethesda, Md.: American Physiological Society, 1983.
3. Valtin, H. *Renal Function: Mechanisms Preserving Fluid and Solute Balance in Health*. Boston: Little, Brown and Co., 1979.
4. Wright, F. S., and Briggs, J. P. Feedback control of glomerular blood flow, pressure, and filtration rate. *Physiol. Rev.* 59:958, 1979.

Pulmonary Circulation

1. Caro, C. G., Pedley, T. J., Schrater, R. C., and Seed, W. A. *The Mechanics of the Circulation*. New York; London: Oxford University Press, 1978. Chap. 15.
2. Grover, R. F., Wagner, W. W., Jr., McMurtry, I. F., and Reeves, J. T. Pulmonary Circulation. In J. T. Shepherd and F. M. Abboud (eds.), *Handbook of Physiology*, Section 2: The Cardiovascular System, Vol. III: Peripheral Circulation and Organ Blood Flow, Part 1. Bethesda, Md.: American Physiological Society, 1983.
3. Martin, L. *Pulmonary Physiology in Clinical Practice*. St. Louis: Mosby, 1987. Pp. 88–128, 147–174.
4. Slonim, N. B., and Hamilton, L. H. *Respiratory Physiology* (5th ed.). St. Louis: Mosby, 1987. Pp. 97–153.

Uterine, Fetal, and Placental Circulations

1. Faber, J. J., and Thornburg, K. L. *Placental Physiology*. New York: Raven, 1983.
2. Gootman, N., and Gootman, P. M. (eds.). *Perinatal Cardiovascular Function*. New York: Dekker, 1983.
3. Heymann, M. A., Iwamoto, H. S., and Rudolph, A. M. Factors affecting changes in the neonatal systemic circulation. *Annu. Rev. Physiol.* 43:371, 1981.

4. Longo, L. D., and Reneau, D. D. (eds.). *Fetal and Newborn Cardiovascular Physiology,* Vols. 1 and 2. New York: Garland, 1978.

5. Meschia, G. Circulation to Female Reproductive Organs. In J. T. Shepherd and F. M. Abboud (eds.), *Handbook of Physiology,* Section 2: The Cardiovascular System, Vol. III: Peripheral Circulation and Organ Blood Flow, Part 1. Bethesda, Md.: American Physiological Society, 1983.

V : Regulation by the Central Nervous System

23 : Functions and Organization of Neural Controls

What the Nervous System Accomplishes

Before learning how something works, one should know what it is for and why it is important. Despite the power and diversity of non-neural mechanisms, control of circulation by the brain is essential for survival. The overall performance of the circulation in unanesthetized animals and humans is dominated by neural controls. Finally, syndromes such as hypertension and edematous states are, to a great extent, disorders of neural regulation. The reason the central nervous system is so important is that it reconciles two opposite requirements, namely, *stability* and appropriate *change*.

Stability

The circulation is not a house of cards. A large measure of stability is provided by the cardiac length-tension relation, the parallel arrangement of organ resistances, autoregulation, and local metabolites. Because of these intrinsic mechanisms, the circulation remains stable in properly supported animals even after the central nervous system is completely destroyed. Though arterial pressure is low in such animals, cardiac output remains sufficient for organ function.

Stability in aneural animals is illusory, for it is possible only if the investigator takes over functions normally performed by the nervous system. *With all feedback loops open, stability cannot be maintained in a changing environment.* For example, if the aneural animal is tilted, blood pools in the dependent parts. The animal dies of this internal hemorrhage, because the animal lacks afferent and efferent pathways for venoconstriction, tachycardia, and increased contractility. If a heat stress is applied, cardiac output is neither increased nor redistributed to the skin, and core temperature rises to lethal levels. Loss of only 10 percent of blood volume (the amount donated at a blood bank) induces fatal hypotension for want of vasoconstriction and cardiac stimulation. Intact animals maintain cardiac output when erect, hold temperature constant in adverse climates, and tolerate loss of 10 percent of blood volume with no change whatever in cardiac output or arterial pressure. Thus it is the central nervous system that provides the stability of vital functions necessary for survival under realistic conditions.

Adaptability

For predator, prey, or pedestrian, survival often depends on large, rapid changes in the same quantities that under basal conditions are held constant by regulatory systems. Constancy and regulation are not synonymous, however. To regulate means "to adjust according to some principle, or to some purpose." Thus cardiac output is regulated according to the principle that it be sufficient to support aerobic metabolism. The cardiac output is held constant at rest because $\dot{V}O_2$ is constant. In exercise, however, it is regulated according to the principle that it increases linearly with $\dot{V}O_2$. Similarly, body temperature at rest is regulated according to the principle that it be about 37°C. In heavy exercise, however, the thermostat is reset, and core temperature is regulated around 40°C. The higher temperature facilitates heat exchange.

Adaptive change is not entirely dependent on the central nervous system. During exercise, the muscle and thoracoabdominal pumps increase venous return. Stretch of the pacemaker increases heart rate, and distension of the ventricle increases stroke volume. Moreover, the rate and extent of exercise vasodilation are almost the same in normal and sympathectomized muscles. Why then is neural control so important in exercise? The answer is obvious when one compares *quantitatively* the performance of an animal with and without its autonomic innervation; see Table 23-1. Dogs were trained to run on a treadmill at a rate slightly below $\dot{V}O_{2max}$. Then the sympathetic chains and adrenals were removed bilaterally. One vagus nerve was cut, and the other was transplanted beneath the skin where it could be blocked with a local anesthetic. After suitable time for recovery and reconditioning, the animals were observed again. Table 23-1 actually underestimates the role of nerves, because many sympathetic fibers to the limbs do not traverse the sympathetic

Table 23-1
Effect of Bilateral Cervical Vagotomy and Excision of the Sympathetic Chains on Average Cardiovascular Responses to Treadmill Exercise in Trained Dogs

	Multiples of Resting Values	
Response	Normal	Denervated
Heart rate	2.2 (Anticipatory)	1.15 (Delayed)
Cardiac output	3	1.45
End-diastolic pressure	0.5	2
Muscle flow	8.5 (Anticipatory)	3 (Rapid)
Arterial pressure	1.4	0.4
$\dot{V}O_2$	24	14

chains and therefore remained intact. The differences, which are detailed in the following paragraphs, are striking nonetheless.

Anticipatory Changes. The autonomic responses that accompany familiar movements are a form of *learned behavior.* As the investigator reached for the switch, and before the treadmill began to move, heart rate increased in normal dogs within three or four beats to a value slightly greater than that during steady exercise. Redistribution of flow to muscle also preceded exercise. These anticipatory changes assure maintenance of aerobic metabolism in the rest-work transition and permit high cardiac output awaiting exercise with little change in arterial pressure. After denervation, cardiac output increased slowly and only after a considerable delay. Though muscle vasodilation was rapid, it did not begin until the animal started to run.

Priorities and Coordination of System Components. Before denervation, arterial pressure rose despite massive vasodilation in muscle, because of increased cardiac output and compensatory vasoconstriction in other vascular beds. "Run now, form urine later" — only the central nervous system can set such priorities and coordinate system components to meet them. After denervation, the right hand, so to speak, did not know what the left hand was doing. The animals sustained a marked fall in arterial pressure, because arterioles in kidney, skin, and splanchnic beds were not "told" to constrict.

Increased Functional Capacity. Before denervation, external cardiac work rose sharply despite lower ventricular end-diastolic pressure. From this we infer that adrenergic nerves shifted the heart to a more advantageous function curve. Greater contractility and faster ventricular relaxation allowed stroke volume to increase even though filling time was greatly reduced by tachycardia. After denervation, heart rate increased hardly at all. The modest increase in stroke volume was purchased at the cost of higher filling pressure, greater wall tension and O_2 consumption, and lowered cardiac efficiency.

After denervation, muscle blood flow was severely limited by low cardiac output and perfusion pressure. Moreover, the distribution of cardiac output was inappropriate. Though intrinsic mechanisms lowered resistance in the working muscles, vasoconstriction failed to divert flow away from the nonworking muscles and the renal, splanchnic, and cutaneous beds. O_2 extraction in the working muscles was therefore maximal, $\dot{V}O_2$ was limited by O_2 delivery, lactic acid accumulated, and the muscles fatigued. The effect on performance — the most important yardstick of all — was obvious. Denervated dogs rapidly became exhausted, sat down, and allowed the treadmill to slide beneath them. After a few such sessions, they refused to run at all. In contrast, normal dogs enjoyed running and could keep it up for hours.

In summary, neural controls are essential for survival because they permit both stability and rapid adaptive change. They allow anticipatory adjustments, set priorities, coordinate components, effect economies, and improve efficiency. These actions increase transport capacity and greatly extend the limits of performance.

A Trip around the Feedback Loop

The adaptive changes just considered are organized within the very same brain structures responsible for voluntary behaviors. However, these structures cannot function in isolation. Neural pathways connect them to centers responsible for reflex regulations that play an essential, though permissive, role by maintaining arterial pressure, cardiac output, and total blood volume within appropriate limits continuously over a lifetime. These long-term regulations are based on closed-loop, negative feedback systems. Figure 23-1 identifies the essential components and their functions. Cardiovascular regulations exhibit complex nonlinear performance characteristics, so the following description is qualitative.

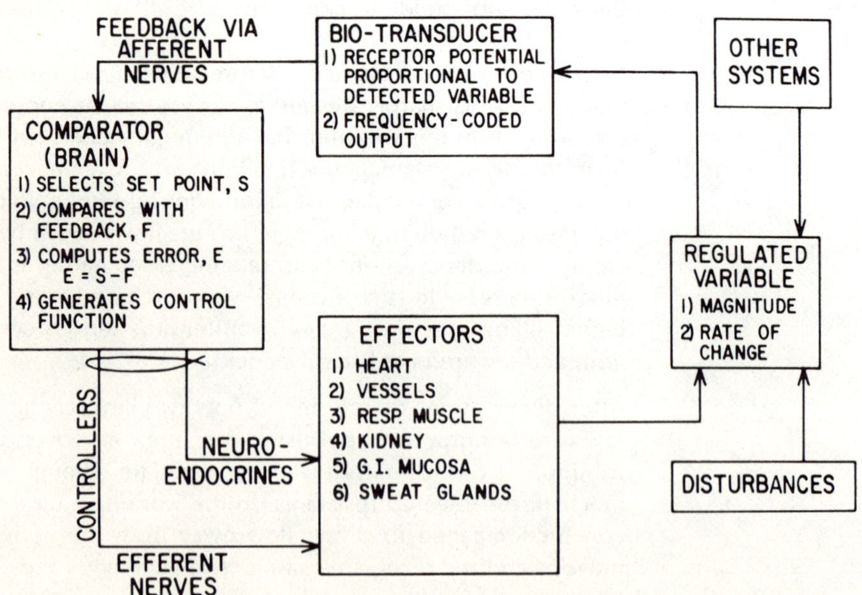

Figure 23-1
General scheme for feedback regulation of a physiological variable.

The brain (box at the left in Figure 23-1) serves as *comparator.* It determines the ideal value or *set point* for the regulation, compares this ideal value with the feedback signal, and computes the error. It then generates a control function (output) to correct the error. The precision of the regulation depends strongly on the accuracy of the computed error, which may not be identical to the real error if there are time lags in the system. Lags may be due to insufficient sensitivity of the receptor to change in the regulated variable, or to delays in neural networks. Delays tend to make the system unstable, because the control function may not be appropriate for the situation at the time it becomes effective, especially if the regulated variable is changing rapidly. Stability can be greatly improved if the brain "knows" not only the magnitude of the regulated variable but also its rate of change. Most mechanoreceptors detect rate as well as magnitude.

The efferent nerves and neuroendocrines act as *controllers;* the mediators they release alter properties of the *effectors*, chiefly heart and vascular smooth muscle. Effectors modify organ function (heart rate, for example) in a way that tends to restore the regulated variable to its ideal value. In general, nerves are required for fast, short-term adjustments, whereas hormones produce slower, more long-lasting effects.

The *gain* of a system component may be defined as how much comes out of the component for a particular input. Perhaps the most important fact to bear in mind about cardiovascular effectors is that their gain is enormous. This is not surprising, for resistance varies inversely as the radius to the fourth power, heart rate can increase threefold, and small changes in length of venous smooth muscle displace large volumes of blood. High effector gain allows fast, accurate response but decreases the margin of stability. Consequently, *circulatory performance is critically dependent on the gain of the receptors* and the properties of the brain. That is why receptor function is emphasized in subsequent chapters. Regulation of arterial pressure, cardiac output, and total blood volume depends on mechanoreceptors. Chemoreceptor reflexes have little effect on circulation except under extreme conditions, and then mostly indirectly, via respiratory afferents.

Specificity and the Role of the Adrenals

Catch-phrases are hard to forget. One hesitates to mention Cannon's notion of "fight or flight," for fear some readers may not have heard it. They conjure up an image of a hissing, hypertensive cat, back bowed, hackles up, pupils dilated, with epinephrine pouring out of its adrenals. Such a massive, generalized autonomic discharge bears no resemblance to normal autonomic behavior. Instead, *specificity* is one of the salient characteristics of both sympathetic and parasympathetic responses under almost all circumstances. Specificity is impossible in the presence of substantial quantities of blood-borne catecholamine. Recall from Chapter 18 that circulating catecholamines have little or no effect on circulation at normal rates of secretion.

In summary, cardiovascular control systems possess powerful but highly specific effectors. Precision of regulation is therefore limited by the receptors and the performance of the brain.

References

1. Abboud, F. M., and Thames, M. D. Interaction of Cardiovascular Reflexes in Circulatory Control. In J. T. Shepherd and F. M. Abboud (eds.), *Handbook of Physiology,* Section 2: Circulation, Vol. III: Peripheral Circulation and Organ Blood Flow, Part 2. Bethesda, Md.: American Physiological Society, 1983.

*2. Grodins, F. S. *Control Theory and Biological Systems.* New York: Columbia University Press, 1963. Pp. 1–26 (for all students), pp. 153–172 (for the mathematically inclined).

24 : Regulation of Arterial Pressure

More than half a century ago Hering showed that tonically active pressure receptors exist and that stimulation of these receptors lowers heart rate and peripheral resistance. The reflex was abolished by cutting the afferent nerve and could be reproduced by electrical stimulation of the central end of the nerve. Thus all the essential elements of a regulatory system were shown to be present. This system proved to be the principal short-term defense of arterial pressure against hemorrage and orthostatic stress. Baroreflexes are also required to "buffer" arterial pressure against changes in cardiac output and peripheral resistance that accompany environmental stress and voluntary behavior. Since the cardiovascular effectors are extremely powerful, the performance of the entire system strongly depends on the properties of the receptors themselves.

The Transfer Function of the Baroreceptors

The baroreceptors are located in the carotid sinus (the junction of the internal and external carotid arteries) and in the aortic arch. An ingenious experiment proved that they respond to stretch and not to pressure per se. A balloon on the end of a catheter was inserted into the carotid sinus; inflation caused hypotension and bradycardia. These responses were abolished when the sinus was enclosed in a plaster cast, and were restored when the cast was removed. The carotid sinus is, in fact, the most distensible part of the arterial system. It consists of thin lamellae of elastic fibers, with little collagen or smooth muscle. The highly branched processes of the baroreceptors are enmeshed in the elastic laminae and are deformed as the vessel is distended.

A general model of a mechanoreceptor is shown in Figure 24-1. The tissue in which the receptor is embedded serves as a *mechanical filter* that determines both the magnitude and rate of strain on the receptor membrane. Strain decreases membrane resistance and allows an inward flow of current, carried largely by Na^+. The corresponding depolarization is called the *receptor potential*. Its principal characteristic is that it is graded by the mechanical stimulus and does not become regenerative. Passive current spread caused by the receptor potential depolarizes the

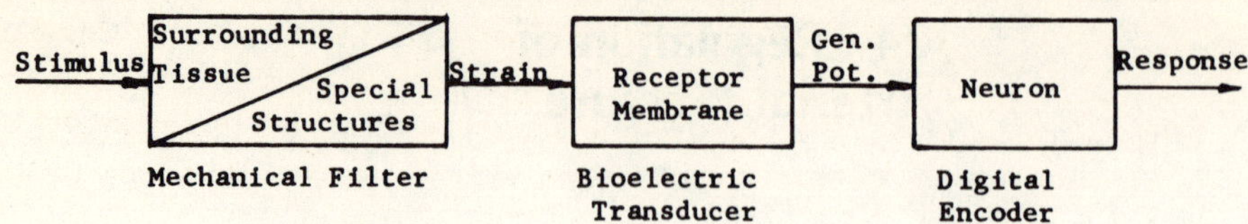

Figure 24-1
Model of a mechanoreceptor. (From W. B. Clarke, Thesis, University of Rochester, 1968.)

contiguous sensory nerve to threshold. The receptor potential in a baroreceptor evoked by a step increase in pressure consists of two distinct components. A large initial depolarization is proportional to the rate of change of pressure (dynamic response). It is followed by a smaller depolarization proportional to the new steady pressure (static response). The static component continues as long as pressure is applied. Both components are encoded as action potential frequencies in the baroreceptor nerves.

What the Baroreceptors Measure

Mean arterial pressure is detected as the static component of receptor discharge. The static response of a single baroreceptor nerve fiber to step changes in carotid sinus pressure is shown in Figure 24-2. No action potentials were recorded until pressure

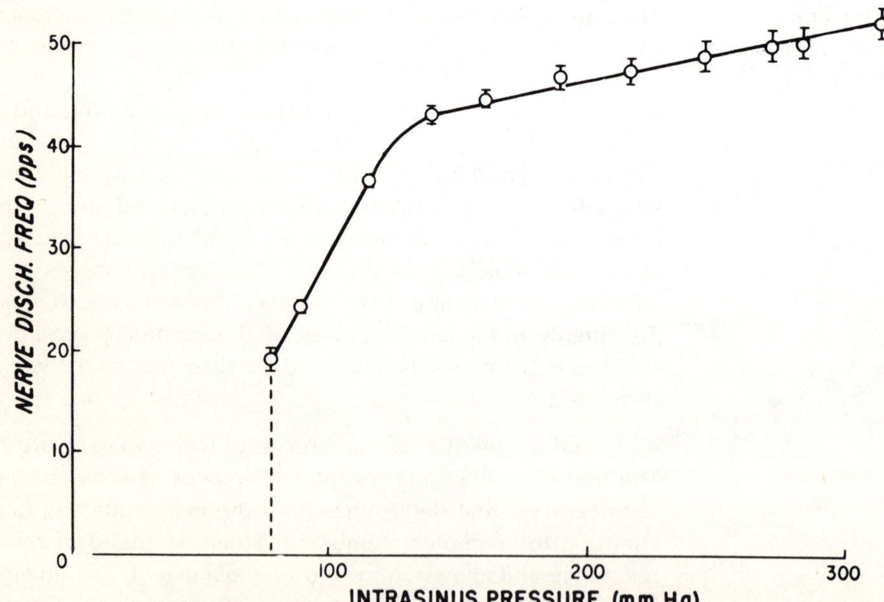

Figure 24-2
Static response of a single fiber to step increments in sinus pressure. The ordinate is in pulses per second. (From W. B. Clarke, Thesis, University of Rochester, 1968.)

reached 75 torr. Other fibers had higher or lower thresholds. Discharge frequency increased steeply and linearly through 140 torr. The change in slope is caused by decreased vessel compliance at higher pressures, as explained on pages 79 to 81. Though a wide range of mean pressures can be detected, the *gain* of the receptors (change in firing rate for a given change in pressure) is greatest at normal pressures. This is also true of the gain of the whole system.

To learn what information is contained in the rate-sensitive component of baroreceptor discharge (dynamic response), pressure was applied to the carotid sinus at known rates. The effect of a large step increase in pressure on discharge frequency in a single fiber is shown in Figure 24-3. The dynamic response peaks when the rate of rise of pressure is maximal and decays in 2 s, leaving a residual discharge. This residual is, of course, the static response. The dynamic response tends to dominate action potential frequency in the baroreceptor afferents, particularly when pulse pressure is augmented by sympathetic drive, or by aortic valve disease.

The baroreceptors detect the rate of fall as well as rate of rise. Consequently, the discharge pattern evoked by a normal heart beat roughly resembles the contour of the pressure pulse, as shown in Figure 24-4. Thus the determinants of pulse pressure — contractility, heart rate, and peripheral resistance — are en-

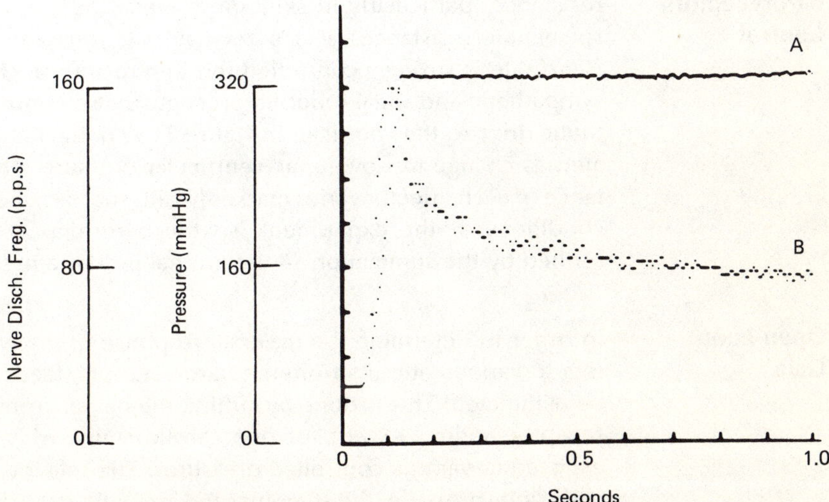

Figure 24-3
Effect of a step increase in carotid sinus pressure from 50 to 330 torr. The pressure recording (trace A) appears as a series of dots during the rapid rise. Trace B is the nerve discharge frequency in pulses per second. (From W. B. Clarke, Thesis, University of Rochester, 1968.)

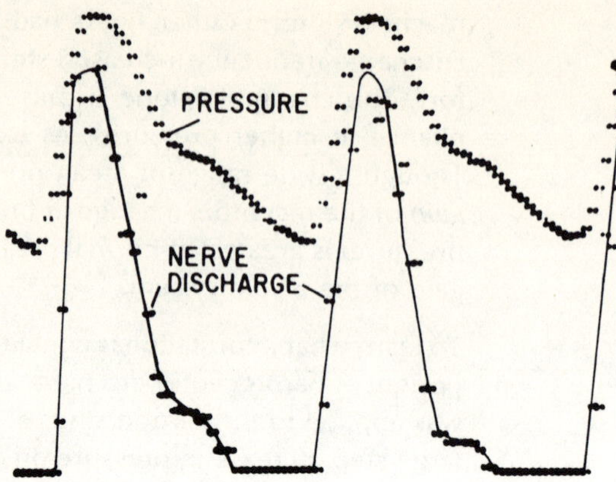

Figure 24-4
Relation between carotid arterial pressure (*upper curve*) and action potential frequency in a single fiber from the sinus nerve. The computer-generated frequency data were connected with a continuous line to clarify the time course of nerve discharge. (Modified from B. N. Christensen, H. R. Warner, and T. A. Pryor. In P. Kedzi [ed.] *Baroreceptors and Hypertension*. Oxford: Pergamon, 1967.)

coded in the pattern of nerve discharge. Information about these controlled quantities is essential for precise regulation of pressure because of the enormous gain of the cardiovascular effectors.

What the Baroreceptors Control

The principal effector engaged in the baroreflex is arteriolar resistance, particularly in skin and skeletal muscle. Renal and splanchnic resistances also participate vigorously in humans. Heart rate is strongly controlled through reciprocal changes in sympathetic and vagal tone. Baroreceptors also control sympathetic drive to the ventricle. In Figure 24-5 contractility is evaluated as change in isovolumic ventricular pressure. The importance of each effector varies markedly with species, and with the conditions of the experiment, so the baroreflex is best described by the summation — the arterial pressure itself.

Open-Loop Gain

In order to determine the maximal response of the whole system to various outputs from the baroreceptors, feedback must be eliminated. This is done by cutting the nerves from all baroreceptor regions except for one carotid sinus, which is then exposed to various controlled pressures. The relation between endosinus pressure (the stimulus) and systemic arterial pressure (the open-loop response) is shown in Figure 24-6. The open-loop gain of the system, defined as change in systemic pressure for a given change in sinus pressure, is shown in the upper panel. It is maximal at normal pressures. The gain of the recep-

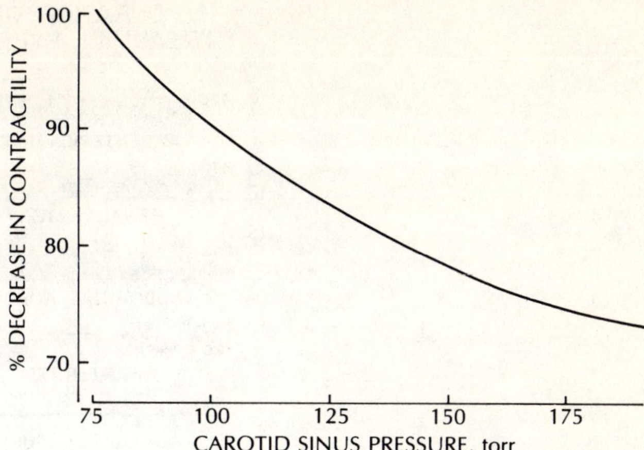

Figure 24-5
Effect of baroreceptor stimulation on strength of ventricular contraction.

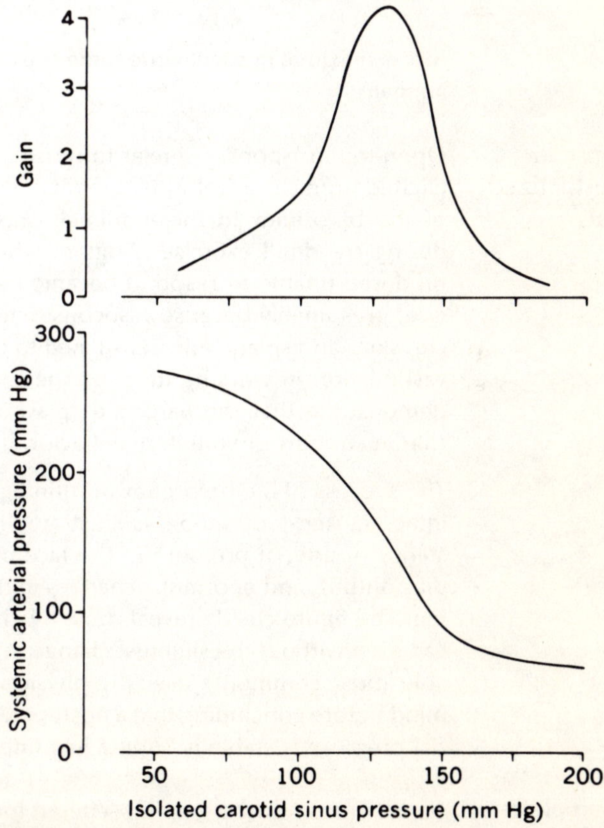

Figure 24-6
Quantitative characteristics of baroreceptor reflex in open-loop mode. (From data of P. I. Korner, *Physiol. Rev.* 51:312, 1971. As modified in Milnor, William R.: The Cardiovascular Control System. In Mountcastle, Vernon B., editor: *Medical Physiology*, Ed. 14, 1980, St. Louis, The C. V. Mosby Co.)

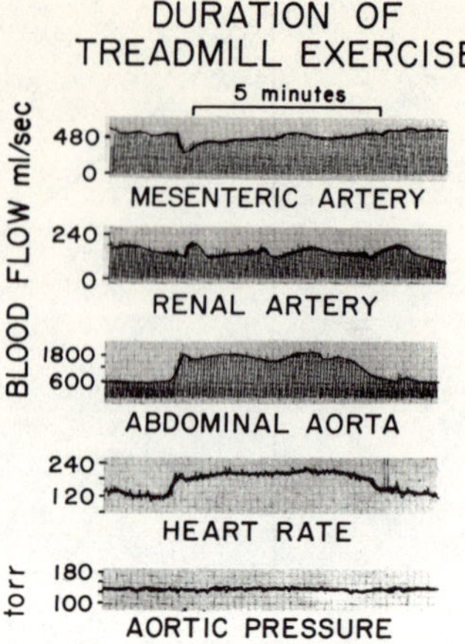

Figure 24-7
Constancy of arterial pressure during treadmill exercise in dogs, despite gross changes in peripheral circulation. (Modified from R. F. Rushmer, *Cardiovascular Dynamics* [2nd ed.]. Philadelphia: Saunders, 1961.)

tors is maximal in exactly the same pressure range in the normal animal.

Response in Unanesthetized Animals

Open-loop responses similar to those in Figure 24-6 have been elicited from chronically instrumented conscious dogs. The gain of the baroreflex in these animals was the same at rest and during treadmill exercise. Dogs in which baroreceptors were rendered unable to respond became hypotensive during exercise, presumably because vasoconstriction in nonworking muscle, skin, and splanchnic beds failed to compensate for massive vasodilation in working muscle. These important observations demonstrate that the baroreflex plays an essential *permissive* role in support of voluntary behavior.

The success of the baroreflex in running dogs with all receptors intact (closed-loop mode) is illustrated in Figure 24-7. The constancy of arterial pressure in the face of tachycardia, high cardiac output, and enormous changes in flow distribution is striking. The figure clearly reveals how much cardiovascular turmoil can exist without the slightest change in the cardiovascular variable most commonly used by physicians. Bear this figure in mind before concluding that a postoperative patient whose arterial pressure is stable is "doing just fine."

The Complete Feedback Loop

An expansion of the general scheme for cardiovascular regulation is shown in Figure 24-8. The reader should take the time to become thoroughly familiar with this key diagram. Central processing of the baroreflex — that is, the functions of the box labelled Brain — is considered in Chapter 26. A good point of

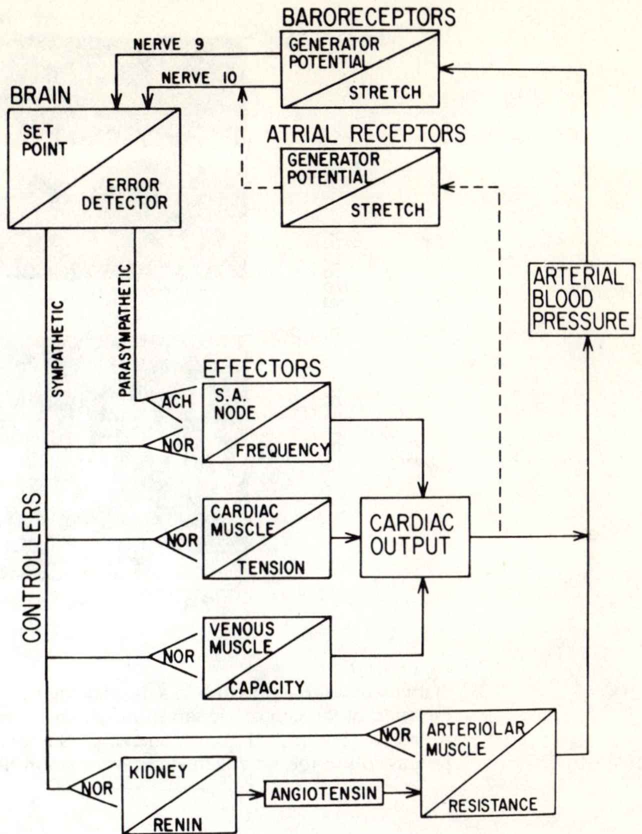

Figure 24-8
Interaction of systems for regulation of arterial pressure and cardiac output. The feedback loop for cardiac output is shown by the dashed lines. (*NOR* = norepinephrine; *ACH* = acetylcholine; *S.A.* = sinoatrial.)

departure is the box labelled Arterial Blood Pressure at right. Pressure and flow regulation are shown together because cardiac output is a major determinant of arterial pressure, and the two variables share the same controllers and some of the same effectors. The feedback loop for cardiac output is indicated by the dashed lines. Pressure and cardiac output can change independently, as in exercise, or concomitantly, as in hemorrhage or orthostatic stress.

The Buffer Action of the Baroreceptors

Baroreceptor afferents are often called *buffer nerves*, because they stabilize arterial pressure against internal as well as external stimuli. To characterize this buffer function, heart rate, arterial pressure, cardiac output, and total peripheral resistance were measured 24 hours a day for several weeks before and after

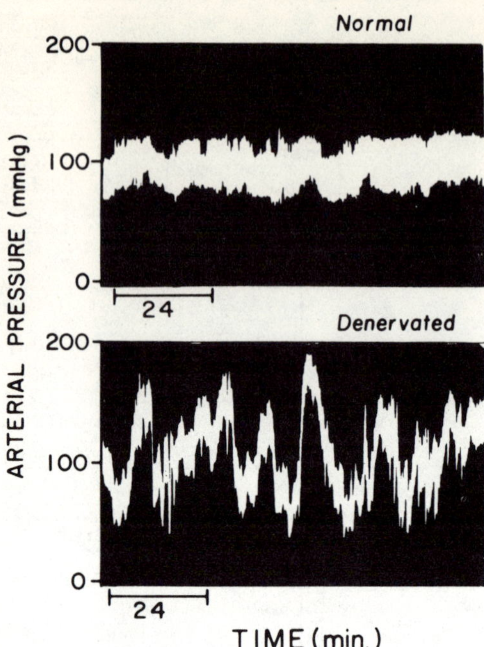

Figure 24-9
Stability of arterial pressure in a normal dog is contrasted with extreme lability after baroreceptor denervation. Animals were unanesthetized. (From A. W. Cowley, Jr., J. F. Laird, and A. C. Guyton, *Circ. Res.* 32:564, 1973. By permission of the American Heart Association, Inc.)

complete baroreceptor denervation. To minimize psychic stimuli, animals were isolated in a quiet room; data were transmitted to investigators outside. The principal result is shown in Figure 24-9. Both dogs were standing quietly without overt excitement, and without any known exogenous stimuli. Nevertheless, arterial pressure in the denervated animal fluctuated between 45 and 180 mm Hg! Presumably, the unbuffered pressure responded to psychic stimuli as the dog thought of cats, fire hydrants, and the investigators. Since hypotension as well as hypertension occurred, mean pressure over the duration of the recording was only slightly greater than normal.

Blood pressure varied even more chaotically during simple behavior such as feeding or changing from the recumbent to standing position. Increases were more prominent than decreases. Consequently, mean pressure during the course of the day would have been high had the animals been exposed to the usual exigencies of life. In sharp contrast, cardiac output was as stable as in the normal dog, indicating that baroreceptors are not essential for regulation of total flow.

Clinical Application

Baroreceptor Function in Hypertension

How is hypertension possible? If stresses or excessive basal tone in vascular smooth muscle raise arterial pressure, the baroreceptors should cause a compensatory decrease in sympathetic tone. Nevertheless, a large component of sympathetic tone persists in experimental renal hypertension. Moreover, if one stretches the sinus in a hypertensive animal, the systemic arterial pressure falls markedly. Thus the control system appears to defend an inappropriately high level of arterial pressure. Electroneurograms from multifiber preparations of the carotid sinus nerve indicate that action potential frequency at any pressure is lower than normal. This indicates a defect in the feedback signal. The most likely explanation is a change in the physical properties of the arterial wall (the mechanical filter) caused by sustained excessive stretch. Actual destruction of some receptors is suggested by recent histological findings. These pathological changes appear to be the *result* of hypertension rather than the initiating or primary *cause*. They nevertheless help to maintain the hypertensive state and contribute to the lability of arterial pressure in some forms of human hypertension. Defective baroreceptor function in hypertension is an excellent example of the dependence of system performance on feedback. In this sense, hypertension in any form is, in part, a disease of regulation.

Clinicians have exploited the above information by installing electronic pacemakers on the sinus nerve. The stimulators deliver bursts of pulses in early systole to stimulate the normal discharge pattern. Results in a few carefully selected patients indicate that arterial pressure can be decreased for long periods, particularly when pacing is accompanied by conventional therapy.

References[1]

1. Clarke, W. B. Static and dynamic characteristics of carotid sinus baroreceptors. Thesis, University of Rochester, 1968.

2. Cowley, A. W., Jr., Laird, J. F., and Guyton, A. C. Role of the baroreceptor reflex in daily control of arterial blood pressure and other variables in dogs. *Circ. Res.* 32:564, 1973.

3. Kunze, D. L. Regulation of activity of cardiac vagal motoneurons. *Fed. Proc.* 39:2513, 1980.

4. Matsuura, S. Depolarization of sensory nerve endings and impulse initiation in common carotid baroreceptors. *J. Physiol.* [Lond.] 235:31, 1973.

[1] References to central processing of the baroreflex are cited in Chapter 26.

*5. Sagawa, K. Baroreflex Control of Systemic Arterial Pressure and Vascular Bed. In J. T. Shepherd and F. M. Abboud (eds.), *Handbook of Physiology*, Section 2: The Cardiovascular System, Vol. III, Part 2. Bethesda, Md.: American Physiological Society, 1983.

6. Sleight, P. *Arterial Baroreceptors and Hypertension*. New York, London: Oxford University Press, 1980.

7. Stephenson, R. B., and Donald, D. E. Reflexes from isolated carotid sinuses of intact and vagotomized conscious dogs. *Am. J. Physiol.* 238:H815, 1980.

25 : Regulation of Cardiac Output and Blood Volume

Cardiac Output

The precise linear relation between cardiac output and $\dot{V}O_2$ during exercise (Figure 13-6) and the constancy of cardiac output at rest strongly suggest that cardiac output is regulated to match $\dot{V}O_2$. An ingenious test of this hypothesis makes use of the fact that cardiac output = stroke volume × heart rate. If the product is actively regulated and heart rate is varied, stroke volume should change to compensate.

Instrumented dogs were trained to run on a treadmill. In each animal a highly reproducible relation between cardiac output and work rate was observed. Pacemakers were then implanted, and after recovery and reconditioning the animals ran again. This time, however, heart rate was fixed between 80 and 240 beats per minute. For each animal the cardiac output was the same (about 7L/min) *regardless of heart rate* when the animal was running at 3 miles per hour. When the treadmill speed was increased to 4 miles per hour, cardiac output increased to about 12 liters per minute, even though heart rate remained constant. From such data we can infer that cardiac output is indeed regulated to match O_2 demand.

If a quantity is regulated, it must be detected. A large body of evidence indicates that the "flowmeter" is a stretch receptor that senses cardiac filling. The most advantageous place for such a receptor would be in the compliant atria, since end-diastolic pressures in atria and ventricles are the same. The atria contain subendocardial receptors much like those in the carotid sinus. Their axons travel in the vagus. Atrial receptors exhibit two distinct discharge patterns; see Figure 25-1.

Type A receptors fire only during atrial systole and signal heart rate. They are distributed throughout both atria, in close relation to cardiac muscle cells. A very different discharge pattern arises from receptors enmeshed in the connective tissue at the origin of the caval or pulmonary veins (type B receptors). Their frequency is maximal just before the AV valves open. Discharge ceases very early in diastole and does not begin again until the next systole. This pattern parallels *atrial volume:* When the ventricle contracts, the atria cannot empty, but venous return con-

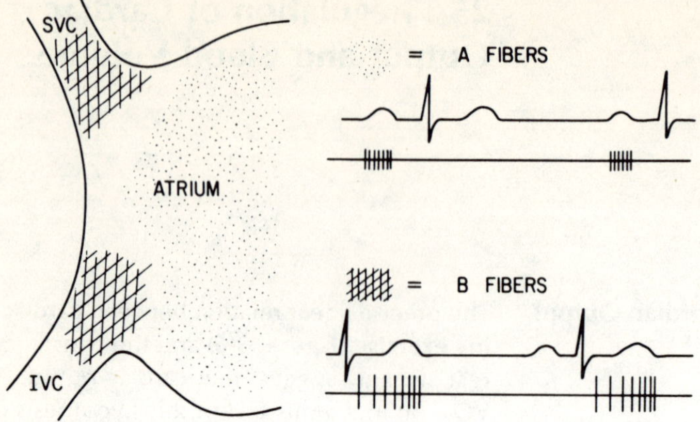

Figure 25-1
Location and time of discharge of atrial type A and type B receptors.

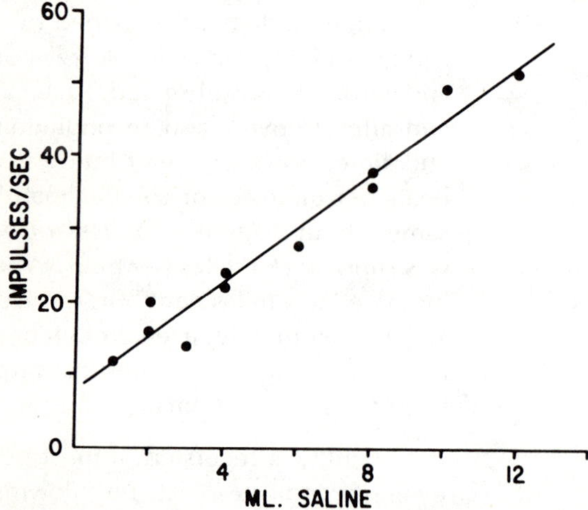

Figure 25-2
Volume in an isolated atrium was varied, and frequency was measured in single type B fiber. (From A. S. Paintal, *J. Physiol.* [Lond.] 120:610, 1953. By permission of Cambridge University Press.)

tinues. The resulting stretch produces a discharge, and rapid emptying in diastole turns the discharge off. The relation between atrial volume and action potential frequency from a type B receptor is precisely linear, as shown in Figure 25-2. Information about stroke volume as well as heart rate is therefore available to the brain.

Stretch of atrial receptors increases heart rate. The extent of the increase is conditioned by sympathetic and vagal tone, as set by the arterial baroreceptors. Heart rate is also affected by unmyelinated ventricular afferents. Where and how the brain inte-

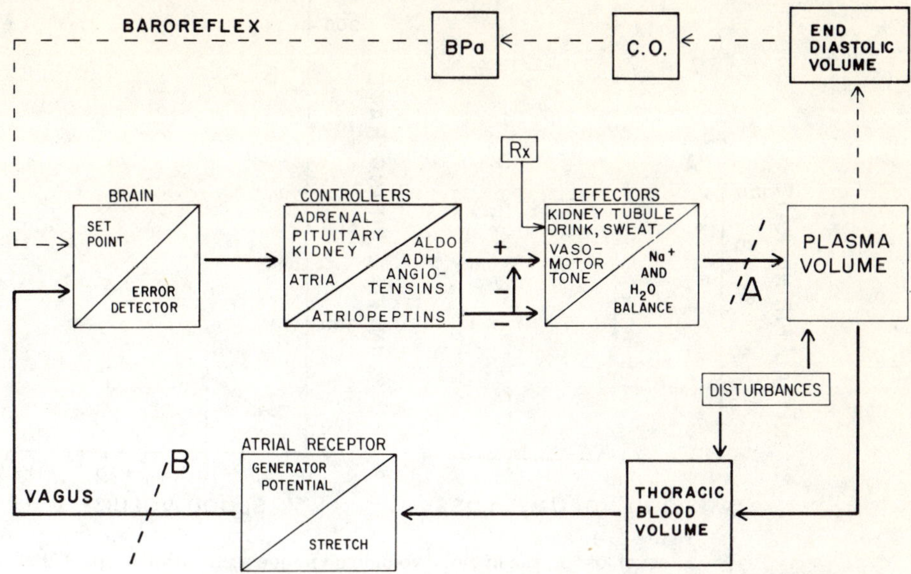

Figure 25-3
Heavy, continuous arrows denote the system that regulates plasma volume. Cardiac output (*C.O.*) and arterial pressure (*BPa*) are affected indirectly. Dashed lines A and B indicate sites at which disease may open the loop. (*ALDO* = aldosterone; *ADH* = antidiuretic hormone.)

grates information from various receptors to compute cardiac output is not known.

Regulation of Blood Volume

In Chapter 12 we learned that blood volume is remarkably constant throughout adult life. Long-term constancy in the face of changing rates of fluid intake and loss implies regulation. The systems shown in Figure 24-8 influence blood volume through control of capillary filtration pressure. If blood volume falls, as in hemorrhage or dehydration, reflex vasoconstriction occurs, and fluid is mobilized from the extravascular compartments. Though volume redistributions are *necessary* for rapid, short-term adjustments, they are not *sufficient*. They must be reinforced by a second line of defense to stabilize the total volume of body fluids. The system responsible for long-term volume regulation is outlined in Figure 25-3. We next consider each component in sequence.

The Atrial Volume Receptor

Atrial stretch varies with thoracic blood volume. Atrial B fibers therefore monitor a representative sample of total blood volume. Notice in Figure 25-4 that a 10 percent reduction in blood volume lowers frequency in an atrial B fiber to half its control value! Threshold for detection is about 2 percent of blood volume (roughly 100 ml). So small a hemorrhage has no effect on

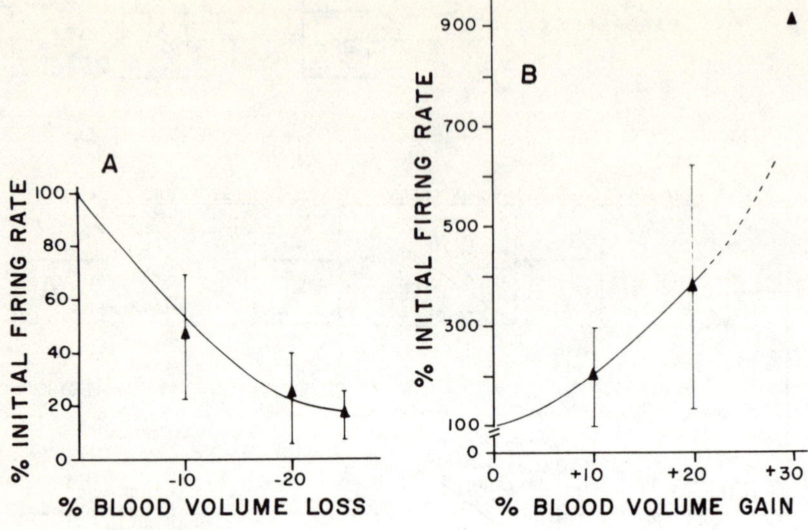

Figure 25-4
Effect of loss or gain in blood volume on frequency in an atrial type B fiber of a dog. (Modified from P. D. Gupta, J. P. Henry, R. Sinclair, and R. Von Baumgarten, *Am. J. Physiol.* 211:1429, 1966.)

mean arterial pressure, pulse pressure, or discharge frequency in arterial baroreceptors, and lowers atrial pressure by less than 1 torr. A 10 percent increase in blood volume doubles receptor discharge (Figure 25-4*B*). A sensitive feedback signal is essential for volume regulation because the gain of the neuroendocrine controllers and the effectors is extremely large.

Controllers and Effectors

The principal effector for long-term volume regulation is the kidney, though drinking behavior, the gastrointestinal tract, and sweat glands also contribute. Controllers that act to conserve salt and water include *antidiuretic hormone (ADH), angiotensins, aldosterone, and atriopeptins.*

Antidiuretic Hormone. Atrial receptors project to the hypothalamus, which controls drinking behavior and release of ADH. The effect of an orthostatic stress on plasma ADH levels in humans is shown in Figure 25-5. The reverse changes in ADH levels occur if the central blood volume is expanded, as in exposure to cold (venoconstriction) or water immersion (venous compression). Readers are doubtless familiar with the water diuresis that accompanies these experiences.

Angiotensins and Aldosterone. The angiotensin-aldosterone system is described in Chapter 18. Production of both hormones is limited by the rate of release of renin, which in turn is strongly influenced by action potential frequency in the renal sympa-

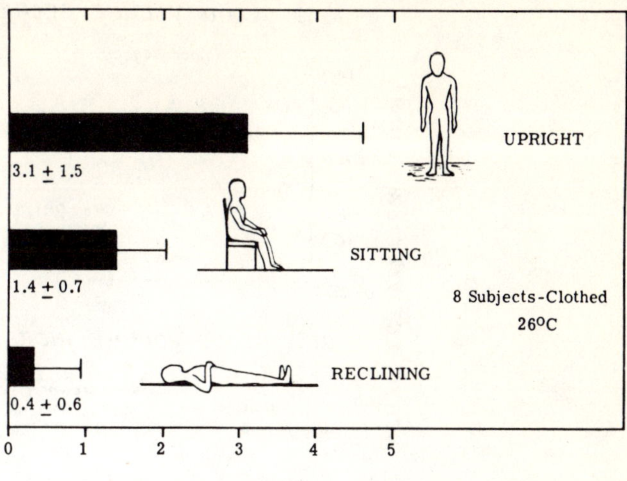

Figure 25-5
Response of plasma antidiuretic hormone (*ADH*) to orthostatic stress. (From W. W. Moore, *Fed. Proc.* 30:1389, 1971.)

thetic nerves. These nerves decrease their firing rate if the atria are distended and increase their activity if blood volume falls, as in hemorrhage; see Figure 25-6. These responses are greatly diminished by cutting the cardiac afferents. Thus atrial volume receptors exert tonic restraint on renal sympathetic discharge. In so doing, they tonically suppress release of renin.

The influence of volume receptors on renin release in humans is shown in Figure 25-7. Immersion in water up to the neck increased atrial transmural pressure 8 to 10 torr. Cardiac volume, determined from x-rays, increased 100 to 300 ml. The open and closed symbols in Figure 25-7 demonstrate that plasma levels of aldosterone fell in parallel with plasma renin when the atria were distended. Angiotensin-mediated control of aldosterone secretion is of the utmost importance, for in dehydration caused by sweating, vomiting, or diarrhea, conservation of salt as well as water is essential. Angiotensins also promote water conservation through direct effects on the renal tubules, by modifying release of ADH, by increasing sympathetic nervous system activity, and by promoting thirst. All the foregoing effects sustain or augment fluid balance, blood volume, and, indirectly, arterial pressure.

The Atriopeptins. Atriopeptins appear to have evolved as antagonists to ADH and the angiotensin-aldosterone system, as explained in Chapter 18. They are capable of producing rapid, profound diuresis and natriuresis, and also inhibit release of renin. Thus atrial mechanoreceptors provide the feedback sig-

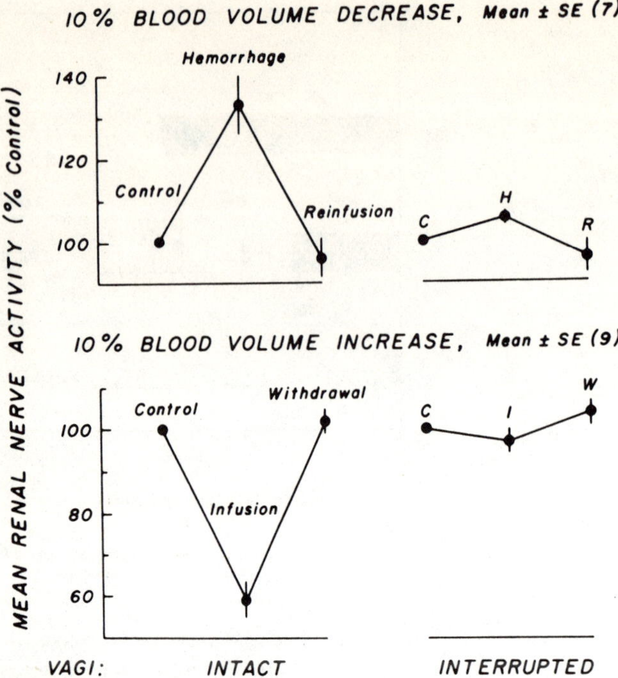

Figure 25-6
Changes in frequency in a small bundle of renal sympathetic nerves before and after interruption of vagal afferents. (From D. L. Clement, C. L. Pelletier, and J. T. Shepherd, *Circ. Res.* 31:824, 1972. By permission of the American Heart Association, Inc.)

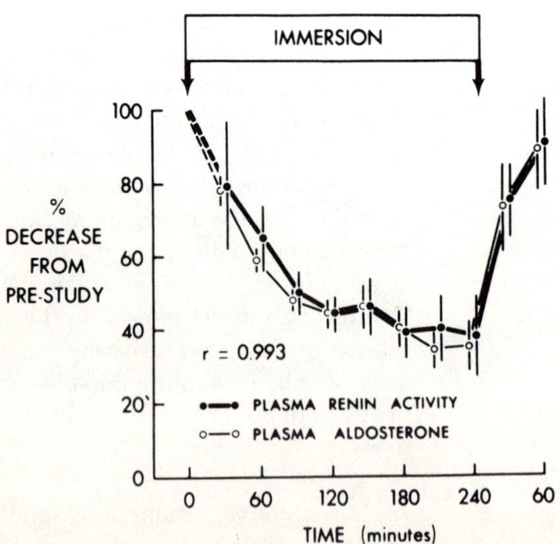

Figure 25-7
In normal humans, immersion expands the central blood volume and suppresses plasma renin activity and aldosterone secretion. (Data of M. Epstein, D. S. Pins, J. Sancho, and E. J. Haber, *Clin. Endocrinol. Metab.* 41:618, 1975.)

nal for reciprocal control of effectors, as shown by the plus and minus signs in Figure 25-3.

Clinical Application

Disorders of Volume Regulation

Plasma protein concentration may be reduced by inadequate diet, liver failure, or loss in the urine. If plasma oncotic pressure drops below a critical value, fluid filters into the interstitium, and plasma volume falls. This decreases discharge from volume receptors; promotes secretion of ADH, angiotensin, and aldosterone; and inhibits release of atriopeptins. Fluid conserved by the kidney cannot be retained in the vascular compartment in the presence of hypoproteinemia. Consequently plasma volume, the regulated variable, remains low, and the effectors continue to be driven by the controllers. Since there are no receptors for extravascular volume, edema fluid simply accumulates until net filtration pressure is balanced by tissue pressure. Thus hypoproteinemia opens the feedback loop in Figure 25-3 at point *A*.

Patients with congestive circulatory failure have large, dilated hearts but respond as though blood volume were reduced. They avidly retain salt and water and accumulate large amounts of edema fluid. This paradox was resolved by measurements of discharge frequency in atrial B fibers. In dogs with cardiac failure (Figure 25-8, *dashed curve*), discharge frequency at 40 cm H_2O (29 mm Hg) was about the same as in normal dogs at 4 cm H_2O. Loss of receptor gain is due to the effect of atrial overdistension on the mechanical filter in which the volume receptors are embedded. The similarity to loss of arterial baroreceptor gain in chronic hypertension is striking. Deprived of tonic restraint from volume receptors, sympathetic discharge to the kidney is high, and excessive amounts of renin and aldosterone are secreted. Low renal blood flow caused by low cardiac output also promotes renin release. In effect, congestive heart failure opens the loop in Figure 25-3 at point *B*. Experiments in dogs indicate that atrial receptor discharge recovers if atrial volume is restored to normal.

Therapy for congestive failure is designed to decrease heart size and eliminate or compensate for overdrive of the effectors. Diastolic volume may be decreased by digitalis, Na^+ reabsorption by the renal tubules may be inhibited with diuretics, and the action of aldosterone may be blocked by competi-

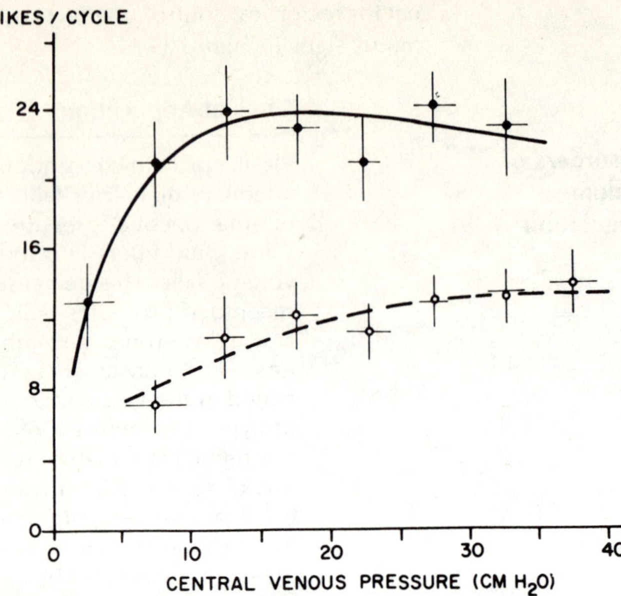

Figure 25-8
Action potential frequency in type B atrial receptors in a normal dog (*filled circles*) and a dog with chronic heart failure (*open circles*). Central venous pressure was increased by volume expansion. (From T. T. Greenberg, W. W. Richmond, R. A. Stocking, P. D. Gupta, J. P. Meehan, and J. P. Henry, *Circ. Res.* 32:424, 1973. By permission of the American Heart Association, Inc.)

tive antagonists. The response to diuretics well illustrates the power of the effectors; up to 10 liters of edema fluid (about 2½ gallons) may be lost in a single day.

References

1. Atlas, S. A., Volpe, M., Sosa, R. E., Laragh, J. H., Camargo, M. J. F., and Maack, T. Effects of atrial natriuretic factor on blood pressure and the renin-angiotensin-aldosterone system. *Fed. Proc.* 2115, 1986.
2. Claybaugh, J. R., and Share, L. Vasopressin, renin, and cardiovascular responses to continuous slow hemorrhage. *Am. J. Physiol.* 224:519, 1973.
3. DiBona, G. F. Neural mechanisms in body fluid homeostasis. *Fed. Proc.* 45:2871, 1986.
4. Epstein, M., Pins, D. S., and Miller, M. Suppression of ADH during water immersion in normal man. *J. Appl. Physiol.* 38:1038, 1975.
5. Gauer, O., and Henry, J. P. Neurohumoral control of plasma volume. *Int. Rev. Physiol.* 9:145, 1976.
6. Greenberg, T. T., Richmond, W. W., Stocking, R. A., Gupta, P. D., Meehan, J. P., and Henry, J. P. Impaired atrial receptor responses in dogs with heart failure due to tricuspid insufficiency and pulmonary artery stenosis. *Circ. Res.* 32:424, 1973.
7. Hintze, T. H., Currie, M. G., and Needleman, P. Atriopeptins: Renal-specific vasodilators in conscious dogs. *Am. J. Physiol.* 248:H587, 1985.

8. Linden, R. J., and Kappagoda, C. T. *Atrial Receptors*. London: Cambridge University Press, 1982.

9. Menninger, R. P., and Frazier, D. T. Effects of blood volume and atrial stretch on hypothalamic single-unit activity. *Am. J. Physiol.* 223:288, 1972.

10. Reid, I. A. Actions of angiotensin II on the brain: Mechanisms and physiologic role. *Am. J. Physiol.* 246:F533, 1984.

11. Saper, C. B., Standaert, D. G., Currie, M. G., Schwartz, D., Geller, D. M., and Needleman, P. Atriopeptin-immunoreactive neurons in the brain: Presence in cardiovascular regulatory areas. *Science* 227:1047, 1985.

12. Seymour, A. A., Marsh, E. A., Mazack, E. K., and Blaine, E. H. Natriuretic and hypotensive responses to synthetic atrial natriuretic factor in conscious hypertensive rats. *Hypertension* 7 (Suppl. 1):35, 1985.

26 : Brain Function and Cardiovascular Control

Cardiovascular regulations are *means,* not ends. Their main function is to provide the stability required for appropriate change in support of behavioral goals. Regulations are necessary but not sufficient for circulatory responses to mating, feeding, fighting, exercise, and the turmoil of "civilized" life. Perhaps the most important idea in this chapter is that *control of circulation is inextricably linked to voluntary and subconscious behavior.*

Mapping the Brain

Brain function must be understood in relation to the properties and locations of neurons and the sites to which their axons project. By use of a stereotaxic device and an appropriate atlas, an electrode can be placed at known locations. One can then stimulate electrically and search with a second electrode for responses evoked elsewhere. Another approach is to interrupt pathways with precisely placed electrolytic lesions. The effect on evoked potentials and cardiovascular responses can be observed, or the course of the degenerating axons can be traced by histologic methods. Finally, the properties of neurons at various sites can be tested by discharging putative mediators from micropipettes. By use of the above methods, sites from which cardiovascular changes can be elicited have been identified at every level of the nervous system from cortex to spinal cord. Nevertheless, transection of the brainstem from above downward has no effect on arterial pressure until the upper medulla is compromised. Transection at the first spinal segment produces bradycardia and profound hypotension. Thus the most essential apparatus for cardiovascular control is located in the medulla.

An Organizational Plan

For many years the medulla was considered "the vasomotor center," with functions almost independent of higher levels of the brain. Recent discoveries make this view untenable. Certain cortical and hypothalamic sites project directly to the spinal cord, without synapsing in the medulla. Others strongly influence the output of the medulla, both tonically and under special circumstances. Conversely, ascending excitatory and in-

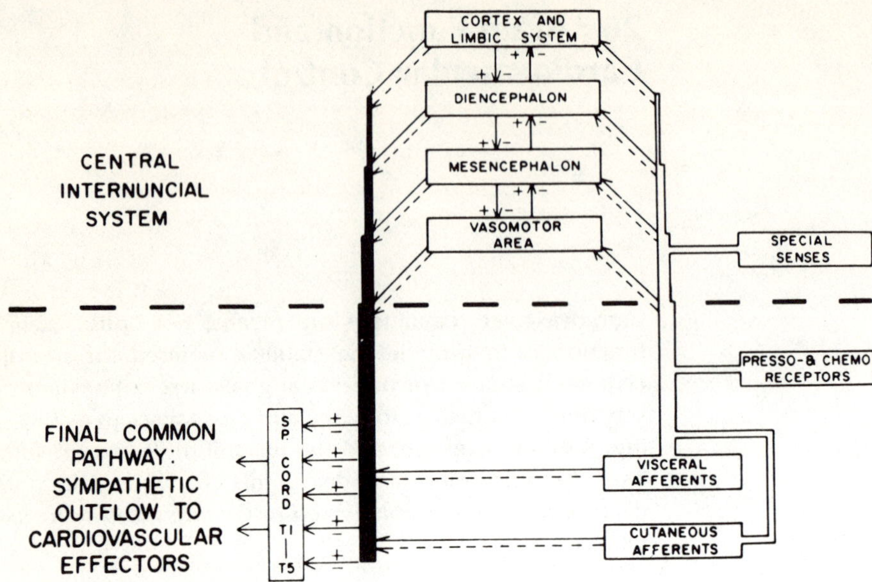

Figure 26-1
Logic diagram of hierarchical organization of cardiovascular control. Notice that all cardiovascular afferents enter the central nervous system above the cord. Solid arrows and plus signs represent excitatory connections; dashed arrows and minus signs mean inhibitory ones. (From C. N. Peiss. In W. C. Randall [ed.], *Nervous Control of the Heart*. Baltimore: Williams & Wilkins, 1965.)

hibitory fibers from the medullary reticular formation modulate discharge from higher centers. These in turn are interconnected by polysynaptic paths. Thus opportunities exist for integration at every level. This admirably flexible arrangement is diagrammed in Figure 26-1. Notice that the last integration site and the *final common pathway* for information leaving the central nervous system via sympathetic nerves is the preganglionic cell in the intermediolateral column of the cord. Each such cell makes numerous synaptic contacts with descending excitatory or inhibitory fibers. In similar fashion, fibers from every level converge on the nucleus ambiguus and dorsal motor nucleus of the vagus in the medulla, the final common path for parasympathetic control of the heart. The net result of all modulating influences is the transmembrane potential and hence discharge frequency of the vagal or sympathetic preganglionic neurons.

The *hierarchic* nature of cardiovascular controls is evident in Figure 26-1. To appreciate the holistic behavior of the intact system it helps to consider neuronal interaction and cardiovascular performance at various levels of organization.

The Spinal Level

The physiology of the all-important spinal preganglionic neurons is largely unknown. To judge from the morphology of vesicles in presynaptic terminals, these neurons are controlled by at least three neurotransmitters. Some spinal preganglionic cells fire spontaneously at 1 to 2 per second, indicating that a small component of sympathetic tone originates in the cord.

The simplest spinal sympathetic reflex consists of four neurons: an afferent fiber in the dorsal root, an interneuron, the preganglionic cell, and the postganglionic cell in the sympathetic chain. The afferent fiber can be somatic or visceral. Spinal reflexes can modify local blood flow and produce modest changes in blood pressure, heart rate, and contractility. Such reflexes are generally localized to a few spinal segments, however, and are heavily damped by supraspinal projections. Damping permits maximal control by the brain.

Clinical Application

High spinal transection is followed by a shocklike state characterized by extremely low sympathetic tone. Cardiovascular and other regulations are abolished because the major receptors are disconnected; see dashed line, Figure 26-1. Consequently, critical variables must be held within tolerances by the investigator or physician. Recovery of humans from spinal shock requires several months. During this interval the spinal preganglionic neurons, deprived of central drive, gradually increase their sensitivity to circulating catecholamines. This *denervation hypersensitivity* increases action potential frequency and restores arterial pressure to near-normal values. Intolerance to hypoxemia and to orthostatic and thermal stress is permanent.

The Medulla and the Baroreceptor Reflex

Origin of Sympathetic Tone

The neurons primarily responsible for sympathetic tone are diffusely distributed in the lateral reticular formation of the rostral two-thirds of the medulla. The effect of electrical stimulation on this region well illustrates the power of the effectors; see Figure 26-2. Arterial pressure went off scale at 240 torr, and heart rate rose to 170 per minute! Hypertension long outlasted the brief stimulus and persisted despite vagal bradycardia evoked by baroreceptors. Identical responses could be elicited from sites

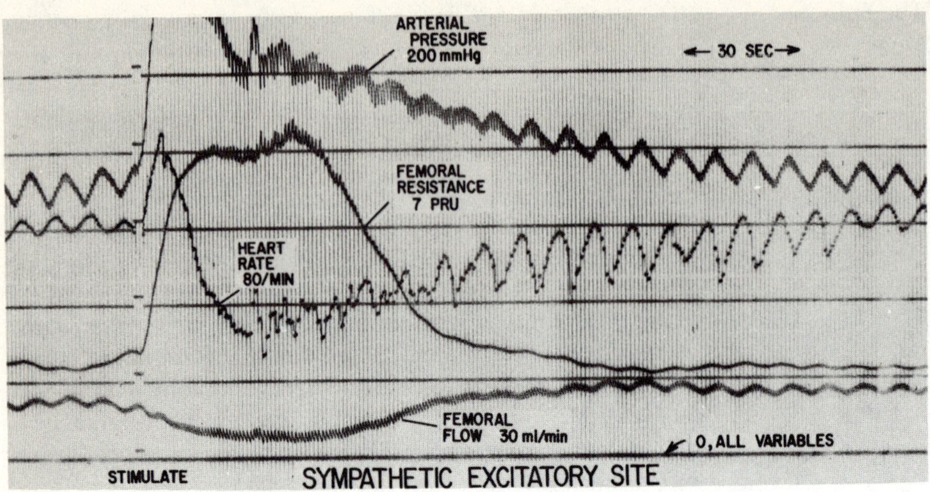

Figure 26-2
Stimulation in rostrolateral medullary reticular formation evokes profound vasoconstriction. Resistance is computed from pressure and flow and displayed as an analog voltage. Note reflexly mediated bradycardia. Elevation of baseline indicates stimulus duration. Responses long outlast stimulus.

separated by many millimeters. The reason a 50-μm electrode can cause massive discharges from diverse locations is that the reticular formation disseminates the excitation. The soma and dendrites of the predominant cell make numerous synaptic contacts, and the axon ramifies widely. Long fibers from the reticular formation ascend to the diencephalon and descend to preganglionic neurons of the cord. Thus the reticular formation provides the anatomical basis for integration of medullary responses with other parts of the nervous system.

Tonic Inhibition of Sympathetic Tone

The sympathetic excitatory neurons are spontaneously active and would produce disastrous responses, like those in Figure 26-2, if they were not tonically inhibited. The inhibitory cells lie near the midline in the caudal one-third of the medullary reticular formation. These cells release an inhibitory transmitter on the sympathetic excitatory neurons. The effect of electrical stimulation of the inhibitory cells is shown in Figure 26-3. The fall in heart rate suggests that cardiac output decreased, the arterial pressure fell 50 torr. Nevertheless, femoral flow doubled, indicating profound vasodilation in the leg, and probably in skin and muscle generally. The extent of vasodilation in other vascular beds depends on the level of sympathetic vasoconstrictor tone before stimulation of the inhibitory neurons.

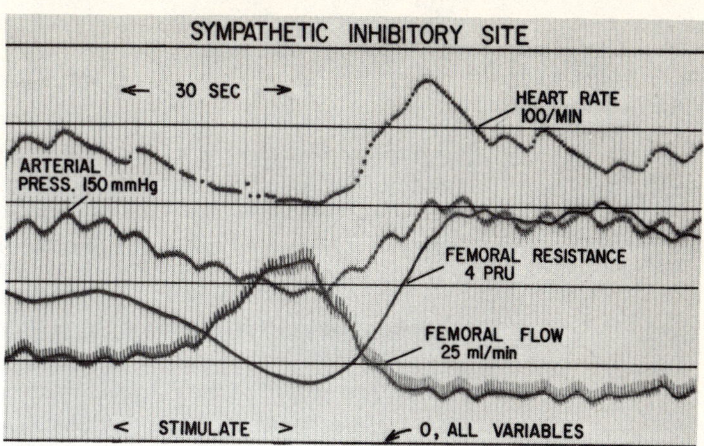

Figure 26-3
Stimulation in caudal medulla close to the midline evokes profound inhibition of sympathetic drive to the heart and vascular smooth muscle. Trace labelled femoral resistance was computed from pressure and flow.

Role of Cardiovascular Afferents

How do the inhibitory neurons "know" how to adjust sympathetic tone? The answer, of course, is from information supplied by the baroreceptors and other cardiovascular afferents. Were it not for this feedback, pressure would fluctuate wildly between the extremes in Figures 26-2 and 26-3. (Recall the lability of the arterial pressure in unanesthetized dogs after baroreceptor denervation.)

All cardiovascular afferents terminate and synapse in the nucleus tractus solitarius in the caudal medulla. Electrolytic lesions in this region produce extreme hypertension and abolish baroreceptor reflexes. The second neuron projects either to the nucleus ambiguus, where it modulates vagal tone, or to sympathetic inhibitory cells in the reticular formation. Some sympathetic inhibitory and excitatory fibers descend to the cord without participating in baroreceptor reflexes. They appear to control vessels in skin and kidney that are not strongly engaged in the regulation of pressure.

Modulation by Higher Centers

Medullary control must be coordinated with cardiovascular changes that accompany behaviors organized at higher levels of the brain. This requires a flow of information to and from the medulla. For example, during exercise, increased cardiac output is essential. However, sympathetically mediated increases in contractility, stroke volume, and heart rate greatly augment the dynamic component of baroreceptor discharge and increase action potential frequency in the sinoaortic nerves. If this feedback were not modified, the sympathetic drive required to sustain high cardiac output would be "switched off." Such maladaptive behavior is prevented by the hypothalamus, which receives baroreceptor input via a fast-conducting pathway. On the basis of this feedback, signals are generated that turn off some of the medullary inhibitory units activated by baroreceptors. More important, hypothalamic projections to the nucleus ambiguus directly inhibit vagal outflow that would otherwise slow the heart.

Medullary responses are strongly influenced by cerebellum, amygdala, and limbic cortex as well as hypothalamus. Conversely, the output of these higher centers is modified by baroreceptor mechanisms in the medulla. It is the lack of baroreceptor restraint of vasomotion initiated from higher centers that accounts for the lability of pressure in unanesthetized animals deprived of baroreceptors. A similar phenomenon appears to contribute to labile hypertension in some humans.

Supramedullary Controls

Integration of visceral and voluntary responses is accomplished mainly in the hypothalamus and limbic system. Stimulation at well-defined sites in these structures elicits cardiovascular changes appropriate to maintenance of body temperature, sleeping, feeding, fighting, exercise, emotion, and sexual activity. These instinctive behaviors are essential for survival of the individual or species. To assure their ready availability, they are prepackaged, like a computer subroutine. The complete pattern of voluntary and visceral response is generated in response to a natural stimulus. Such patterns are the result of neuronal interaction at all levels of organization, even though recognizable fragments can be elicited by electrical stimulation of discrete sites. Some examples of behaviorally linked circulatory patterns are given below.

Temperature Regulation

The anterior hypothalamus contains the principal receptors for temperature regulation. They can be stimulated electrically, or by means of a small probe that can be warmed or cooled (thermode). In dogs, warming the receptors causes panting, sweating, increased cardiac output, cutaneous vasodilation, and splanchnic vasoconstriction; cooling causes cutaneous vasoconstriction and shivering. Note that panting and shivering require voluntary muscles.

Homeotherms, especially humans, rely heavily on behavioral as well as physiological mechanisms to maintain body temperature. We would rather wear a sweater than shiver. Behavioral and physiological thermoregulation require the same hypothalamic sites, as shown by ingenious experiments on monkeys with chronically implanted thermodes. The animals were trained to adjust ambient temperature to a comfortable level. They did this by pulling a chain to introduce hot or cool air into an environmental chamber. When the anterior hypothalamus was warmed, the monkeys selected cool air and mobilized physiological responses to heat, even though body temperature fell. Thus a small hypothalamic site coordinates highly specific cardiovascular changes with respiration, muscle activity, sweating, and goal-oriented voluntary behavior.

Alerting, Exercise, Fighting, and Stress

One can hardly improve on Folkow and Neil's imaginative account of responses triggered by danger or emotionally charged situations:[1]

> Imagine a gazelle grazing, which hears a twig crackle under the foot of a predator. The immediate somatomotor response is perhaps only an alerting reaction, but at the same time the full-fledged cardiovascular-hormonal changes are put into action—being probably already present in the predator, lurking in the grass. Another cautious move from his side and the gazelle explodes into an all-out flight response, his cardiovascular system being already prepared to give the nutritional supply needed.
>
> It has sometimes been argued that not much could be gained by such anticipatory cardiovascular adjustments: the muscular effort would—so goes the argument—be virtully as good without it. This overlooks the fact that a split-second gain, though of little use in comfortable civilized life, may determine whether the gazelle escapes the killer; quite an important "marginal" gain for the gazelle. Beyond doubt, this cardiovascular-hormonal anticipatory adjustment is of the utmost importance for survival in the animal kingdom, and not infrequently for man as well.

A major component of the alerting reaction is active sympathetic vasodilation (ASVD) in skeletal muscle. Resistance begins to fall in 2 to 4 s and increases flow in resting muscle severalfold. The anatomical pathways are sympathetic, but the vasodilator response can be blocked by atropine, which suggests that the final mediator released on vascular smooth muscle may be acetylcholine. Responses that accompany vasodilation include tachycardia, increased contractility and stroke volume, and vasoconstriction in the cutaneous, splanchnic, and

[1]From B. Folkow and E. Neil, *Circulation*. New York; London: Oxford University Press, 1971. Pp. 345–348, by permission.

renal vascular beds. Arterial pressure may increase or decrease slightly, depending on how vasodilation in the whole skeletal muscle mass is balanced by vasoconstriction elsewhere, and by increased cardiac output. Thus, ASVD and associated circulatory changes make it possible for our gazelle, head turned toward the perceived danger but otherwise stationary, to have an almost maximal cardiac output yet near-normal arterial pressure. Moreover, cardiac output is already redistributed to skeletal muscle. Once the gazelle begins its flight, contraction per se maintains vasodilation in active muscles. At the same time vasoconstriction occurs in the inactive muscles. Fibers responsible for this highly specific vasoconstriction arise in the motor cortex and pass without synapsing directly to the cord.

ASVD originates in the motor cortex. It also can be produced by electrical stimulation of the amygdala, a major relay station for fibers from the phylogenetically old limbic cortex. The limbic system is largely responsible for mood, emotional states, and instinctive, nonverbal behavior, which suggests that ASVD may be induced by stress or emotional stimuli. As in Folkow and Neil's example, stress often coexists with exercise. Fibers responsible for ASVD converge at the hypothalamus and descend directly to the cord without synapsing in the medulla. Thus ASVD does not participate in baroreflex regulation of blood pressure.

ASVD has been demonstrated in nonhuman primates, and a comparable phenomenon exists in humans; see Figure 26-4. The subject was suddenly led to believe that he was bleeding profusely. The stimuli were therefore fear, anxiety, and a sense of helplessness. As in animals, vasodilation was confined to muscle, accompanied by tachycardia, sympathetically mediated, and blocked by atropine. Notice especially that arterial pressure remained nearly constant, and that flow to the skin (*open circles*) did not change significantly even though flow to muscle (*filled circles*) rose sixfold. This specificity stands in sharp contrast to the massive, diffuse responses characteristic of the medullary level of organization (Figures 26-2 and 26-3).

The relation of ASVD to natural behavior was studied in chronically instrumented cats. When confronted with a barking dog, they remained immobile but prepared for action with tachycardia, renal vasoconstriction, and ASVD. When faced with a hostile cat, muscle flow and heart rate decreased. *The psychic significance of the confrontation determined the cardiovascular outcome*. This important result reminds us that fear and anxiety are entirely different emotions from anger. The range of emotional expression is enormous, especially in hu-

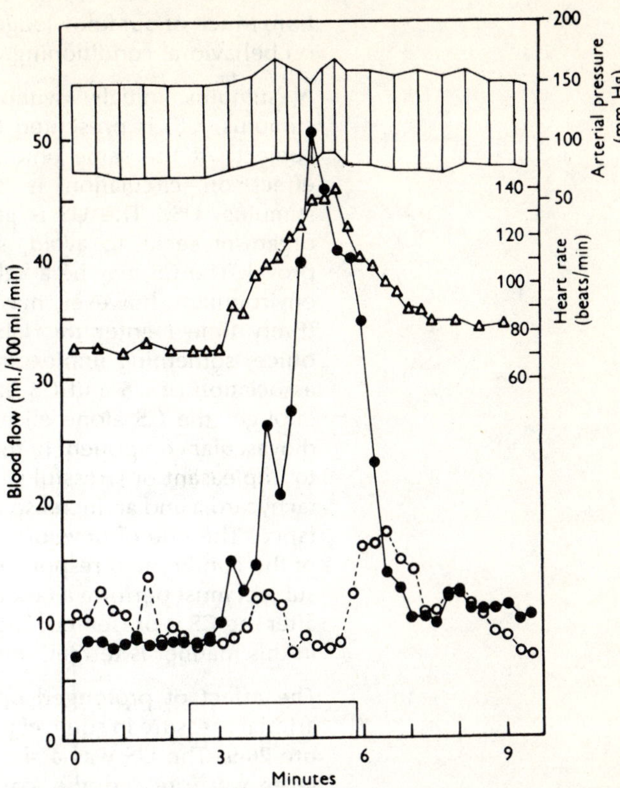

Figure 26-4
A person was exposed to severe emotional stress during the time indicated by rectangle. ASVD was evoked in the forearm (mainly muscle, *filled circles*) but not in the hand (mainly skin, *open circles*). Triangles indicate heart rate. (From D. A. Blair, W. E. Glover, A. D. M. Greenfield, and I. C. Roddie, *J. Physiol.* [Lond.] 148:633, 1959. By permission of Cambridge University Press.)

mans, and the cardiovascular responses engendered by emotion are correspondingly diverse.

If cats were allowed to fight, ASVD occurred in the limbs used for striking. However, when the animals were in repose, limb movement was not accompanied by ASVD; a background of highly specific emotional stress is necessary to activate this special vasodilator mechanism.

Clinical Application

Cardiovascular Conditioning and Diseases of Anxiety

Thus far we have been concerned with cardiovascular responses during conscious, short-term, goal-oriented behavior in response to external stimuli. There is good reason to believe that subconscious, internal stimuli influence both behavior and circulation. Much of our knowledge of this subject is based on behavioral conditioning.

A stimulus initially without effect (conditional stimulus, CS) is presented to an animal or human subject. At the same time a stimulus that has an effect on circulation is applied (unconditional stimulus, US). The US is generally something the organism seeks to avoid, such as pain or disapproval. The CS may be a light or sound. The entire environment, however, may be a very efficient CS. (Every time I enter this laboratory, house, boss's office, something unpleasant happens.) When the association of US and CS has been repeated often enough, the CS alone elicits a response. The cardiovascular component of the conditioned response to unpleasant or stressful stimuli generally includes tachycardia and an increase in total peripheral resistance. The rate of development and the magnitude of the conditioned response can be increased if the subject must perform a task in order to avoid the US after the CS is presented. Engagement of the subject in this manner is termed operant conditioning.

The effect of prolonged operant conditioning on arterial pressure in squirrel monkeys is shown in Figure 26-5. The US was a shock, the CS a light. If a lever was pressed the correct number of times within 20 s, the light was extinguished and a shock was avoided. The light appeared on a fixed schedule, 12 hours a day. At first, heart rate and arterial pressure rose only during the stress caused by appearance of the light. Muscle and coronary flows rose about 50 percent, whereas cutaneous, splanchnic, and renal flows decreased 20 to 40 percent. Total peripheral resistance rose about 20 percent, and in similar experiments renin release was enhanced.

As conditioning continued, the animals became increasingly hyperexcitable and hostile. Large increases in arterial pressure occurred when they were cleaned or fed. Within three to four months, systolic and diastolic pressures became elevated throughout the day, not just during stress. Hypertension was accompanied by bradycardia significant for a squirrel monkey. Time required for development of sustained hypertension could be reduced by decreasing the time allowed for lever pressing. Thus the conditioned response depended on the intensity of the stress.

Frontal lobectomy is required to extinguish cardiovascular responses to an anxiety-producing

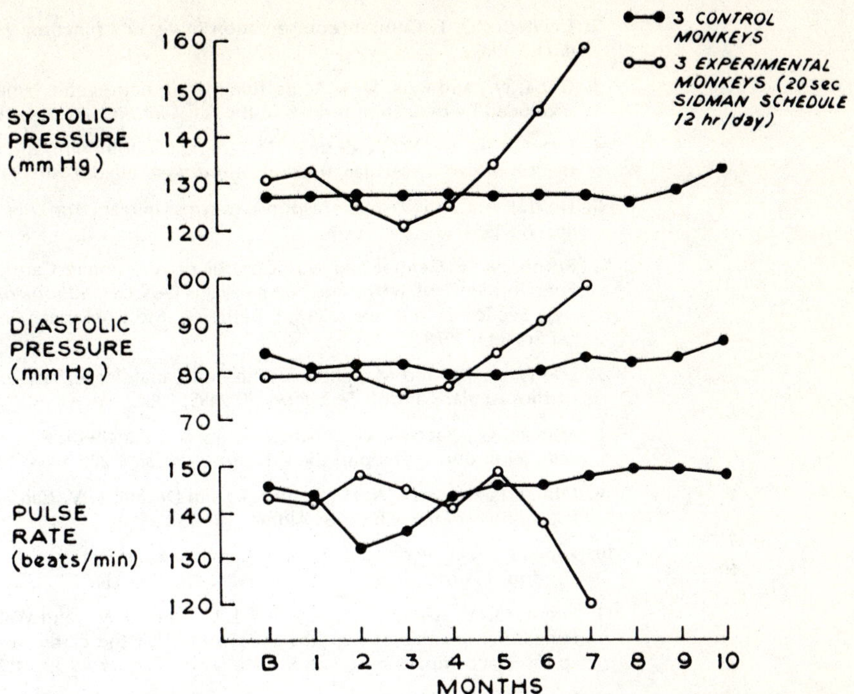

Figure 26-5
Effect of operant conditioning on mean arterial pressure and heart rate in squirrel monkeys. Each data point is the mean of 700 observations per month in each of 3 animals. (From R. P. Forsyth, *Psychosom. Med.* 31:300, 1969.)

stimulus permanently, which indicates that the cortex plays the primary role. This is of the utmost importance because of the symbolizing and associative functions of the cortex, especially in humans. For example, in human subjects word symbols for the US or CS often induce larger and longer-lasting cardiovascular responses than the physical stimuli themselves. Moreover, with time, the CS becomes generalized; symbols the subject associates with the CS also induce a response. The implications for psychosomatic illness are obvious.

A quantitative psychophysiology of cardiovascular behavior is rapidly emerging from studies such as those described in this chapter. This new knowledge should play a major role in understanding and controlling hypertension and other ills engendered by the tensions of modern life.

References

1. Adair, J. R., and Manning, J. W. Hypothalamic modulation of baroreceptor afferent unit activity. *Am. J. Physiol.* 229:1357, 1975.

2. Cechetto, D. F. Central representation of visceral function. *Fed. Proc.* 46:17, 1987.

3. Doba, N., and Reis, D. J. Acute fulminating neurogenic hypertension produced by brainstem lesions in the rat. *Circ. Res.* 32:584, 1973.

4. Engel, B. T., and Schneiderman, N. Operant conditioning and the modulation of cardiovascular function. *Annu. Rev. Physiol.* 46:199, 1984.

5. Herd, J. A. Cardiovascular response to stress in man. *Ann. Rev. Physiol.* 46:177, 1984.

*6. Korner, P. I. Central Nervous Control of Autonomic Cardiovascular Function. In R. M. Berne and N. Sperelakis (eds.), *Handbook of Physiology,* Section 2: The Heart, Vol. I. Bethesda, Md.: American Physiological Society, 1979.

7. Loewy, A. D., and McKeller, S. The neuroanatomical basis of central cardiovascular control. *Fed. Proc.* 39:2495, 1980.

8. Mancia, G., Baccelli, G., Adams, D. B., and Zanchetti, A. Vasomotor regulation during sleep in the cat. *Am. J. Physiol.* 220:1086, 1971.

9. Obrist, P. A., Black, A. H., Brener, J., and DiCara, L. V. *Cardiovascular Psychophysiology.* Chicago: Aldine, 1974.

*10. Randall, W. C. *Nervous Control of Cardiovascular Function.* New York; London: Oxford University Press, 1984. Pp. 307–434.

11. Smith, O. A., Astley, C. A., DeVito, J. L., Stein, J. M., and Walsh, K. E. Functional analysis of hypothalamic control of the cardiovascular responses accompanying emotional behavior. *Fed. Proc.* 39:2487, 1980.

12. Snyder, D. W., Nathan, M. A., and Reis, D. J. Chronic lability of arterial pressure produced by selective destruction of the catecholamine innervation of the nucleus tractus solitarii in the rat. *Circ. Res.* 43:662, 1978.

Appendixes

Appendix 1 : Abbreviations and Symbols

The abbreviations that follow are necessary to read the physiological literature. Each is defined in the text when first introduced.

Electrophysiology

E_m	=	Transmembrane potential
$E_{K^+}, E_{Na^+}, E_{Ca^{++}}$	=	Equilibrium potential for K^+, Na^+, or Ca^{++}
C_m	=	Membrane capacity
$I_{K^+}, I_{Na^+}, I_{Ca^{++}}$	=	Transmembrane current carried by K^+, Na^+, or Ca^{++}
I_{si}	=	Slow inward current carried mainly by Ca^{++} and to some extent Na^+
$P_{K^+}, P_{Na^+}, P_{Ca^{++}}$	=	Permeability to K^+, Na^+, Ca^{++}
$g_{K^+}, g_{Na^+}, g_{Ca^{++}}$	=	Conductance for K^+, Na^+, Ca^{++}
SA	=	Sinoatrial
AV	=	Atrioventricular
ECG	=	Electrocardiogram

Hemodynamics

P	=	Pressure
torr	=	Unit of pressure equal to 1 mm Hg
kP	=	kilopascal; 10^3 newtons/meter^2; international unit of pressure = 7.5 torr
$\dot{Q}$	=	Rate of volume flow
R	=	Resistance
PRU	=	Peripheral resistance unit; torr/ml $\cdot$ min^{-1}
C	=	Conductance
C_F	=	Capillary filtration coefficient
C.O.	=	Cardiac output
Re	=	Reynolds number
T	=	Tension
η	=	Viscosity
HCT	=	Hematocrit ratio
C.D.	=	Capillary density
ICD	=	Intercapillary distance
PCWP	=	Pulmonary capillary wedge pressure

Blood-Gas Transport; Metabolism

According to standard convention for respiratory physiology, *P*, *C*, *V*, and *S* stand for partial pressure, content of gas per volume of blood, volume, and saturation, respectively. An overbar denotes a mean, and a dot indicates a rate. Capital letters are used to indicate alveolar air, and lowercase letters refer to blood.

PO_2	=	O_2 partial pressure
PAO_2	=	PO_2 in alveolar air
PaO_2	=	PO_2 in arterial blood
PvO_2	=	PO_2 in venous blood
$P\bar{v}O_2$	=	PO_2 in mixed venous blood from right ventricle or pulmonary artery
$P_{cap}O_2$	=	PO_2 in capillary
PtO_2	=	PO_2 in tissue

Similarly for CaO_2, $C\bar{v}O_2$, and SaO_2, $S\bar{v}O_2$, etc.

Hb	=	Hemoglobin
Vol %	=	ml gas per 100 ml blood
ATP	=	Adenosine triphosphate
ADP	=	Adenosine diphosphate
Pi	=	inorganic phosphate
2,3-DPG	=	2,3-diphosphoglycerate
$\dot{V}A$	=	Rate of alveolar ventilation
$\dot{V}O_2$	=	Rate of O_2 consumption
E	=	Extraction
MET	=	Unit of physical exercise; 1 MET = $\dot{V}O_2$ at rest

Cardiovascular Control

Ach	=	Acetylcholine
Nor	=	Norepinephrine
AI, AII, AIII	=	Angiotensin I, II, or III
ADH	=	Antidiuretic hormone
Aldo	=	Aldosterone
ASVD	=	Active sympathetic vasodilation
CS	=	Conditional stimulus
US	=	Unconditional stimulus
CNS	=	Central nervous system

Appendix 2 : Normal Values for Cardiovascular Variables[1]

Variable	*Mean*	*Range*	*Units*
ECG intervals			ms
P		80–100	
P–Q		120–200	
QRS		60–100	
Q–T at			
40 beats/min	450		
80 beats/min	350		
120 beats/min	280		
180 beats/min	230		
Arterial blood pressure, humans[2]			torr
Age 1 week			
Systolic	66	46–84	
Diastolic	45	28–58	
Age 3–5 years			
Systolic	98	77–118	
Diastolic	56	50–71	
Age 15 years			
Systolic	115	90–147	
Diastolic	66	54–80	
Age 30 years			
Systolic	125	96–150	
Diastolic	76	57–95	
Age 50 years			
Systolic	135	97–172	
Diastolic	83	61–106	
Age 70 years			
Systolic	145	93–197	
Diastolic	82	52–112	
Right ventricular end-diastolic pressure			Less than 6
Left ventricular end-diastolic pressure			Less than 12

[1] Modified from P. L. Altman and D. S. Dittmer (eds.), *Biological Handbooks: Respiration and Circulation*. Bethesda, Md.: F.A.S.E.B., 1971.
[2] Data based on 3600 children, 7500 adults.

Variable	*Mean*	*Range*	*Units*
Pulmonary artery pressure			
Age < 1 week			
Systolic	49	16–80	
Diastolic	22	0–42	
Age 1–5 years			
Systolic	20	8–25	
Diastolic	7	5–12	
Adult			
Systolic	21	11–30	
Diastolic	9	5–16	
Pulmonary capillary wedge pressure (PCWP)	9	4–15	torr
Ventricular ejection fraction	0.67	0.6–0.8	
[3]Cardiac output, humans, at rest			L/min
Newborn	~1		
Age 10	5.5	3.3–7.7	
Age 20	6.5	5.5–7.5	
Age 35	6.6	6.0–7.2	
Age 45	5.3	5.0–5.7	
Age 55	4.6	4.2–5.0	
Age 65	4.3	3.7–4.9	
Age 75	4.0	3.5–4.5	
Cardiac output, humans, maximum exercise			L/min
Age 20–25 sedentary	22.8	20.5–25.0	
Age 20–25 trained	36.0	27.8–42.0	
Age 55 sedentary	17.0	13.4–20.6	
Age 55 trained	26.8	22.0–31.0	
Heart rate during maximum exercise, humans			beats/min
Age 20–25 sedentary	193	189–205	
trained	190	170–206	
Age 50–55 sedentary	173		
trained	170	147–191	
Oxygen consumption, humans			L/min
Age 20–25, at rest	0.27	0.21–0.40	
Age 20–25			
Work, kg · m/min			
290	0.91	0.8–1.0	
540	1.43	1.25–1.75	
1250	3.05	2.6–3.2	

[3]To calculate cardiac index (C.O./m^2), compute body surface area (*S.A.*) in meters squared, as follows:

$S.A. = 0.0097\,(H + W) - 0.545$,

where H = height in centimeters and W = weight in kilograms.

Variable	*Mean*	*Range*	*Units*
Age 65			
At rest	0.25	0.091–0.32	
At work, kg · m/min			
290	0.96	0.78–1.32	
540	1.46	1.45–1.86	
Age 20–25, maximum work			L/min
Sedentary	3.4	2.7–3.8	
Trained	5.6	4.7–6.2	
Age 50–55, maximum work			
Sedentary	2.2	1.8–2.6	
Trained	3.6	2.7–4.2	
Cardiac output, dog			L/min
Anesthetized, 25 kg	2.7	2.0–3.2	
Unanesthetized basal, 25 kg	3.3	1.8–4.4	
Running, 5 mph	12.1	12.1–12.5	
Regional blood flow			Percent cardiac output
At rest			
Cerebral	13		
Coronary	4		
Renal	21		
Muscle	20		
Splanchnic	22		
Skin	9		
Maximum exercise			
Cerebral	3		
Coronary	4		
Renal	1		
Muscle	88		
Splanchnic	1		
Skin	3		
Cardiovascular expansion factors, young adults			Multiples of resting value
Heart rate	2.5–3		
Cardiac output	4–6		
Muscle blood flow	18–20		
Coronary blood flow	3–5		
Whole-body AV difference	3.5–5		
Capillary density, dog			
Skeletal muscle	2–3		
Heart	2–4		
Hemoglobin			g/100 ml
Adult men	16	14–17.5	
Women 20–40 years	14.1	11.8–17.0	
Hematocrit			%
Adult men	47	40–54	
Women 20–40 years	43	37–47	

Variable	*Mean*	*Range*	*Units*
SaO_2	96.6	94.7–98.2	%
PaO_2	96	86–105	torr
PCO_2	40	31–46	torr
pHa	7.443	7.419–7.497	
Arteriovenous O_2 difference, humans			vol %
$CaO_2 - C\bar{v}O_2$, at rest	4.7	3.2–5.5	
Cerebral	6.4	5.4–7.6	
Coronary	11.5	10.5–12.5	
Renal	1.3	1.0–1.5	
Splanchnic	4.1	2.3–6.2	
Skin and resting muscle	4.3	3.3–5.2	
$CaO_2 - C\bar{v}O_2$, trained, maximum work	17.2	15.7–18.6	
Total blood volume, humans	77	73–80	ml/kg lean wt
Thoracic blood volume: see Table 12-1, p. 114			
Plasma volume, humans	42	36–48	ml/kg
Total body water	55		% body weight
Interstitial fluid volume	12		% body weight
Plasma protein	7.3	6.8–82	g/100 ml
Serum albumin	4.6	4.2–5.4	g/100 ml

Appendix 3 : Oxydissociation Curve of Human Blood at pH 7.4 and 37°C

SO_2 %	PO_2 torr	SO_2 %	PO_2 torr	SO_2 %	PO_2 torr	SO_2 %	PO_2 torr	SO_2 %	PO_2 torr
1	1.9	30	19.2	70	36.9	94	69.4	98.5	129
2	3.4	35	21.0	75	40.4	95	74.2	99	159
4	5.7	40	22.8	80	44.5	95.5	77.3	99.5	225
6	7.5	45	24.6	85	49.8	96	81.0	99.8	350
10	10.3	50	26.6	90	57.8	96.5	86.0	99.9	500
15	13.1	55	28.7	91	60.0	97	91.6	99.95	700
20	15.4	60	31.2	92	62.7	97.5	99.6		
25	17.3	65	34.0	93	65.7	98	111		

Modified from P. L. Altman and D. S. Dittmer (eds.), *Biological Handbooks: Respiration and Circulation*. Bethesda, Md.: F.A.S.E.B., 1971.

Note: A nomogram for *estimating* saturation, given PO_2, temperature, and pH, or for *estimating* PO_2, given saturation, temperature, and pH, appears in the text cited above. Such estimates can be seriously in error, because they do not take account of other modifiers, such as 2,3-DPG.

Appendix 4 : Approximate Energy Cost (in MET) of Various Activities

Light or moderate work (1.5–3.0 MET)	Sitting at desk	
	Driving a car	
	Using hand tools, light assembly work	
Moderate work (2.5–4.5 MET)	Standing quietly, working at own pace or at moderate rate using light hand tools	
	Stocking shelves	
	Carrying trays, dishes	
	Light housework	
	Gas station mechanic	
Heavy work (>4.5 MET)	Lifting and carrying objects	*Energy Cost (MET)*
	9–20 kg	5.0
	20–29 kg	6.0
	30–38 kg	7.5
	39–45 kg	8.5
	Painting, paperhanging	5.0
	Carpentry	6.0
	Pneumatic tools (jackhammers, drills)	6.0
	Shovel, pick	8.0
	Moving, pushing objects 75 lb or more	8.0
Leisure activities		*MET*
	Bicycling	3–8
	Bowling	2–4
	Dancing	3–7
	Golf, walking	5–7
	Jogging	7–10
	Tennis	4–9
	Walking, level	2–5
	Walking, stairs	6–8
	Skiing, downhill	5–8
	Squash	8–12

Appendix 5 : Problems

Suggested Approaches

Cardiovascular physiology is a *practical* subject for both physicians and bioscientists. The problem sets allow you to determine whether you can actually use the material. An hour spent problem solving is worth days of rereading and underlining! The following suggestions may be helpful.

How to Begin

The key to each of the problems is in deciding what the *main issue* is. Then you can select the proper quantitative relationships on which to base your thinking; some examples include the Na^+ inactivation curve, the ventricular function curve, the Fick principle, the oxyhemoglobin dissociation curve, and Starling's filtration principle. These and others allow you to set limits on possible changes and to estimate factors of safety or physiological reserves. With such estimates in mind, you can think about mechanisms and attempt diagnostic or therapeutic judgments.

Expectations

One reason detailed answers are not provided is that *there often is no single correct answer.* The transition from physics and chemistry courses can be a culture shock! It is essential to reconcile oneself to this kind of insecurity; clinicians and investigators frequently cannot be sure their reasoning is correct. The former deal with incomplete data and uncontrolled situations, and the latter try to discover what no one else knows. One also must become accustomed to making estimates of quantities that cannot be measured. The accuracy of such estimates will reflect your understanding of the physiology involved.

The problems are of graded difficulty. Some are designed to test your grasp of facts. These are straightforward and not unlike problems you have encountered in other courses. Though facts are essential they are not sufficient, for facts are merely tools. After you possess them you must learn to use them skillfully. To that end, more complex problems, including some clinical ones, are provided. *Organization* of facts and concepts is essential for such problems.

Organizational Techniques

Clinicians and investigators are routinely faced with large amounts of information — facts, data, and concepts. These are related through interdependence, or dependence on common variables, and are further related causally and temporally. For example, Problem 16c involves analysis of O_2 supply and O_2 demand in a hypertrophied heart. An adequate answer includes application of cardiac mechanics, hemodynamics, fluid balance, O_2 transport, coronary circulation, and cardiovascular control. Such complexity requires deliberate cultivation of organizational techniques.

Lists may be necessary at first, *but they are not sufficient,* even when items are ranked according to their importance for the problem at hand. Your main task is to recognize the *interaction* of the variables and concepts you have identified. In Problem 16c, for example, heart rate has major consequences for both O_2 supply and O_2 demand. Wall tension, another key variable, is not only the principal determinant of demand, but a determinant of supply as well. A technique well suited to physiology is the logic diagram; Figure 11-1, page 104, is an example. In the case of Problem 16c one might set up a dichotomy of determinants of supply and demand:

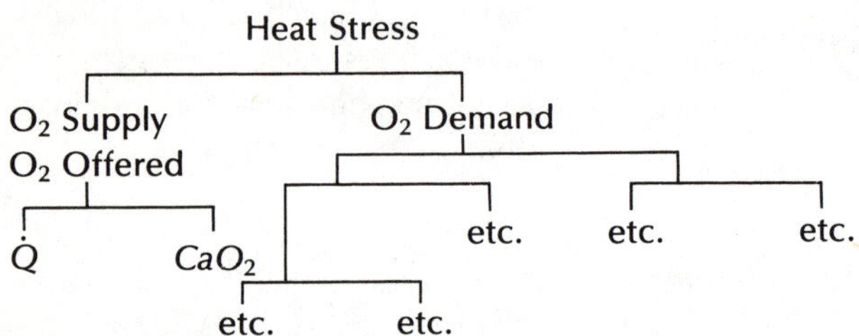

An array of dependencies is particularly useful in comparing two situations — heat stress and emotional stress in Problem 16c. The chief limitation is that temporal and causal relationships are not shown directly. You can develop these in words, or as a systems diagram. Use of a systems diagram to identify positive feedback in disease is illustrated in Figure 7-8.

Apart from technique, the most essential ingredient for success is practice. By all means try to do the problems independently. The specific suggestions in Appendix 6 should be consulted only after you have gone as far as you can on your own, and as a guide in checking your written answers.

Cardiac Electrophysiology (Chapters 2 through 6)

1. The recordings in Figure P-1 were made in an anesthetized dog during an intravenous infusion of KCl.
   a. High, narrow T waves and well-defined S–T segments are the first manifestations of hyperkalemia in the ECG; see

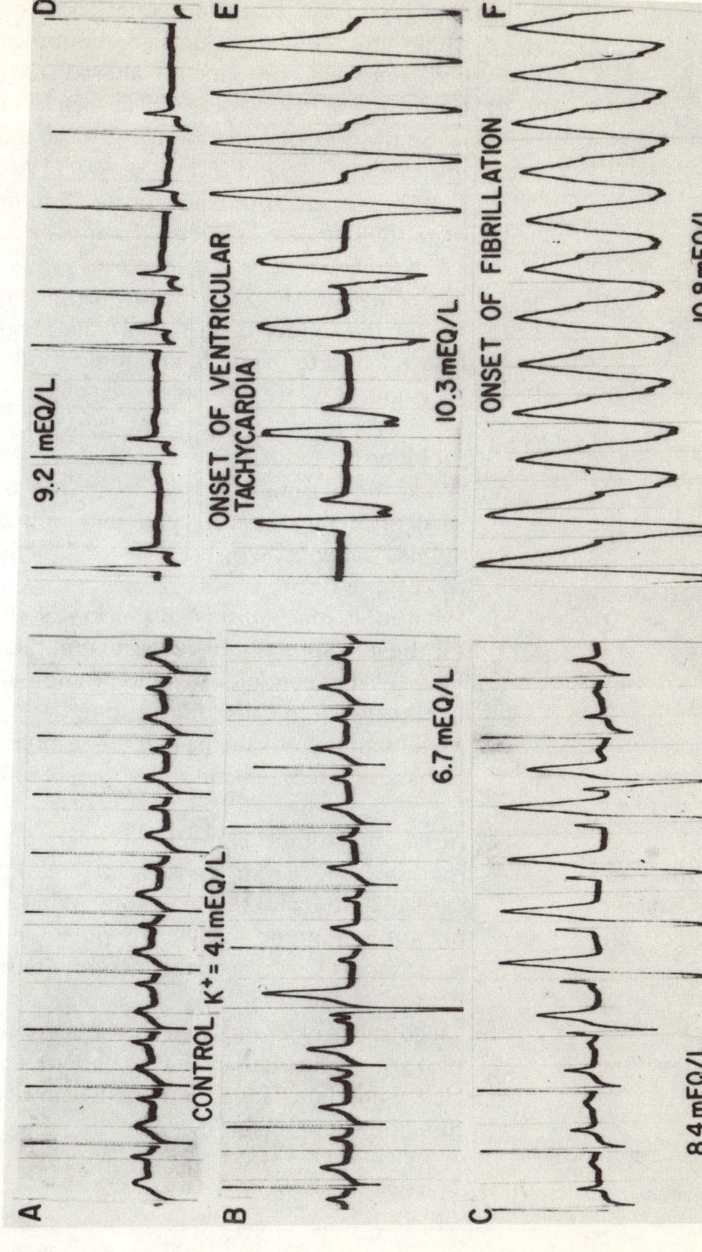

Figure P-1
Electrocardiograms recorded in an anesthetized dog during an intravenous infusion of KCl.

B, C, and *D* in Figure P-1. What are the corresponding changes in the action potential and electrograms of a single fiber? What can be said about the summation of electrograms to produce the altered ECG?

b. Calculate the resting potential at each level of plasma K^+, using the Nernst equation (p. 17), 140 mEq per liter for intracellular K^+, and 26 mV for RT/F. Would you expect E_K to be a good approximation of E_m in hyperkalemia?

c. Mark the calculated values of E_m *directly on Figure 3-5* (p. 33). Now account for the increases in Q–T interval from *A* to *D* in Figure P-1, and the further increase from *D* to *E*.

d. Explain the sudden drop in heart rate between *C* and *D* in Figure P-1 in terms of E_m and ionic conductances in the AV node. How are the ionic mechanisms responsible for slow AV conduction different from those identified in Problem 1c?

e. When the plasma $[K^+]$ is 10 to 12 mEq per liter, a very small further increase will generally induce fibrillation, as in this "patient." Why does electrical activity deteriorate so abruptly?

f. What ionic mechanisms and electrical changes account for the development of ventricular fibrillation in *E* in the figure? What conditions would promote the tendency of hyperkalemia to cause fibrillation?

g. How might hyperkalemia and the resulting electrical disturbances affect tension development and contractility?

Cardiac Mechanics and Hemodynamics (Chapter 1 and Part II)

2. a. Atrial fibrillation (AF) is often converted to normal sinus rhythm (NSR). From the data in Table P-1 calculate the cardiac output and stroke volume. What additional information is required to calculate pulmonary and systemic resistances? Use reasonable assumptions to obtain estimates.

b. Calculate stroke work before and after conversion, and plot your estimated and calculated values on Figure 1-7.

c. How were the changes in hemodynamics and ventricular function brought about?

Table P-1

Rhythm	Heart Rate	$\dot{V}O_2$ (ml/min)	$CaO_2 - C\bar{v}O_2$ (ml/100 ml)	Pulmonary Arterial Pressure (torr)	Systemic Arterial Pressure (torr)
Fibrillation	68	190	5.3	18	84
Normal rhythm	83	240	4.3	18	82

Table P-2

Posture	Whole Body $\dot{V}O_2$ (ml/min)	Whole Body $CaO_2 - C\bar{v}O_2$ (ml/100 ml)	Femoral $CaO_2 - CvO_2$ (ml/100 ml)
Supine	0.21	3.5	2.8
70° tilt	0.26	5.7	9.2

Table P-3

Catheter Site	Pressure (Systolic/ diastolic, torr)	Mean Pressure (torr)	O_2 Content (ml/L blood)
Vena cava			100
Right atrium		3	97
Right ventricle	40/3	17	99
Pulmonary artery	40/10	24	127
Pulmonary vein			142
Aorta	110/35	63	142

3. Refer to Figure 8-5, page 83.
   a. How does the pulse wave velocity compare with red cell velocity in the aorta (Figure 8-7)? Why are the two velocities so different?
   b. What is the main determinant of arterial pressure during vagal arrest?
   c. Why is the difference between the *mean* central and peripheral arterial pressures so small?

4. A healthy young man participated in an experiment on a tilt table. Measurements were made when he was supine and at 3 minutes after he was tilted 70 degrees from the horizontal. During the tilt, both legs hung passively (non-weight-bearing). The results are shown in Table P-2.
   a. Estimate *change* in flow to a leg, assuming its $\dot{V}O_2$ remained constant.
   b. How much of this change is due to vasoconstriction in the leg?
   c. Consult Figure 1-7, page 12, and Figure 12-3, page 118. What physiological and environmental factors determine whether or not fainting occurs in such an experiment?

5. a. The data in Table P-3 were obtained in a 3-year-old child by cardiac catheterization. Arterial O_2 capacity was 146 ml per liter, arterial O_2 saturation was 97%, and $\dot{V}O_2$ was 95 ml per minute. Calculate the systemic and pulmonary flows, and resistances. (In certain congenital cardiac defects systemic and pulmonary flows are not equal.)

Table P-4

Variable	Control		Epinephrine		Angiotensin		Saline	
Heart rate (beats/min)	156		140		128		136	
Cardiac output (L/min)	1.0		1.8		0.8		1.7	
Stroke volume (ml/beat)								
BPa systolic/diastolic	174/124		180/85		222/192		190/100	
and mean (torr)		136		105		204		142
Rt. atrial pressure (torr)								
Lt. atrial pressure (torr)	4		3		30		9	
Stroke work (g · m)								
Resistance (PRU)								

b. Determine the magnitude of shunt flow from your calculations, and the location of the shunt from O_2 content and arterial pressures in different parts of the circuit. Bear in mind that minor differences in O_2 content are expected because of experimental error.

c. What features of the pulmonary circulation account for its low vascular resistance?

6. Catheters were placed in the aorta, left atrium, and pulmonary artery of a dog. Cardiac output was determined by dilution of indocyanine green. The circulation was perturbed by injecting epinephrine and angiotensin, and by infusing 500 ml of saline rapidly intravenously. Results are shown in Table P-4.
   a. Complete the table, using your best judgment about right atrial pressures.
   b. How did each of the perturbations affect ventricular function and vasomotor tone? By what mechanisms?
   c. What factors contributed to changes in pulse pressure?

7. a. Refer to Table 13-1, page 134. What fraction of total muscle blood flow during light exercise was due to redistribution of cardiac output in the normal person and in the patient with mitral valve stenosis?
   b. What symptoms other than dyspnea and orthopnea might the patient with mitral stenosis have experienced because of maldistribution of cardiac output?

Integration of Hemodynamics, Transport, and Control

8. Additional aspects of this protocol will be considered in subsequent problems, so it will help to keep a record of your answers. *Note to graduate students:* Do not be put off because the data were collected in a hospital instead of a laboratory. Consider this an experiment designed by nature.

A 55-year-old clerk was admitted for cardiac evaluation. About six months previously, he began to notice easy fatigability and breathlessness during exertion and emotional upheavals. The worst episode occurred after an argument with his son; it was accompanied by coughing and mental confusion and lasted about 30 minutes. Climbing hills or stairs, mowing his lawn, and working in his garden became progressively more difficult. Six weeks before admission he began to have spells of waking up at night gasping for breath and having to sit up or walk around to get relief. He was more comfortable sleeping with an extra pillow, which also reduced the number of these spells.

Physical findings. The patient was comfortable sitting up, but his respiratory rate increased when he was asked to lie flat for part of the examination. His heart rate was 74 per minute, and his arterial pressure was 140 torr systolic and 40 torr diastolic (140/40). The left ventricle was hypertrophied and hyperdynamic. A loud systolic murmur heard at the base of the heart radiated into the carotid arteries, and an early diastolic murmur was heard at the left sternal edge. The aortic valve closure sound was inaudible. The patient's chest was clear except for slight congestion at the lung bases. Cardiac enlargement and evidence of interstitial edema at the lung bases were seen on x-ray.

The night of admission, the hospital air conditioning system failed, and the patient's room became humid and extremely hot (31.1°C). He awoke about 2:00 A.M. with severe breathlessness, cough, and wheezing. Although he sat up, his symptoms rapidly progressed. His heart rate was 90 per minute, arterial pressure 150/25, and temperature 39.5°C. He became confused and began to produce pink, frothy sputum. An ECG showed S–T segment and T-wave changes indicative of extensive subendocardial ischemia. An arterial sample drawn before administration of oxygen revealed the following: PaO_2 = 42 torr, SaO_2 = 78%, $PaCO_2$ = 35 torr, pHa = 7.45. He was treated in the intensive care unit with O_2, positive pressure ventilation, sedation, intravenous digitalis, diuretics, and extremity tourniquets, with gradual improvement. Two days later his aortic valve was replaced, and he eventually returned to work symptom-free.

a. Quantitative thinking based on rough-and-ready estimates is essential in clinical medicine. For example, use Appendix 4 to estimate the patient's reserve of $\dot{V}O_2$, and Figure 13-6, page 131, to estimate his cardiac output reserve at various times.
b. Mark directly on Figure 1-4, page 8, your estimate of end-diastolic pressure when the patient was symptom-free at rest, during the argument with his son, and during acute

pulmonary edema. Bear in mind that much of the ejected volume was "regurgitated" back into the ventricle in diastole. What factors did you take into account in arriving at your estimate?

c. What factors influenced ventricular afterload during the argument and during heat stress? Did afterload influence preload and ejection fraction?

d. Draw directly on Figure 1-7 ventricular function curves for the patient's left ventricle when he was symptom-free at rest, during the argument with his son, and on admission to the intensive care unit. Interpret your curves in terms of the patient's reserves of contractility. (Similar plots are used routinely for hemodynamic monitoring in the operating room and in intensive care units.)

e. Draw directly on Figure 1-6 a systolic elastance (contractility) line and pressure-volume loop for the patient's heart when symptom-free at rest, using given values and your estimate of ejection fraction.

f. Explain orthopnea, ease of fatigue, low aortic diastolic pressure, high pulse pressure, and the origin of the systolic murmur.

g. Explain the rationale for the following treatments: upright position, sedation, extremity tourniquets to produce venous congestion, positive pressure ventilation, digitalis.

9. A 20-kg child was fed a diet deficient in protein. He had a potbelly and grossly swollen legs. His serum albumin was 1.5 g per 100 ml. If π_{cap} = 6 torr, and C_F for the body as a whole is 0.006 ml/min · torr per 100 g, consider how the determinants of transcapillary filtration apply to this child.

10. A 28-year-old waitress was troubled by swelling of the legs below the knees. The swelling disappeared at night and reaccumulated rapidly in the morning, then more slowly while at work throughout the day. She was thyrotoxic ($\dot{V}O_2$ 35 percent above normal) and required a large cutaneous blood flow to dissipate heat. What mechanisms other than heart failure could account for the characteristics of the edema?

11. Construct a step diagram like Figure 17-1 for each of the following situations:

a. Congenital venoarterial shunt, PaO_2 half normal.
b. Chronic hemolytic anemia, [Hb] half normal.
c. Chronic mitral valve stenosis, cardiac output half normal.
d. Chronic ventricular hypertrophy, cardiac capillary density half normal.

e. For a to d above, list the principal compensations.
f. For a to d above, list the remaining reserves.
g. For a to d above, list the dangers to which persons are exposed *because* they have used reserves.

12. Reread Problem 8 and review your answers.
    a. Use your ventricular function curves to evaluate P_{cap} and fluid balance at the bases of the lungs during the patient's argument with his son and on admission to the intensive care unit.
    b. Interpret the blood gas values. Why did the situation warrant use of the intensive care unit?

13. List ways in which the feedback loops in Figure 24-8 (p. 249) could be opened or modified, and predict how the interventions you listed would affect system performance.

14. A patient with hepatic cirrhosis had 12 liters of fluid removed from his abdomen by paracentesis. Laboratory data: plasma protein 8.2 g per 100 ml, serum albumin 3.2 g per 100 ml, protein content of ascitic fluid 3.2 g per 100 ml. He was treated with a diet that contained only 34 mEq of Na^+ per day (!) and with diuretics. Nevertheless, over the next year he gained 23 pounds of edema fluid, mostly as ascites. The concentration of protein in blood remained the same, but the ascitic fluid albumin decreased to 1.5 g per 100 ml.
    a. What factors are responsible for accumulation of ascites? About how high was intra-abdominal pressure?
    b. Consult Figure 25-4. What neuroendocrine mechanisms contributed to fluid retention? Would you expect the patient's blood volume to be normal?

15. Refer to Problem 6 and Table P-4. Account for changes in heart rate, arterial pressures (systolic, diastolic, mean, pulse), contractility, and peripheral resistance induced by each treatment. Consider both afferent signals and efferent responses in your answer.

16. Reread Problem 8 and review your answers.
    a. What mechanisms were responsible for increased cardiac output and flow redistribution when the patient was subjected to heat stress? Specify the locations, pathways, and interactions of the neurons thought to be involved. Why did core temperature rise despite cutaneous vasodilation?
    b. Was the cardiac output low, normal, or high when acute heart failure developed?
    c. Compare the determinants of myocardial O_2 supply and demand when the patient argued with his son and during heat stress.

d. What mechanisms account for the change in the patient's mental acuity during acute heart failure?
e. What factors contributed to the subendocardial localization of cardiac ischemia?
f. Construct a systems diagram of the sort shown in Figure 7-8, page 76 to illustrate the positive feedback and interaction of variables that produced acute heart failure during heat stress.
g. If the patient had refused surgery, what would you have tried to accomplish by use of drugs? (No knowledge of pharmacology is required; consider unnamed drugs as "magic wands.") How would you have used your knowledge of physiology to formulate specific discharge instructions?

Appendix 6 : Specific Suggestions for Solving Problems

Problem 1

a. Relate information in Figures 5-4 and 6-1 and associated text.
b. See pages 23 and 24, Figure 2-5, and Figure 5-4.
c. Review text related to Figures 3-4 and 3-5.
d. Recall that nodal action potentials depend on I_{si}, whereas Na^+ is responsible for phase 0 depolarization in the rest of the heart; see page 24. Characteristics of I_{si} are given on pages 26 and 55.
e,f. Notice the steep slope of the Na^+ inactivation curve in Figure 3-5. Consider also the interaction of K^+ and Ca^{++} (p. 53) and how this interaction might affect contractility, arterial pressure and coronary flow. These interactions could influence electrical homogeneity.
g. Bear in mind that I_{si} controls tension in an individual fiber, and conduction determines how tension is summed in the fiber population.

Problem 2

The first step in evaluating a hemodynamic problem is to calculate the resistance. In doing so, remember that the numerator is ΔP. You will have to use your judgment in selecting appropriate values of end-diastolic pressure. In thinking about mechanisms, recall that the atria give the ventricles a quick stretch just before they contract. This "booster pump" permits a larger stroke volume and ejection fraction and greater mechanical efficiency. End-diastolic volume also becomes more constant from beat to beat after conversion.

Problem 3

See pages 80 to 81 and 97 to 98.

Problem 4

You can calculate *change* in flow to the leg, but not flow per se. Remember the leg flow is also affected by cardiac output. What cannot be accounted for by change in cardiac output is due to change in resistance in the leg.

Problem 5

Remember that the Fick principle is a statement of conservation of mass (p. 123). Therefore differences in inflow and outflow concentrations must be balanced by flow. What anatomical structure could raise O_2 content between right ventricle and pulmonary artery, and lower systemic arterial diastolic pressure?

Problem 6

a. The completed table describes changes in contractibility, afterload, and preload. The *initial* effect of each stress is on one of those three variables. The overall effect is the algebraic sum of the initial change and the reflex responses it generates.

b. See pages 10 to 12, 176 to 177, 182, and 244 to 246.

c. See pages 79 to 80.

Problem 7

Assume that decreases in renal, splanchnic, and cutaneous flows are taken up entirely by the working muscles. Notice especially the qualitative difference between the normal subject and the patient in respect to skin flow.

Problem 8

a. If symptoms limit performance, the $\dot{V}O_2$ required for that task approaches $\dot{V}O_{2_{max}}$.

b–e. The thick, hypertrophied left ventricle is less compliant than normal. Also, the total stroke volume greatly exceeds the volume that contributes to external work. The regurgitant volume — and hence preload — varies inversely with peripheral resistance. Factors that influence wall tension and efficiency are considered on pages 13 to 14, 192 to 194. O_2 supply and demand is also important; see Table 19-2.

f. Review the determinants of blood pressure, pages 78 to 80. Low diastolic pressure is not solely a mechanical phenomenon; reflex vasodilation initiated by the high pulse pressure also plays a role (p. 245). Use the formula for the Reynolds number (pp. 87 to 88) in thinking about murmurs.

g. Treatments are designed to decrease preload and afterload and to increase efficiency and contractility. You can develop the specifics.

Problem 9

Set up the equation for transcapillary flow of filtrate (p. 139). Notice that if normal values of P_{cap}, P_{IF}, and π_{IF} are used, the predicted flow will soon exceed the total plasma volume! Swelling will stop when $\Delta P = 0$. Figure 14-3 shows how this is accomplished. The determinants of ΔP are different for the abdomen, hands, and feet. Abdominal fluid is called ascites; its origin is considered on page 217.

Problem 10

How might the heat produced by hypermetabolism affect arteriolar and venous tone in skin? What are the consequences of posture and vasodilation for P_{cap}? See pages 149 to 150, and pages 220 to 222.

Problem 11

If you need help you had best reread Chapter 17 in its entirety; pay particular attention to the oxydissociation curve as a means of quantifying your thinking.

Problem 12

a. See pages 193 to 194. Time is almost always important in physiology; were the two stresses of equal duration?

b. CO_2 is much more diffusible than O_2, so the partial pressures of the two gases can change in opposite directions. The fall in PCO_2 means that hypoxemia occurred despite hyperventilation. Loss of the plateau of the dissociation curve and positive feedback makes pulmonary edema life-threatening on a time scale of minutes.

Problem 13

Consider physical and pharmacological treatments that change gain as well as those that interrupt the feedback signal or block system components. Notice that the vagus is both afferent and efferent.

Problem 14

a. Recall Problem 9; ascites formation stops when the extracapillary hydrostatic pressure balances P_{cap}. Hepatic cirrhosis is considered on pages 217 to 218.

b. All feedback systems require an error signal, but it can be very small if system gain is large. Inattention to diet and change in responsiveness to diuretics may also have contributed to ascites in this patient.

Problem 15

An important concept in physiology is that *every response is also a stimulus* for reflexly mediated change. For example, the initial tachycardia in Figure 26-2 is the direct response to electrical stimulation of sympathetic nerves. The associated increases in mean pressure, pulse pressure, and rate of change of pressure are powerful stimuli to the baroreceptors. The reflexly mediated response is profound vagal bradycardia despite continued sympathetic drive. Apply the same thinking to Problem 15.

Problem 16

a. See pages 220 to 222, Table 13-1, and pages 268 to 269. Recall that heat stress can increase cardiac output two- to threefold in a normal person. How does this compare with the expansion factor for cardiac output you estimated for this patient? Based on your analysis of Problem 7, could arterial pressure be maintained if skin flow were greatly increased without a large increase in cardiac output?

b. Cardiac failure may be defined as insufficient cardiac output to deal with metabolic needs — in this case, temperature regulation. Thus failure may exist despite high cardiac output relative to the statistical norm. Criteria and characteristics of cardiac failure are considered on pages 14 to 15.

c–f. Organizational suggestions in Appendix 5 include hints about how to deal with this problem. O_2 demand is dominated by wall tension, as affected by determinants of preload and afterload. The latter could be vastly different in heat stress and emotional stress. Other factors include heart rate, hypertrophy, external work (calculated for total stroke volume including the regurgitant volume), and body temperature itself. Supply is dominated by determinants of flow, especially aortic diastolic pressure and the coronary vasodilator reserve. Heart rate and the ΔP for subendocardial flow are also important. Though quantitative data are unavailable, determinants of transcapillary and intracellular O_2 gradients should be considered. The effect of hypertrophy on the capillary reserve could be a major factor in this situation. In contrast, hypoxemia reduced O_2 offered (flow times O_2 content) by only 20 percent, because of the plateau of the dissociation curve. Though hypoxemia was not insignificant, it should be treated as a secondary factor in the pathogenesis of acute heart failure in this patient. If O_2 and other treatments had been unavailable, however, hypoxemia could have become a major problem in short order.

g. Your answers to 15c to 15f contain all the information you need. Therapeutics is straightforward when you have thoroughly analyzed the physiology.

Index